Ankylosing Spondylitis and *Klebsiella*

Alan Ebringer

Ankylosing Spondylitis and *Klebsiella*

Springer

Alan Ebringer B.Sc., M.D.,
FRCP, FRACP, FRCPath
Professor of Immunology
King's College London

Honorary Consultant
Rheumatologist
Middlesex Hospital
UCH School of Medicine
King's College London
Division of Life Sciences
London, SE1 8WA, UK
United Kingdom

ISBN 978-1-4471-4299-7 ISBN 978-1-4471-4300-0 (eBook)
DOI 10.1007/978-1-4471-4300-0
Springer London Heidelberg New York Dordrecht

Library of Congress Control Number: 2012949895

Printed on acid-free paper

Springer is part of Springer Science+Business Media (www.springer.com)

This book is dedicated to the memory of the late Dr. A.C. Boyle (1918–1998), Chief Consultant Rheumatologist at the Middlesex Hospital, who served with Field Marshal Slim in Burma. During his service overseas, his wife was killed by a flying bomb.

He trained many rheumatologists in the UK and emphasised that public speaking should be an attribute of consultants.

Trainees were expected to give a 10-min talk, as long as it was not on a medical topic. We learned about Wagner's heroes, stock exchange and trips down the Amazon. One budding Consultant Rheumatologist gave a learned talk on 'joints' in Chippendale furniture and Hepplewhite chairs.

When he was approached that we could probably explain HLA-B27 in ankylosing spondylitis, his answer was 'utter poppy-cock' and promptly provided the funds, hospital facilities and patients to set up an 'Ankylosing Spondylitis Research Clinic of the Middlesex Hospital'.

When the first results came, linking Klebsiella to his ankylosing spondylitis patients, he declined to be on the paper with the gruff reply 'Nonsense, nobody would believe it'.

To Wendy, Andrew and Lawrence

Acknowledgements

The discovery of a new link between a disease and the environment depends on many individuals who by their efforts and insight have helped to establish this association.

First of all I would like to thank and acknowledge the work of the two Research groups, one from the Westminster Hospital in London and the other one from Los Angeles in the United States who by their discovery of a link between ankylosing spondylitis and HLA-B27 have made it possible for us from King's College and the Middlesex Hospital to study 'B27 disease'. Especially I would like to thank Dr. D.C.O. James of the Westminster group who helped us in tissue typing patients for HLA-B27 and provided access to tissue typed healthy control subjects.

Secondly I would like to acknowledge the help we have received from my medical colleagues in the Department of Rheumatology at the Middlesex Hospital, now part of the University College London Hospital in helping to set up the 'Ankylosing Spondylitis Research Clinic of the Middlesex Hospital' which ran from 1974 till 2002. Especially I would like to thank Dr. A.C. Boyle, Dr. Mary Corbett, Dr. M. Shipley and Prof. D. Isenberg who were bemused by the idea that a bowel microbe could be involved in ankylosing spondylitis but gave unstinting support and help over the years. My brother Dr. Roland Ebringer was an enthusiastic supporter who ran the clinic from 1974 till 1980 when he returned to Australia to practise rheumatology. Professor G. Panayi and Dr. A. Trull from the Department of Rheumatology at Guy's Hospital also collaborated in some of these early studies. One also requires the help of skilled and dedicated nursing staff. Sisters Abigail Olaleye, Avery Davis, Jean Heath and Evelyn Williams by their concern and sympathy for the patients helped to ensure a smooth and efficient outpatient research clinic.

Thirdly I would like to thank the skilled laboratory work of many research workers and Ph.D. doctoral fellows, initially from Queen Elizabeth College and later from King's College who were responsible for the excellent results that eventually saw the light of day in refereed publications. Without their efforts we would not have been able to help the patients in the 'AS Research Clinic of the Middlesex Hospital' and define the concept of 'B27 disease'. I would like to thank Dr. H. Avakian, Dr. P. Cowling, Dr. Jane Welsh, Dr. M. Baines, Dr. C. Wilson, Dr. M. Childerstone,

Dr. Teresa Ptaszynska, Dr. Shiva Khalafpour, Dr. G. Robinson, Dr. T. Rashid, Dr. P. Cunningham, Dr. Mariam Ghuloom, Dr. Faranak Shodjai-Moradi, Dr. Khatereh Ahmadi, Dr. Ilham Abuljadayel, Dr. M. Fielder and Dr. H. Tiwana who struggled brilliantly with 'coded runs' when they did not know which samples came from patients and which belonged to healthy blood donor subjects. In the earlier years, Don Robinson, Professor of Biochemistry, and John Pirt, Professor of Microbiology, at Queen Elizabeth College encouraged us academically and financially in our studies into the biochemical and microbiological aspects of autoimmune diseases.

Dr. C. Wilson Ph.D., FRCPath and Dr. Tasha Rashid M.B.Ch.B., M.Phil., were with us for over 20 years and provided outstanding medical and microbiological expertise. Research does not grow in a vacuum and requires financial support. Over the years we have been helped by the Matilda Poole Research Fund of the Middlesex Hospital, Medical Research Council, Science Research Council, Nuffield Foundation, Arthritis Research Council, Government of Bahrain and the American Friends of King's College.

Fourthly I would like to express my gratitude to the many patients who explained to me the varieties of pains and symptoms which they endured over the years and helped us in defining the concept of 'B27 disease'. The outstanding feature of their contribution was the recurring complaint or disappointment that the early stages of their disease went unrecognised for so many years and sometimes even decades.

The imputation or suggestion that these pains were not worthy of attention, or worse the product of a nervous or neurotic disposition, sometimes bordering on outright malingering, was not kindly accepted by this large population of sufferers with 'B27 disease'.

Finally I would like to thank and acknowledge three of my former patients who suggested that this book should be written. Ms. Judith Beard who was followed for 28 years, Mr. George McCaffery who provided financial support for the internet website 'Kick-AS' and popularised in cyberspace the idea of a 'Low Starch Diet' for patients with ankylosing spondylitis and Ms. Carol Sinclair who discovered the low starch diet by herself and wrote a book about it. This book would not have been possible without the support of all these people but the errors of omission or commission as well as the opinions expressed are all my own.

Contents

Chapter 1
Ankylosing Spondylitis as a Scientific Problem

1.1 Ankylosing Spondylitis: An Introduction

Ankylosing spondylitis is an arthritic disorder characterised by chronic inflammation affecting the lumbar spine, large peripheral joints and eventually producing generalised severe stiffness and rigidity, involving ribs and neck. It also occasionally affects the eyes.

There are over 30 million people in the world who suffer from this incapacitating disease, but the number of affected individuals may be higher if early stages or 'formes frustes' are included.

The disease is not only a health problem for the affected individual but is also a social burden to society in the costs involved in caring and treating such patients.

Extensive research studies have been carried out over the last one hundred years to try and characterise the onset and cause of this disease.

Predisposing genetic factors have been discovered over the last 30 years which could throw some light on the origin of this debilitating condition.

1.2 Clinical Features of Ankylosing Spondylitis

The onset of the disease is often insidious, and the patient may complain of transient muscular pains, stiffness, tiredness, malaise and fatigue before any joint symptoms appear.

Some patients present with acute episodes of pain involving the buttocks, lumbar spine, ribs and large joints such as hips, knees and ankles.

A major feature is 'early morning muscle stiffness' whereby the patient finds great difficulty in getting out of bed and often describes that they are so stiff they have to 'roll out of bed'. It is almost a diagnostic symptom of the disease. Muscular stiffness is a prominent symptom in the mornings and especially after periods of inactivity.

Aches in buttocks may be initially transient; in a matter of months, they become more persistent. In some patients, the pain may come on very acutely and be so

A. Ebringer, *Ankylosing Spondylitis and Klebsiella*,
DOI 10.1007/978-1-4471-4300-0_1, © Springer-Verlag London 2013

severe as to suggest a crush fracture or injury to the spine. Sometimes the pain is deep in the gluteal region often described as dull, but even if severe, it is difficult for the patient to localise it accurately. It may extend upwards towards the iliac crest, down to the thigh and knee, the trochanteric region and occasionally towards the groin (Hart 1980).

Often the lumbar pains are on one side, and some days later they are prominent on the other side. Buttock pains changing from one side to the other are commonly described by ankylosing spondylitis patients.

The presence of back pain, especially in a young adult, usually the commonest presenting symptom, must not be dismissed and merits careful clinical assessment. The characteristics of the pain should be assessed in terms of its mode of onset, side, severity, periodicity, aggravating factors such as pain on coughing, decreasing pain and stiffness on exercise and reduced chest expansion (Calin et al. 1977).

As the disease progresses, it involves the hip joints, knees and ankles. Heel pains may occur and shoulders become involved, occasionally even the temporomandibular joints.

The multifaceted manifestations of this disease reflect different patterns with each individual sufferer and must be distinguished from other possible causes such as diffuse idiopathic skeletal hyperostosis (DISH) also known as Forestier's disease, brucellosis, fluorosis, osteomas, Whipple's disease, polyvinyl chloride intoxication, ochronosis, tylosis, vitamin D-resistant hypophosphataemic rickets or relapsing polychondritis (Dixon and Macleod 1980).

Probably in ankylosing spondylitis in more than in any other condition there is an unfortunate 'delay to diagnosis' sometimes lasting 5–10 years, where the patient visits one specialist after another until eventually a diagnosis is made. Often the patient is greatly relieved that his or her backache symptoms have an objective and rational explanation and no longer has to suffer the accusation of 'malingering' or being a neurotic.

During active phases of the disease, a low-grade fever may be present with a normocytic anaemia and an elevated erythrocyte sedimentation rate. As the disease advances, muscle spasms give rise to flexion deformities in the joints. Later, permanent and irreversible changes occur leading to a fixed, rigid spine.

1.3 Radiological Features of Ankylosing Spondylitis

Sacroiliitis is characterised by a gamut of features varying from marginal sclerosis to complete obliteration.

The first changes in the vertebral bodies are erosions at the site of attachment of the annulus fibrosus.

Calcification of the spinal ligaments occurs, ultimately resulting in the classical 'bamboo appearance'.

Vertebral bodies lose their concave anterior configuration, appear 'square' and can have shiny corners, also known as Romanus lesions.

The apophyseal joints may become obliterated, and on the antero-posterior view of the lumbar spine are seen as two parallel continuous 'railroad tracks' (Percy and Lentle 1980).

1.4 The Disability of Ankylosing Spondylitis

Ankylosing spondylitis, as it progresses, is an extremely disabling and debilitating disease. Backache is severe and unremitting, requiring increasing doses of analgesic drugs. The spine becomes progressively rigid and when it reaches the neck, the patient finds it difficult to turn, cross the street, and generally it reduces the capacity for walking or even sitting.

The patient cannot open doors, drive a car, hold a spoon or go to the toilet without encountering serious difficulties in daily living.

There are approximately 0.6–2.4 million individuals in the USA affected by ankylosing spondylitis, and this implies a severe burden of morbidity, mortality and disability involving medical, physical, social and financial complications (Helmick et al. 2008).

1.5 The Social and Financial Costs of Ankylosing Spondylitis

Ankylosing spondylitis is a musculoskeletal disorder with a high prevalence throughout the developed world having a clinical course which progressively degrades the patient's quality of life and reduces his or her life expectancy.

In a German study, mean direct costs of ankylosing spondylitis was 13,513 Euros per patient per year which was close to the rheumatoid arthritis costs of 15,637 Euros. When costs due to disability were included, the financial costs per ankylosing spondylitis patient rose to 29,647 Euros (Huscher et al. 2006).

Similar results were reported from the USA, Canada, Netherlands and Sweden.

In a study from Spain, involving 601 ankylosing spondylitis patients, the mean costs per patient per year were 20,328 Euros (Range: 5,000–75,000), and the costs increased significantly with worsening disease and in particular diminishing physical function. Almost a quarter of patients had to stop working because of the disease. (Kobelt et al. 2008).

The therapy of ankylosing spondylitis involves not only the use of non-steroidal anti-inflammatory drugs, methotrexate, sometimes steroids but also newer biological preparations which place an exorbitant financial strain on health providers and society in general. Many of these drugs have undesirable side effects.

The general principle in such a therapy is to reduce the intensity of the inflammation once it has started in a patient.

Inflammation is the body's response to injury. The question arises: 'What has been responsible for the tissue injury?' In other words, what is the primary cause which sets off ankylosing spondylitis?

A possible way as to how to answer such a question may be to look for previous successful solutions in finding the cause of a disease, and no better example is provided than by rheumatic fever.

1.6 Molecular Mimicry and Rheumatic Fever

The prototype of an autoimmune disease evoked by an external agent and operating through the mechanism of 'molecular mimicry' is rheumatic fever.

It usually occurs some 2–4 weeks after an upper respiratory tract infection by Lancefield group A *streptococci.* Some *streptococci* have been found to have antigens which cross-react with cardiac myosin, and others resemble some molecular sequences found in the basal ganglia of the brain. When someone develops tonsillitis by this microbe, the resultant antibodies will not only attack the *streptococcal* bacteria but also the heart and the brain. Thus anti-*streptococcal* antibodies produce rheumatic fever and Sydenham's chorea by acting as cytopathic autoantibodies. It would appear that rheumatic fever and Sydenham's chorea are autoimmune diseases caused by an infection.

Other diseases operate by a similar mechanism. Some 20–30 million individuals in South America, especially Brazil, are infected by the protozoan parasite *Trypanosoma cruzi.* Patients with Chaga's disease have antibodies which react with both antigens present on the surface of the parasite as well as with cardiac endothelium and myocardium giving rise to a myocarditis which pathologically resembles rheumatic fever. Thus, it would appear that even parasites can be triggers or causative agents of an autoimmune disease (Ebringer et al. 2003).

It is not inconceivable that a similar mechanism may operate in ankylosing spondylitis.

1.7 The Properties of the Ankylosing Spondylitis Problem

To investigate a 'scientific problem', it is relevant to note the properties of the problem which define the puzzle or question. It is these properties that provide possible answers for the scientific enquiry. The philosopher of science Karl Popper has always emphasised that in trying to solve a scientific problem one must generate hypotheses which can then be tested experimentally. For such hypotheses to be labelled as scientific they must prohibit certain results. If such prohibited results are obtained, then the theory is found to be invalid or has failed in explaining the 'scientific problem'.

We then must produce new hypotheses to tackle the problem under investigation. So scientific research proceeds by a succession of conjectures or guesses and refutations.

The properties of the ankylosing spondylitis problem would appear to be the following:

1. *Sex ratio*: Ankylosing spondylitis is found 3–4 times more frequently in men than women.
2. *Early age of onset*: The age of onset in ankylosing spondylitis is between the ages of 20 and 30 years. In some patients, it starts even in their teens. This clearly distinguishes this disease from rheumatoid arthritis where the age of onset is in the 40's and 50's and occurring more frequently in women.
3. *Family studies*: It has been known for a long time that there is a familial aggregation of ankylosing spondylitis, and this suggests somehow that there is a genetic link associated with the development of the disease.
   Since the disease does not start till the teens or twenties, clearly an environmental element is involved with the onset of ankylosing spondylitis.
4. *Genetic links*: Ankylosing spondylitis is found more frequently in individuals belonging to HLA-B27 group. Over 90 % of ankylosing spondylitis patients belong to the HLA-B27 group whilst the frequency of this antigen in the general population of the UK or the USA is about 8 %.

It is proposed to use these properties of the ankylosing spondylitis problem to investigate the possible cause of this disease by research workers associated with the King's College Immunology Unit in London.

1.8 King's College Immunology Unit

The Women's Department of King's College London opened in 1885 and in 1915 moved to Campden Hill road, Kensington.

In 1953, it received a royal charter and was named Queen Elizabeth College after the Queen Mother.

The college distinguished itself in teaching and research in microbiology, biochemistry, physiology and nutrition. In 1972, an Immunology Unit was set up within the departments of biochemistry and microbiology with an interest in research into genetic and environmental factors in rheumatic diseases, especially ankylosing spondylitis and rheumatoid arthritis. Many students and doctoral candidates passed through the unit, and two stayed for over 20 years, Dr. Clyde Wilson Ph.D., MRCPath and Dr. Taha Rashid MBChB, M.Phil.

In 1985, Queen Elizabeth College remerged with King's College and moved to the Waterloo Campus in Stamford street on the South Bank.

Ankylosing spondylitis has been a research interest of the unit since 1974 when Dr. D.C.O. James, who was involved in the discovery of the link between HLA-B27 and ankylosing spondylitis, suggested a collaborative study and that he would tissue type any patients attending the 'Ankylosing Spondylitis Research Clinic of the Middlesex Hospital'.

A leading American research worker has stated that the chronic inflammatory reaction in ankylosing spondylitis is the result of an interaction between bowel bacteria involving immunological and inflammatory processes (Taurog et al. 1994). It is the aim of this book to try and identify the origin of such immunological and inflammatory processes.

References

Calin A, Porta J, Fries JFF. The clinical history as a screening test for ankylosing spondylitis. J Am Med Assoc. 1977;237:2613–4.

Dixon ASJ, Macleod M. Diagnostic problems and differential diagnosis. In: Moll JMH, editor. Ankylosing spondylitis. London: Churchill Livingstone; 1980. p. 151–62.

Ebringer A, Rashid T, Wilson C. Molecular mimicry as the basis of new theory of autoimmunity. In: Zouali M, editor. Frontiers in autoimmunity. Burke: IOS Press; 2003. p. 79–99.

Hart FD. Clinical features and complications. In: Moll JMH, editor. Ankylosing spondylitis. London: Churchill Livingstone; 1980. p. 52–68.

Helmick CG, Felson DT, Lawrence RC, Gabriel S, Hirsch R, Kwoh CK, Liang MH, Kremers HM, Mayes MD, Merkel PA, Pillemer SR, Reveille JD, Stone JH. Estimates of prevalence of arthritis and other rheumatic conditions in the United States. Arthritis Rheum. 2008;58:15–25.

Huscher D, Merkesdal S, Thiele K, Zeidler H, Schneider M, Zink A. Costs of illness in rheumatoid arthritis, ankylosing spondylitis, psoriatic arthritis and systemic lupus erythematosus in Germany. Ann Rheum Dis. 2006;65:1175–83.

Kobelt G, Sobocki P, Mulero J, Gratacos J, Pocovi A, Collantes-Estevez E. The burden of ankylosing spondylitis in Spain. Value Health. 2008;11:408–15.

Percy JS, Lentle B. Radiological and scintigraphic features. In: Moll JMH, editor. Ankylosing spondylitis. London: Churchill Livingstone; 1980. p. 76–86.

Taurog JD, Richardson JA, Croft JT, Simmons WA, Zhou M, Fernandez-Sueiro JL, Balish E, Hammer RE. The germfree state prevents development of gut and joint inflammatory disease in HLA-B27 transgenic rats. J Exp Med. 1994;180:2359–64.

Chapter 2
History of the Origin of Ankylosing Spondylitis

2.1 Introduction

There is always a continuous debate about the origin and early detection of a disease. This is inevitable as diagnoses and labels change over time, and this problem also occurs with ankylosing spondylitis. Multiplicity of diagnostic labels is certainly a problem with ankylosing spondylitis, and in a recent review of this condition, it was described by 20 different names over the last two centuries (Benedek 2009).

Diseases associated with infections may eventually progress to an overt rheumatological disorder as occurs in 'Gram-negative reactive arthritis'.

Palaeohistorical evidence provides only limited material on which to make a diagnostic assessment, and therefore the hunt for the first sighting of a disease becomes a rather problematic enterprise.

2.2 Ankylosing Spondylitis and the Egyptian Pharaohs

It has been suggested that among the pharaohs of the eighteenth and nineteenth dynasty there were at least three rulers who may have had ankylosing spondylitis based on radiological examinations: Amenhotep II, Ramses II the Great and his son Mereptah (Feldtkeller et al. 2003).

However a reappraisal by Canadian radiologists proposed that the findings suggested 'diffuse idiopathic skeletal hyperostosis' (DISH) and not ankylosing spondylitis in the skeleton of Ramses II (Chem et al. 2004).

A. Ebringer, *Ankylosing Spondylitis and Klebsiella*,
DOI 10.1007/978-1-4471-4300-0_2, © Springer-Verlag London 2013

2.3 Ankylosing Spondylitis in the Middle Ages

A comprehensive review of 560 adult skeletons, with at least part of the vertebral column intact, on remains gathered from various churches and cemeteries including the bones of 7 Saxon bishops interred in Wells Cathedral were examined by a group from Bristol (Rogers et al. 1985).

Nearly half of the skeletons examined had some degree of spinal osteophytosis, but despite the large number of specimens examined, only two cases of spondyloarthritis could be identified.

A medieval adult male skeleton from Bath Abbey showed axial changes including bilateral ankylosis of sacroiliac joints and ankylosis between T7 and L1. Spinal syndesmophytes were asymmetrical and predominantly anterior lateral.

'Diffuse idiopathic skeletal hyperostosis' (DISH) was found in 2.3 % of specimens and this is similar to the rate found in Finnish patients (Julkunen et al. 1968).

2.4 Ankylosing Spondylitis and Realdo de Colombo

Probably the first suggestive sighting of an ankylosing spondylitis skeleton occurred in Italy. Realdo de Colombo was an assistant to Andreas Vesalius and later became Professor of Anatomy in the University of Padua. The University is one of the oldest in Europe having been founded in 1222. In 1559, Realdo de Colombo produced anatomical descriptions of two skeletons typical of ankylosing spondylitis in his book *De Re Anatomica*.

Spinal kyphosis could not have been a rare occurrence in those times since the surgeon Johannes Scultetus (1595–1645) described horrendous contraptions to straighten a kyphotic patient.

2.5 Connor's Observations in France

The first definite description of ankylosing spondylitis may be credited to Bernard Connor (1666–1695) who described an unusual skeleton.

Bernard Connor was born in county Kerry in Ireland, attended the medical schools of Paris, Montpellier and Rheims, where he received his M.D.

Whilst demonstrating anatomy in France, he came across a most peculiar skeleton, found in a graveyard in Rheims, in which the sacrum and the 15 lowest vertebrae and adjoining ribs form one continuous bone.

Connor fully realised the importance of his discovery and reported it in three languages; in French in a letter published in Paris to Sir William de Waldegrave in 1691 (Fig. 2.1), in Latin published in Oxford and in English in his Rheims thesis which was published by the Royal Society in 1695.

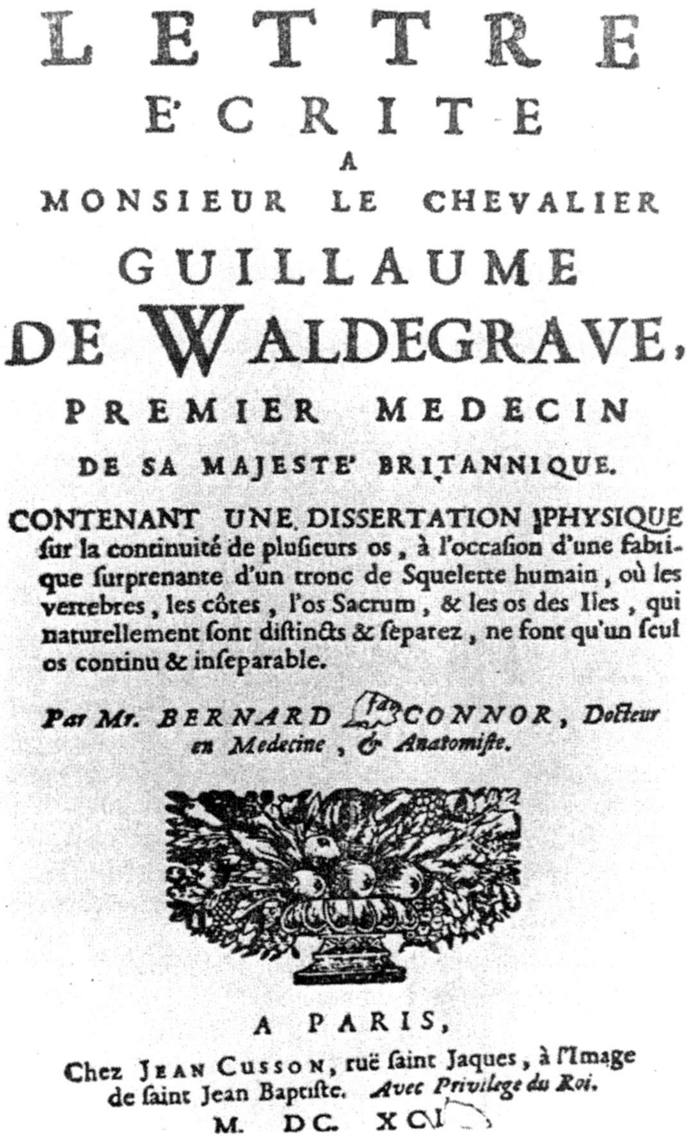

LETTRE
E'CRITE
A
MONSIEUR LE CHEVALIER
GUILLAUME
DE WALDEGRAVE,
PREMIER MEDECIN
DE SA MAJESTE' BRITANNIQUE.
CONTENANT UNE DISSERTATION PHYSIQUE sur la continuité de plusieurs os, à l'occasion d'une fabrique surprenante d'un tronc de Squelette humain, où les vertebres, les côtes, l'os Sacrum, & les os des Iles, qui naturellement sont distincts & separez, ne font qu'un seul os continu & inseparable.

Par Mr. BERNARD CONNOR, *Docteur en Medecine, & Anatomiste.*

A PARIS,
Chez JEAN CUSSON, ruë saint Jaques, à l'Image de saint Jean Baptiste. *Avec Privilege du Roi.*
M. DC. XCI

Fig. 2.1 Title page of letter from Connor to Sir William Waldegrave (Courtesy of the Editor, *Journal of History of Medicine*, as quoted by E. Bywaters)

He surmised that the man must have had difficulty in walking or turning and in view of his fused ribs could only have abdominal or diaphragmatic breathing. Connor died rather young, but he had made a significant contribution to the history of rheumatology and medicine.

2.6 The Eighteenth Century in Europe

A second human spine similar to Connor's was discovered in Coburg in Germany by three students whilst on a botanical excursion, and the find was promptly published by their Professor Johann Sebastian Albrecht in 1748.

2.7 The Nineteenth Century in London

There were several descriptions of ankylosing spondylitis in the nineteenth century in London:

1. *Sir Benjamin Brodie's case*
   Sir Benjamin Brodie (1783–1862) described in 1850, a case of a man whose disease started when he was 27 years old, becoming completely rigid within 6 years, had a long continued rheumatism of the spine, with a 'hoop-like' deformity and occasionally suffering from inflammation of the eyes.
   This would appear to be the first reported case of uveitis in a patient with ankylosing spondylitis.
2. *Charles Fagge's case*
   The first correlation of clinical and pathological findings was by Charles Fagge (1838–1883), a clinician at Guy's Hospital who in 1877 described a man of 34 years, with a cough, a rigid curved spine and fixity of the ribs, breathing exclusively with his abdomen (Fagge 1877). 'His dorsal vertebrae formed one large rounded curve, with little or no movement. He had but slight power of moving his neck; the ribs also seemed quite fixed'. When he did the autopsy, he found not only ankylosis of the vertebral bodies, but also fixed apophyseal joints, ribs and a rigid right hip joint as well as upper lobe fibrosis, bronchiectasis and a cardiac valve lesion.
3. *W. Sturge's case*
   In 1858, W. Sturge (1850–1919) gave a detailed description of a man of 26, with a fixed spine and chest, starting at the age of 18 with back pain, urethritis and iritis. Clearly, this is an early sighting of Reiter's disease.

2.8 Bechterew in St. Petersburg

Vladimir Bechterew (1857–1927) was a neurologist who in 1982 described three patients: a mother and daughter and a man who had sometime in the past incurred some trauma to his back.

These were his conclusions:

> Based on the clinical data we may assume that we are dealing with a chronic process of the vertebrae that develops independently and leads to ankylosis. It also probably leads to a diffuse, chronic inflammation of the epidural connective tissue. One must also consider that

> the presentation of our cases resembles spondylitis deformans. The process on the one hand leads to expanding intervertebral rigidity and on the other pressure on the nerve roots.
> This sufficiently explains the rigidity or stiffness of the vertebral column, as well as the sensory symptoms of the spinal nerve roots, the weakness and mild atrophy of the neck and back muscles, as well as the weakness of the muscles of upper extremities that is sometimes observed (Bechterew 1899).

Athough Bechterew favoured a neurological explanation for the disease, a myelopathy, his observation of a mother and daughter being affected, suggested to him that there was also a genetic predisposition to the condition.

2.9 Strűmpell in Erlangen and Berlin

Adolph Strűmpell (1853–1925), in 1897, described two patients with complete ankylosis of the spine and of both hip joints. He also emphasised that lumbar lordosis in a rigid spine was a prominent feature and published dramatic photographs of such patients.

Strűmpell suggested the disease should be labelled in more descriptive terms as 'chronic inflammation of the large joints and vertebral column', without mentioning the neurological features favoured by Bechterew.

2.10 Pierre Marie and Léri in France

It is now generally agreed that Pierre Marie (1853–1940) has given the most detailed and characteristic clinical description of ankylosing spondylitis (Bywaters 1983) and coined the word 'spondylose rhizomélique'. He gave detailed descriptions of six male patients.

He worked as an assistant to Jean Marie Charcot at the Salpêtrière Hospital before becoming Professor of Neurology.

Léri, Marie's assistant, described the full pathological characteristics of ankylosing spondylitis after he had carried out autopsies on two of Pierre Marie's patients. His conclusions anticipated modern developments.

> 'La spondylarthrite ankylosante est une maladie avec certaines propriétés: C'est un trouble trophique à développement lent, sans doute parfois diathésique et probablement souvent infectieux ou toxin infectieux (Léri 1926).'

A prophetic statement anticipating the HLA-B27 discoveries of the 1970s.

2.11 Buckley's Observations in the 1930s

Charles Buckley said in 1935, 'The cause of ankylosing spondylitis is an infection of low virulence, acting for prolonged period and sensitising certain tissues' (Buckley 1935).

2.12 The Heart and Ankylosing Spondylitis

Original studies of heart disease in ankylosing spondylitis included six cases of aortic incompetence, but this was attributed to probable antecedent rheumatic fever.

However, association between ankylosing spondylitis and aortic incompetence occurred serendipitously in 1956, when the first 100 patients into whom Charles W Hufnagel had inserted a prosthetic aortic valve were reviewed, and it was found that five had ankylosing spondylitis, a frequency which was recognised to be far greater than could be attributed to chance (Schilder et al. 1956).

2.13 Diagnostic Help from Physics

Roentgen had developed X-rays in 1896. The first spines showing ankylosing spondylitis were taken by Beneke in 1897.

Since that time refinements and new developments in diagnostic methods, such as magnetic resonance imaging and computerised tomography, have assisted in characterising the early stages of the disease (Sieper et al. 2002).

2.14 Conclusion

Although the recognition of advanced ankylosing spondylitis with patients having rigid spines took some time to be of interest to anyone else but specialised rheumatologists, immunology threw a bombshell into this field by the pre-eminent discovery of HLA-B27 in 1973.

References

Bechterew W. Neue Beobachtungen und pathologische-anatomische Untersuchungen űber Steifigkeit der Wirbelsäule. Deut Ztschr Nervenheilk. 1899;15:45–57.

Benedek TG. How did ankylosing spondylitis become a separate disease? Clin Exp Rheumatol. 2009;27 Suppl 55:S3–9.

Buckley CW. Ankylosing spondylitis. In: Reports on chronic rheumatic diseases. London: Lewis; 1935. p. 77–89.

Bywaters E. Historical perspectives in the aetiology of ankylosing spondylitis. Br J Rheumatol. 1983;27 Suppl 2:1–4.

Chem RK, Schmit P, Fauré C. Did Rameses II really have ankylosing spondylitis ? A reappraisal. Can Assoc Radiol J. 2004;55:211–7.

Fagge CH. A case of simple synostosis of the ribs to the vertebrae and of the arches and articular processes of the vertebrae themselves and also of one hip joint. Trans Pathol Soc Lond. 1877;28:201–6.

Feldtkeller E, Lemmel EM, Russell AS. Ankylosing spondylitis in the Pharaohs of ancient Egypt. Rheumatol Int. 2003;23:1–5.

Julkunen H, Pyorala K, Lehtaurirta F. Hyperostosis of the spine in relation to age and hyperglycaemia in men aged 30–60. Ann Med Intern Fenn. 1968;57:1–7.

Léri A. Études sur les affections de la colonne vertébrale. Paris: Masson; 1926.

Rogers J, Watt I, Dieppe P. Paleopathology of spinal osteophytosis, vertebral ankylosis, ankylosing spondylitis and vertebral hyperostosis. Ann Rheum Dis. 1985;44:113–20.

Schilder DP, Harvey WP, Hufnagel CA. Rheumatoid spondylitis and and aortic insuffciency. N Engl J Med. 1956;255:358–61.

Sieper J, Braun J, Rudwaleit M, Boonen A, Zink A. Ankylosing spondylitis: an overview. Ann Rheum Dis. 2002;61(Suppl III):iii8–18.

Chapter 3
The Discovery of HLA-B27 in Ankylosing Spondylitis and Related Disorders

3.1 The Tissue Typing Unit at the Westminster Hospital

In the early 1970s, following Dr. Christian Barnard's momentous first cardiac transplantation in the world, the field of organ transplantation acquired a new resonance, and tissue typing units were formed in many hospitals.

The 'tissue typing laboratory' at the Westminster Hospital in London was set up by Dr. D.C.O. James, the haematologist, to assist the cardiac surgeon Mr. Charles Drew in his cardiac transplantations.

Dr. James then looked for a suitable project in which the 'Tissue Typing Laboratory' could be used to investigate HLA frequencies in various diseases.

3.2 HLA-B27 in Ankylosing Spondylitis

An international symposium on the 'Pathogenesis of HLA-B27 Associated Diseases' was held at the Middlesex Hospital on 12–13 April 1983.

Dr. James described the work carried out in the 'Tissue Typing Laboratory' of the Westminster Hospital. He writes:

> I recalled many families in my native Wales being affected by rheumatism. Could immunogenetic studies be carried out in such patients.
>
> I wrote to the then Consultant Rheumatologist at the Westminster Hospital Dr. Frank Dudley Hart and asked him for some information on HLA and rheumatism. He wrote back "I am afraid I have no information about HLA and rheumatism but you are welcome to take blood samples from my patients."
>
> Thereupon I contacted his registrar Dr. Roger Sturrock who duly sent an assortment of blood specimens taken at random from rheumatic patients. Not surprisingly, the HLA results showed no predominant feature and were very disappointing to us. The fact that the two samples from ankylosing spondylitis patients had HLA-B27 held no message for us at the time.
>
> I next remember mentioning my quest for a disease having a familial tendency with a rheumatological background to my colleague Professor John Hobbs, who immediately remarked "Why not have a word with Dr. Derrick Brewerton, I am sure he will be interested".

A. Ebringer, *Ankylosing Spondylitis and Klebsiella*,
DOI 10.1007/978-1-4471-4300-0_3, © Springer-Verlag London 2013

Dr. Derrick Brewerton was then Consultant in the Department of Physical Medicine and had studied patients with ankylosing spondylitis.

I contacted him, and as he recalls: "It was lunch in the common room at Westminster Hospital on a hot summer day in 1971. Over the salad, we decided to investigate the frequency of HLA antigens in ankylosing spondylitis."

A small series of blood samples from these patients duly arrived from Dr. Brewerton and I well recall what happened.

My research colleague, Miss M.F.P. Caffrey, who had tissue typed these specimens appeared with the results.

"There is something important here' she said, 'almost all these specimens have B27".

My initial surprise was shared by Derrick Brewerton himself.

Was it a technical error, was it a spurious result due to the disease process itself or was it something due to the drug therapy?

Having convinced ourselves that the results were not spurious, the first and best known investigation shows that, out of a series of 75 controls, 4 % had HLA-B27 but that 72 patients with ankylosing spondylitis out of 75 - that is 96 % had the HLA-B27 antigen.

Our very first laboratory orientated report appeared in "Nature" (Caffrey and James 1973) and our second report, appeared three months later in the "Lancet" (Brewerton et al. 1973a).

This became a citation classic, that is one of the most cited publication in this field (James 1983).

At the same the American group published their tissue typing studies on ankylosing spondylitis patients carried out in Professor Terasaki's Laboratory in Los Angeles (Schlosstein et al. 1973).

3.3 Acute Anterior Uveitis and HLA-B27

Some 30 % of ankylosing spondylitis patients develop an episode of uveitis during their lifetime.

The Westminster group investigated a group of ophthalmological patients with acute anterior uveitis.

HLA-B27 was identified in 26 out of 50 patients suffering from acute anterior uveitis, but only 2 out of 50 of the control subjects possessed the HLA-B27 antigen (Brewerton et al. 1973b).

Here was definite evidence that not only ankylosing spondylitis but also uveitis travelled together with this genetic marker HLA-B27.

Clearly this represented a link whereby both ankylosing spondylitis and acute anterior uveitis had a common denominator or property which was associated with this HLA molecule.

Further studies were required to determine whether HLA-B27 was the predisposing gene for ankylosing spondylitis or was it only a marker for a secondary gene associated by 'linkage disequilibrium'.

3.4 HLA-B27 in Reiter's Disease and Reactive Arthritis

Reiter's disease or 'la maladie de Fiessinger-Leroy', as it is known in France, is a condition associated with a triad of symptoms: urethritis, conjunctivitis and arthritis. It was described following the unhygienic conditions under which soldiers living in trenches, during the First World War, succumbed to this disease. The implication was clear; it was a condition associated with some bacterial infection.

In a further study from the Westminster Hospital, HLA-B27 was found in 25 out of 33 patients with Reiter's disease (76 %), in 9 out of 33 patients with non-specific urethritis but in only in 2 out of 33 controls (Brewerton et al. 1973c)

In a Finnish study, HLA-B27 was identified in 43 out of 49 patients with Yersinia arthritis (88 %) and in 36 out of 40 Reiter's disease (90 %). HLA-B27 is present in 14 % of the general Finnish population (Aho et al. 1974).

These two studies clearly demonstrate that there is a link between HLA-B27 and conditions that are associated with some form of infection.

3.5 HLA-B27 as the Predisposing Gene

The following features appeared to favour a direct role for HLA-B27 in the pathogenesis of ankylosing spondylitis:

(a) The prevalence of ankylosing spondylitis depends on the racial background of the population and follows to a large extent the distribution of HLA-B27 in the general population.
(b) The association between HLA-B27 and ankylosing spondylitis transcends racial and geographical barriers.
(c) In families with multiple cases of ankylosing spondylitis, one observes that the disease almost invariably segregates with HLA-B27.
(d) No stronger association has been observed with any other HLA group belonging to A, B, C or DR loci.
(e) HLA-B27 negative ankylosing spondylitis patients have a somewhat later age of onset and have a lower incidence of uveitis compared to HLA-B27 positive patients.

Ankylosing spondylitis may be considered as a final common pathway arrived through a multitude of factors which includes genetic susceptibility and environmental determinants (Khan 1988).

3.6 Geography of HLA-B27

HLA-B27 is present throughout the world with some notable exceptions.

HLA-B27 is virtually absent among the genetically unmixed, native populations of South America, Australia, African Bantus and Sans Bushmen.

In striking contrast there is a very high prevalence of HLA-B27 among the native peoples of circumpolar arctic regions of Eurasia and North America.

The frequency of HLA-B27 in Canadian Inuit population is 25 %, among the Inuit-Eskimos of Greenland it is 30 % and among the Siberian Chukchi Inuits it is 40 % (Khan 1998).

However, the highest frequency of HLA-B27 is among the Haida Indians living on Queen Charlotte Island of British Columbia where it approaches 50 %, and definite ankylosing spondylitis has been reported to occur in 4 % of the adult male Haida population (Gofton et al. 1975).

A striking South-to-North gradation in the frequency of HLA-B27 occurs in European populations: Southern Europeans 2–6 %, Western Europeans 6–9 %, Slavic populations 7–14 % and Ugro-Altaic (Finland, Estonia, Hungary) populations 12–16 %.

The frequency of HLA-B27 in northern Norway and northern Sweden is 10–16 % and that of ankylosing spondylitis is 1.4 % but whether this reflects an admixture of Lapland populations is unclear.

The risk for ankylosing spondylitis in HLA-B27 positive first-degree relatives of ankylosing spondylitis patients is much greater than among the HLA-B27 population at large, and this suggests a shared factor either of genetic or environmental origin.

3.7 General Discussion and Conclusions

The discovery of the link between HLA-B27 and ankylosing spondylitis would appear to be a scientific puzzle similar to the problem of 'immune response genes' described in experimental animals.

The solution in experimental animals was that there was a similarity or 'molecular mimicry' between the animal equivalent of the human HLA and the environmental antigen.

Since there is already an excellent precedent in the case of rheumatic fever and Sydenham's chorea with its link to *streptococcal* upper respiratory tract infection, it would not be too far fetched to suggest that there is an environmental bacterial agent which resembles HLA-B27.

Such a hypothesis is reinforced by the demonstration that Reiter's disease and *Yersinia* reactive arthritis are also linked to HLA-B27.

This book describes an attempt to solve the problem of the link between HLA-B27 and ankylosing spondylitis.

3.8 The Middlesex Hospital in London[1]

The first Middlesex Hospital opened in 1745 as the Middlesex Infirmary in Windmill street London W1. The second Middlesex Hospital opened in 1757 in Mortimer street and was incorporated by an Act of Parliament in 1836. The new building was opened in 1935, by the Duke of York, later to become King George VI.

[1] History of the Middlesex Hospital previously appeared in *Rheumatoid Arthritis and Proteus*, with permission.

The hospital lobby contained four large paintings, entitled 'Acts of Mercy' by Frederick Cayley Robinson, completed in 1920. After the merger of the Middlesex Hospital with University College Hospital in 1994, the paintings were acquired by the Wellcome Collection.

The Middlesex Hospital was where Dr. WSC 'Will' Copeman had his early appointment as Senior Consultant in Rheumatology in the Arthur Stanley Institute before he wrote his *Textbook of Rheumatic Diseases*.

Professor Eric Bywaters, the doyen of academic rheumatologists, graduated from the Middlesex Hospital.

The post-war services in rheumatology were provided by Dr. Oswald Savage. The Department of Rheumatology at the Middlesex Hospital was founded by Dr. Archibald Cabbourn Boyle, known as 'Bill', and was located in Arthur Stanley House, after it merged with the Arthur Stanley Institute, in Tottenham street, next to the main hospital.

Arthur Stanley House was opened by Her Majesty the Queen in 1965 and became a centre dedicated to the care of rheumatic patients.

The building also contained a physiotherapy and rehabilitation section as well as a Department of Immunology, under Professor Ivan Roitt.

Bill Boyle was a gifted teacher, and by the time of his retirement, he had had a hand in training one third of the rheumatologists in the UK and many from overseas, especially Australasia.

Dr. Mary Corbett was appointed as a second Consultant in Rheumatology and started longitudinal studies on rheumatoid arthritis, known as 'Rheumatoid Arthritis Prospective Studies' or RAPS for short.

She emphasised that early treatment was paramount to prevent the development of irreversible bony changes and deformities. She approved the studies on antibodies to *Proteus* which were carried out on her rheumatoid arthritis patients attending the weekly 'Gold Clinic'.

Professor David Isenberg was appointed Professor of Rheumatology for the merged Middlesex-University College Hospitals and collaborated in some studies in both ankylosing spondylitis and rheumatoid arthritis patients carried out by the King's College group. Dr. Michael Shipley was appointed Consultant in Rheumatology and provided clinical advice for the 'Ankylosing Spondylitis Research Clinic' and support in running two international symposia held at the Middlesex Hospital in 1983 and 1987. Professor Jonathan Edwards contributed to the international symposia and showed that chemical ablation of B cells led to improvement in patients with rheumatoid arthritis.

3.9 The 'Ankylosing Spondylitis Research Clinic of the Middlesex Hospital'

In 1973, two seminal observations were published, one from the Westminster Hospital in London and the other one from Terasaki's group in Los Angeles, that over 95 % of patients with ankylosing spondylitis carried the major histocompatibility marker, HLA-B27, whilst it was present in only 8 % of the general population. Clearly, here was a puzzle that required some form of explanation.

Dr. D.C.O. James, the immunologist involved in the discovery of HLA-B27 at the Westminster Hospital, came to the immunology lectures at Queen Elizabeth College, now part of King's College, and discussed this problem.

We had previously shown that 'high' and 'low' immune responses in inbred animals could be explained by 'molecular mimicry' between H-2, which is the mouse equivalent of human HLA, and an external, environmental antigen (Ebringer and Davies 1973).

The suggestion from our group was that there was probably some form of 'molecular mimicry' between an unknown microbe and HLA-B27.

This was based on the precedent of rheumatic fever and Sydenham's chorea being caused by anti-*streptococcal* antibodies following an upper respiratory tract infection such as tonsillitis.

It was decided to study this question, and Dr. Bill Boyle was approached with the suggestion that this could be investigated in an 'Ankylosing Spondylitis Research Clinic'. He gave his approval and supported the clinic with financial resources. The clinic was started by my brother, Dr. Roland Ebringer who was in charge of the clinical studies till 1980 when he returned to Australia.

The immunological studies were carried out at Queen Elizabeth College and the clinical studies at the Middlesex Hospital. Some 900 ankylosing spondylitis patients were seen at the clinic between 1975 and 2002 when the clinic was closed.

In 1975, molecular mimicry was demonstrated between the bowel microbe *Klebsiella* and HLA-B27. Faecal studies showed that *Klebsiella* microbes could be isolated from active ankylosing spondylitis patients and later elevated levels of antibodies to *Klebsiella* could be demonstrated by several techniques.

When 2 years later, Professor Stastny from Dallas showed that rheumatoid arthritis patients were found more frequently in carriers of HLA-DR4; it was considered that the same explanation might apply to this observation as it did for *Streptococcus* and rheumatic fever or *Klebsiella* and ankylosing spondylitis.

Dr. Mary Corbett gave her approval that her rheumatoid arthritis patients could be investigated by the same methods as the patients in the 'Ankylosing Spondylitis Research Clinic'.

These results showed that rheumatoid arthritis is caused by a urinary tract infection by *Proteus* bacteria and the investigations are described in my monograph *Rheumatoid Arthritis and Proteus* published by Springer in November 2011.

References

Aho K, Ahvonen P, Lassus A, Sievers K, Tiilikainen A. HL-A in reactive arthritis. A study of Yersinia arthritis and Reiter's disease. Arthritis Rheum. 1974;17:521–6.

Brewerton DA, Hart FD, Nicholls A, Caffrey M, James DCO, Sturrock RD. Ankylosing spondylitis and HL-A 27. Lancet. 1973a;i:904–7.

Brewerton DA, Nicholls A, Caffrey M, Walters D, James DCO. Acute anterior uveitis and HL-A 27. Lancet. 1973b;ii:994–6.

Brewerton DA, Nicholls A, Oates JK, Caffrey M, Walters D, James DCO. Reiter's disease and HL-A 27. Lancet. 1973c;ii:996–8.

Caffrey MFP, James DCO. Human lymphocyte antigen association in ankylosing spondylitis. Nature. 1973;242:121.

Ebringer A, Davies DAL. Crossreactivity between synthetic TGAL and transplantation antigens in CBA mice. Nature (New Biol). 1973;74:144–7.

Gofton JP, Chalmers A, Price GE, Reeve CE. HLA 27 and ankylosing spondylitis in B.C. Indians. J Rheumatol. 1975;2:166–8.

James DCO. HLA-B27 in clinical medicine – historical reflections on the discovery of the disease association. Br J Rheumatol. 1983;22 Suppl 2:20–4.

Khan M. Genetics of HLA-B27. Br J Rheumatol. 1988;27 Suppl 2:6–11.

Khan M. A worldwide overview: the epidemiology of HLA-B27 and associated spondyloarthritides. In: Calin A, Taurog JD, editors. The spondyloarthritides. Oxford: Oxford University Press; 1998. p. 17–26.

Schlosstein L, Terasaki PI, Bluestone R, Pearson CM. High association of an HLA antigen W27, with ankylosing spondylitis. N Engl J Med. 1973;288:704–6.

Chapter 4
Molecular Mimicry Between HLA-B27 and *Klebsiella* Bacteria Investigated by Using Rabbit Antisera

4.1 Introduction: The Problem of HLA-B27 in Ankylosing Spondylitis

Many diseases are associated with HLA antigens. For instance, rheumatoid arthritis is found more frequently in individuals possessing HLA-DR1 and HLA-DR4 antigens.

The strongest and best documented association shows that individuals who carry HLA-B27 have a high risk of developing ankylosing spondylitis.

The high frequency of HLA-B27 in these patients could be explained either by a susceptibility gene closely linked to HLA-B27 or to direct involvement of the HLA-B27 molecule through 'molecular mimicry'.

Since the mechanism of molecular mimicry was found to operate in rheumatic fever and also in drug-induced acquired haemolytic anaemia, it was decided to use this approach in studying the problem of HLA-B27 in ankylosing spondylitis.

The suggestion is being made that an external, infectious agent possesses structures or chemicals which stereochemically resemble the HLA-B27 molecule.

In the following experiments, we have sought to demonstrate possible similarities between HLA-B27 lymphocytes and Gram-negative bacterial antigens.

4.2 Rabbit Immunisations

Several rabbits have been immunised with various antigens (Table 4.1).

Rabbit A was immunised with lymphocytes obtained from 83 healthy bone marrow donors attending the 'Westminster Hospital Tissue Typing Unit' and who were HLA-B27 positive. The cells were separated by the Ficoll-Triosil method (Boyum 1968) and injected in multiple subcutaneous sites with Freund's complete adjuvant on 12 occasions over a period of 3 months.

A. Ebringer, *Ankylosing Spondylitis and Klebsiella*,
DOI 10.1007/978-1-4471-4300-0_4, © Springer-Verlag London 2013

Rabbit B was immunised on eight occasions over a period of 4 months. The lymphocytes were obtained from three patients with ankylosing spondylitis attending the 'Ankylosing Spondylitis Research Clinic of the Middlesex Hospital', all having the tissue type A2,X/B27,X. The cells were separated, as previously described and injected into the rabbit with Freund's complete adjuvant.

Rabbits C and D were immunised with 2 × 10^6 lymphocytes, on 4 occasions, over a period of 70 days, without adjuvant from a subject having tissue type A1,A11/B12,B27.

Rabbit E was injected concurrently with 2 × 10^6 lymphocytes on 4 occasions, over a period of 70 days, without adjuvant from a subject having the tissue type A1,A2/B8,B21.

Rabbit I was immunised with ultraviolet light inactivated, whole *Klebsiella pneumoniae* microorganisms, with complete Freund's adjuvant, obtained from patient number 100, attending the 'Ankylosing Spondylitis Research Clinic of the Middlesex Hospital'.

Rabbit II was immunised with an ultrasonicate preparation (KSP=*Klebsiella* sonicate preparation) of *Klebsiella pneumoniae* microorganisms obtained from the same patient 100, attending the 'Ankylosing Spondylitis Research Clinic of the Middlesex Hospital'.

Other rabbit antisera were raised similarly against *Streptococcus pyogenes* (QEC D10), C3000 *Escherichia coli* (ML 30), *Salmonella typhimurium* (QEC B22) as well as against ØX 174 virus (Miles Laboratories), tobacco mosaic virus (Kindly provided by Dr. S. Chant from Chelsea College), horse spleen ferritin (2 × crystallised, Miles Laboratories), rat γ-globulin (precipitated by half saturated ammonium sulphate) and keyhole limpet haemocyanin (KLH; Calbiochem. Ltd).

4.3 Immunodiffusion Experiments

Microorganisms were obtained from the National Collection of Type Cultures (NCTC) (Colindale), from the Queen Elizabeth College (QEC) collection of microorganisms or isolated from patients attending the 'Ankylosing Spondylitis Research Clinic of the Middlesex Hospital' (Table 4.1).

Table 4.1 Rabbit immunisations

Animal	Antigen	Period of immunisation
Rabbit A	Lymphocytes from 83 healthy bone marrow donors positive for HLA-B27	3 months
Rabbit B	Lymphocytes from 3 ankylosing spondylitis patients whose tissue type was A2,X/B27,X	4 months
Rabbits C and D	Immunised with 2 × 10^6 lymphocytes from subject with tissue type A1,A11/B12,B27	70 days
Rabbit E	Immunised with 2 × 10^6 lymphocytes from subject with tissue type A1,A2/B8,B21	70 days

Bacterial broth cultures were set up from nutrient agar plates and microorganisms harvested after 18–24 h, washed three times with phosphate buffered saline (PBS; pH 7.2, 0.15 M), suspended in 25 ml PBS to Brown Opacity 10, resuspended to 2 ml, ultrasonicated (MSE 25) for five 1-min bursts (amplitude 13–16 μm peak to peak), centrifuged and the supernatants used for immunodiffusion.

Ouchterlony plates containing 1 % purified agar (Oxoid) to a depth of 1 cm and 0.1 % sodium azide were prepared, wells cut and filled, allowed to stand overnight at 22 °C, examined through transmitted light and precipitin lines stained with 0.0125 % cadmium chloride (Crowle 1961).

4.4 Haemagglutination Method

Sheep erythrocytes in Alsever's solution (Oxoid Ltd) were coated with lipopolysaccharide (LPS) extract prepared from *Klebsiella pneumoniae* microorganisms by the phenol water-extraction method (Westphal et al. 1952).

Erythrocytes at a concentration of 4 % in PBS were incubated at 37 °C for 1 h with 40 μg of *Klebsiella* LPS, washed three times in PBS and resuspended to a final concentration of 1 %.

Doubling dilutions of 20-μl amount of test antisera, decomplemented at 56 °C for 20 min, were prepared with PBS containing 0.5 % normal rabbit serum in haemagglutination plates. Equal amounts of cell suspensions were added to each well, incubated at 37 °C for 1 h, then overnight at 4 °C and the highest dilution showing agglutination read as the end point.

Rabbit red cells were coated with *Klebsiella* LPS or *Klebsiella* trichloroacetic acid (TCA) extract (Staub 1967) and then resuspended to a concentration of 1 % in PBS. Doubling dilutions of non-heat inactivated 200 μl amounts of rabbit sera were prepared in PBS containing up to 1 % bovine serum albumin (BSA) and 40-μl amount of coated red cell suspension added. Plates were then incubated and read as before.

Human blood group B red cells were coated with ultrasonicates of *Enterobacter aerogenes* microorganisms prepared as for immunodiffusion, washed once with PBS, resuspended to a concentration of 1 % in PBS and haemagglutination assay carried out as before.

4.5 Bacterial Agglutination

Enterobacter aerogenes microorganisms, cultured as described previously, were adjusted to Brown Opacity 4 and stored at 4 °C.

Doubling dilutions of antisera in PBS were prepared to a volume of 250 μl, an equal volume of bacterial suspension added, transferred to agglutination Dreyer tubes (G.W.S. 60 × 7 mm), incubated at 37 °C for 4 h and overnight at 4 °C. Tubes were examined under diffuse light, compared to bacterial suspension without added serum and the highest antiserum dilution resulting in visible agglutination recorded as the end point.

4.6 Radio-Binding Assay with *Klebsiella* Sonicate Preparation (KSP)

Klebsiella pneumoniae microorganims grown on MacConkey plates were harvested, washed twice with cold PBS (4 °C), resuspended in 20 ml (1.3×10^{13} microorganisms) and ultrasonicated.

Supernatant was filtered through Sephadex G25 (medium), dialysed against distilled water, lyophilized and the residue dissolved in PBS ($E_{1\,cm}^{1\%}$ at 280 nm was 11.8).

Klebsiella sonicate preparation (KSP) was labelled with $Na^{125}I$ (specific activity 15 μCi/μg by the chloramine-T method (Greenwood et al. 1963).

Antigen and sera were diluted in a 0.1 M phosphate buffer, pH 7.4, containing 0.015 M sodium azide, 0.1 M sodium chloride and 0.4 % w/v BSA. To a 50 μl amount of assay buffer in LP3 plastic tubes (Luckhams), 50 μl buffer containing 3 ng of KSP-^{125}I was added, and a 50 μl amount of serum dilution (test) or 50 μl amount of assay buffer (blank) was also added, then incubated at 37 °C for 30 min and overnight at 4 °C with 50 μl co-precipitating donkey anti-rabbit IgG (1:10) (Wellcome Reagents). Precipitate was washed twice and radioactivity measured in a well-type gamma counter (Packard 578). Binding was expressed as percentage of the total radioactivity and calculated according to the formula:

$$\text{Percentage bound}(\%B) = \frac{\text{Test cpm} - \text{Blank cpm}}{\text{Total cpm} - \text{Blank cpm}} \times 100$$

4.7 Lymphocytotoxicity Assay

Lymphocytes were prepared by Ficoll sedimentation from 10 ml fresh, heparinised blood, taken from either HLA-B27-positive AS patients or healthy HLA-B27-negative controls.

Cells were washed three times, resuspended in McCoy's medium with 10 % foetal calf serum to a concentration of 2×10^6 cells/ml.

Terasaki plates containing 2 μl of serum were added with 2 μl of cell suspension, incubated for 1 h at 37 °C, then 2 μl of rabbit complement (cryopreserved in liquid nitrogen) and incubated for a further 2 h at 22 °C. Cells were stained with trypan blue and viability assessed by direct-light microscopy using an inverted microscope.

Tests were performed under code, in duplicate and expressed to the nearest 5 %. If background cell death exceeded 20 %, tests were repeated.

Table 4.2 Microorganisms used in immunodiffusion studies with rabbit A

Microorganism	Culture reference number
Alcaligenes faecalis	NCTC 415
Bacillus megaterium	QEC 54
Bacillus subtilis	QEC 56
Chlamydia (Group D)	Inst. Ophthalmology
Enterobacter aerogenes	NCTC 10006
Enterobacter aerogenes	NCTC 10336
Enterobacter cloacae	NCTC 9529
Enterobacter cloacae	NCTC 10005
Escherichia coli	ML 30
Klebsiella aerogenes	NCTC 9644
Klebsiella pneumoniae	NCTC 5056
Klebsiella pneumoniae	AS patient 1
Klebsiella pneumoniae	AS patient 2
Klebsiella pneumoniae	AS patient 3
Klebsiella pneumoniae	AS patient 4
Mycobacterium smegmatis	NCTC 8150
Proteus mirabilis	NCTC 6197
Proteus vulgaris	NCTC 10020
Pseudomonas aeruginosa	QEC B15
Pseudomonas aeruginosa	NCTC 8203
Pseudomonas fluorescens	NCDO 750
Salmonella typhimurium	QEC B22
Sarcina lutea	QEC C7
Serratia marcescens	QEC B8
Shigella sonnei	QEC B21
Staphylococcus aureus	QEC C18
Streptococcus agalactiae	QEC D11
Streptococcus faecalis	QEC D2
Streptococcus lactis	NCTC 6681
Streptococcus pyogenes	QEC D10
Yersinia enterocolitica (serotype 3)	Ahvonen P12 22a P46

4.8 Results of Immunodiffusion Experiments

Serum from rabbit A after immunisation with HLA-B27 lymphocytes produced precipitin lines against extracts from 4 microorganisms out of 31 tested (Table 4.2).

Precipitin lines were observed against two different strains of *Enterobacter aerogenes* (NCTC 10006 and NCTC 10336), one out of four *Klebsiella pneumoniae* strains isolated from faecal cultures obtained from patients with ankylosing spondylitis (AS) and *Yersinia enterocolitica* serotype 3.

Serum obtained from rabbit B after immunisation with HLA-B27/X lymphocytes produced precipitin lines against extracts from *Klebsiella pneumoniae* and *Shigella sonnei* (Table 4.3).

Table 4.3 Results of immunodiffusion experiments with sera obtained from rabbit B before and after immunisation with HLA-B27/X lymphocytes

Microorganism	Reference number	Before immunisation	After immunisation
Escherichia coli	ML 30	−ve	−ve
Klebsiella pneumoniae	MX 100	−ve	+
Salmonella typhimurium	QEC-B22	−ve	−ve
Shigella sonnei	QEC-B21	−ve	+

A plus sign indicates the presence of a precipitin line

Table 4.4 Haemagglutination titres of sera obtained from animals immunised with *Klebsiella* microorganisms (rabbit I), *Klebsiella* sonicate preparation (KSP) (rabbit II) and human HLA-B27 lymphocytes (rabbits A and B)

			Titre (reciprocal dilution)	
Animal	*Klebsiella* antigen	Erythrocyte	Before immunisation	After immunisation
Rabbit I	LPS	Sheep	4, 8	2,048; 2,048; 2,048
Rabbit I	LPS	Rabbit	8, 8, 16	1,024; 1,024; 1,024
Rabbit I	TCA	Rabbit	8, 8, 8	4,096; 4,096; 4,096
Rabbit II	LPS	Sheep	2, 8	2,048; 2,048
Rabbit II	TCA	Rabbit	16, 16	1,024; 1,024
Rabbit A	LPS	Sheep	4, 4	128; 128
Rabbit A	TCA	Rabbit	2, 8, 8	32; 32; 64
Rabbit B	LPS	Sheep	16, 16, 4	512; 512; 512
Rabbit B	LPS	Rabbit	64, 64, 64	1,024; 1,024; 1,024
Rabbit B	TCA	Rabbit	128, 128, 128	1,024; 1,024; 1,024

Uncoated erythrocytes gave a titre of 8 or less

4.9 Haemagglutination Results

The results of the haemagglutination studies using rabbit antisera are summarised in Table 4.4.

Rabbits A and B, immunised with HLA-B27 lymphocytes, showed increased haemagglutinating activity against sheep or rabbit red cells coated with *Klebsiella* LPS ($t=8.50$, $p<0.001$) or *Klebsiella* TCA ($t=4.02$, $p<0.02$) extracts, and these differences are statistically significant when compared to serum obtained from the same rabbit before immunisation.

Furthermore, serum from rabbit A agglutinated human blood group red cells coated with an ultrasonicate preparation of *Enterobacter aerogenes* to a titre of 1,024, whilst serum from the same rabbit obtained before immunisation gave a titre of 16. Similar preparations of *Klebsiella pneumoniae* could not be coated on to sheep, rabbit or human red blood cells.

Rabbit antisera obtained after immunisation with *Streptococcus pyogenes*, *Escherichia coli*, *Salmonella typhimurium*, ØX 174 virus, tobacco mosaic virus and the antigens horse spleen ferritin, keyhole limpet haemocyanin and rat γ-globulin, all failed to show haemagglutinating activity against sheep red blood cells coated with *Klebsiella* LPS extract above a titre of 16.

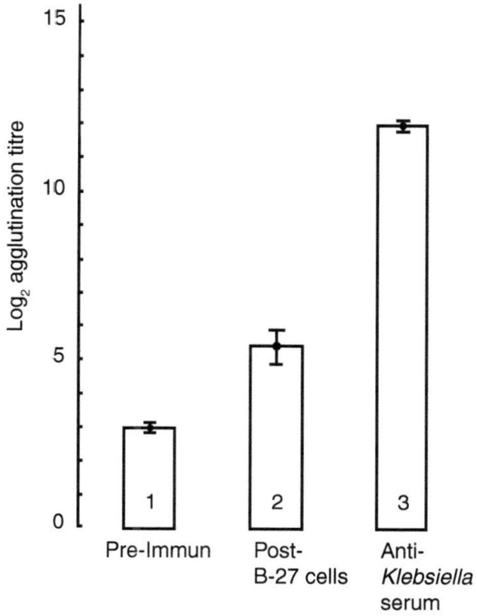

Fig. 4.1 Agglutination of *Enterobacter aerogenes* microorganisms by sera obtained from rabbit A before (1) and after (2) immunisation, respectively, with HLA-B27 lymphocytes. A rabbit antiserum to *Klebsiella pneumoniae* (3) agglutinated *Enterobacter aerogenes* microorganisms up to a dilution of 1/2,048

4.10 Bacterial Agglutination Results

The results of bacterial agglutination tests using the motile, flagellate microorganism *Enterobacter aerogenes* are summarised in Fig. 4.1.

Serum obtained from rabbit A, after immunisation with HLA-B27 lymphocytes, agglutinated *Enterobacter aerogenes* to a greater extent than did serum obtained from the same rabbit before immunisation ($t = 2.28$, $p < 0.025$). However, studies with the non-motile microorganism *Klebsiella pneumoniae* failed to show any significant bacterial agglutination, even with rabbit *Klebsiella* antiserum.

Ankylosing spondylitis patients were examined for the presence of the three microorganisms detected in the pilot study with serum obtained from rabbit A, namely, *Enterobacter aerogenes*, *Klebsiella pneumoniae* and *Yersinia enterocolitica*. Only *Klebsiella pneumoniae* was found more frequently in patients with active ankylosing spondylitis, and further studies were confined to this microorganism (Welsh et al. 1980).

4.11 Results of Radio-Binding Assay with *Klebsiella* Sonicate Preparation (KSP)

Sera from rabbits A and B, which were immunised with HLA-B27 lymphocytes, showed higher percentage binding of KSP-^{125}I compared to a pooled control serum obtained from three unimmunised rabbits at every dilution tested above 1/200 (Fig. 4.2).

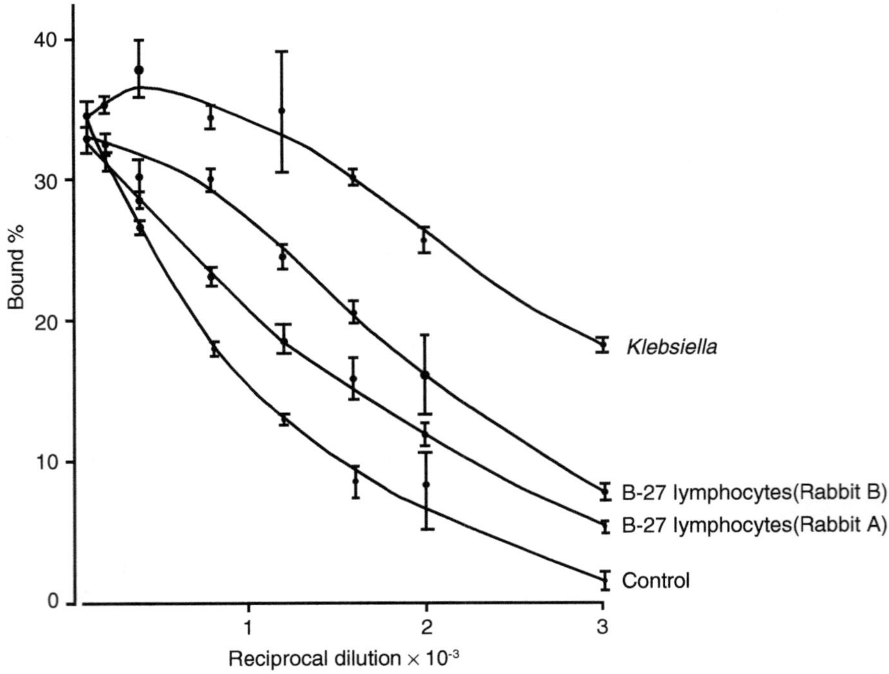

Fig. 4.2 Comparison of rabbit antisera raised against HLA-B27 lymphocytes (A and B), *Klebsiella pneumoniae* microorganisms and pooled serum from three unimmunised rabbits (control) in a *Klebsiella*SP-^{125}I-binding assay. Each point is a mean of quadruplicate estimations, and bars represent standard errors of the mean

At a dilution of 1/800, serum from rabbit A had a binding titre of 22.6±0.3 % (mean±standard error) (t=11.68, p<0.001), whilst rabbit B had a titre of 24.4±0.8 % (t=7.79, p<0.001) when compared to a titre of 17.8±0.3 % for the pooled control serum.

Studies at dilutions 1: 100, 1: 250, 1: 500 and 1: 1,000 on sera obtained from rabbits C and D, before and after immunisations with HLA-B27 lymphocytes, without adjuvant, showed a small but definite increase (p<0.05) in binding *Klebsiella* SP-^{125}I compared to sera obtained from rabbit E before and after immunisation with an equal quantity of non-B27 lymphocytes which did not show any increased binding.

4.12 Cytotoxicity Results

Rabbit anti-*Klebsiella* sonicate preparation (KSP) was more cytotoxic for HLA-B27 positive lymphocytes obtained from ankylosing spondylitis patients than for lymphocytes obtained from healthy, non-B27 control subjects (Fig. 4.3).

Control sera obtained from two unimmunised rabbits had no cytotoxic activity against either B27 positive or B27-negative lymphocytes.

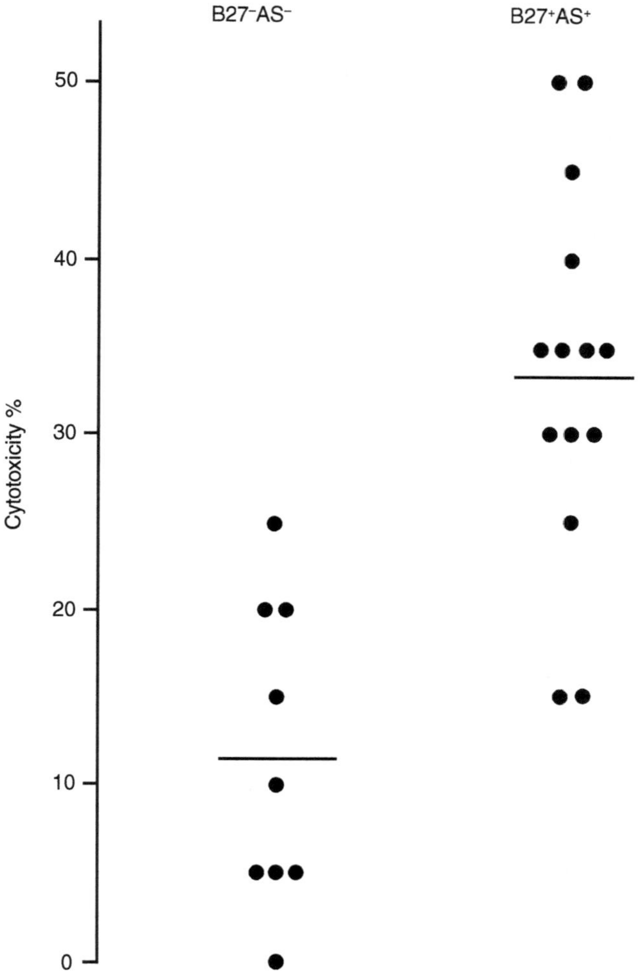

Fig. 4.3 Percentage of lymphocytes killed after incubation with rabbit anti-*Klebsiella* SP serum. Each point represents the mean of duplicate experiments from one individual after subtraction for background cell death. Serum obtained from the same rabbit before immunisation with *Klebsiella* SP had no cytotoxic activity

4.13 Discussion and Conclusions

Rabbits immunised with HLA-B27 positive lymphocytes, obtained either from healthy bone marrow donors or ankylosing spondylitis patients, have been shown to produce antisera which have immunological activity against the Gram-negative microorganisms *Klebsiella pneumoniae*, *Enterobacter aerogenes*, *Shigella sonnei* and *Yersinia enterocolitica*. These microorganisms share common enterobacterial antigens. Two of these microbes are closely related, except that *Enterobacter aerogenes* is motile whilst *Klebsiella pneumoniae* is non-motile.

Furthermore, two of these microorganims, *Shigella sonnei* and *Yersinia enterocolitica*, have been implicated as causative agents of 'reactive arthritis' (Aho et al. 1975).

In haemagglutination studies, the rabbit HLA-B27 lymphocyte antisera raised with Freund's complete adjuvant have been shown to agglutinate, up to a titre of 1/512, sheep and rabbit red cells coated with *Klebsiella* extracts prepared by several different methods. Other rabbit antisera, also raised with Freund's complete adjuvant against a variety of protein antigens, viruses and microorganisms including *Salmonella typhimurium* and *Escherichia coli*, did not exceed a haemagglutination titre of 1/16 when tested with *Klebsiella* LPS-coated sheep red blood cells.

It is thus unlikely that non-specific adjuvant effects could have been responsible for the elevated titre produced by sera obtained from rabbits immunised with HLA-B27 lymphocytes.

Enterobacter aerogenes microorganisms reacted both by haemagglutination and bacterial agglutination against these rabbit HLA-B27 lymphocyte antisera.

However, *Klebsiella pneumoniae* failed to agglutinate in these assays, and this could have been due to the absence of flagellae in these microorganisms.

Increased binding to *Klebsiella* extracts by these rabbit HLA-B27 lymphocyte antisera was shown not only in the IgM-dependent haemagglutination assay but also in the IgG-dependent radio-binding assay.

Lymphocytoxicity experiments have demonstrated that rabbit antisera raised against *Klebsiella pneumoniae* have greater cytotoxic activity against HLA-B27 lymphocytes obtained from ankylosing spondylitis patients than for non-B27 lymphocytes obtained from healthy subjects.

Although these observations are compatible with cross-reactivity between HLA-B27 lymphocytes and some antigens present in several species of Gram-negative microorganisms, such as *Klebsiella* or *Yersinia*, the cross-reactive peptides involved need to be identified.

When rabbits are immunised with human lymphocytes, antibodies will also be produced against the non-specific, xenogeneic membrane components, and these could readily mask any specific antibodies against HLA antigens.

One possible way to eliminate the problem of heterophil interaction is to study allogeneic sera having specificity for defined HLA antigens, such as tissue typing sera.

In conclusion, it would appear that rabbits immunised with human HLA-B27 lymphocytes produce sera with immunological activity against some Gram-negative microorganisms, including *Klebsiella pneumoniae*, but the peptides or antigens responsible for this cross-reactivity have not been identified.

References

Aho K, Ahvonen P, Alkio P, Lassus A, Sairanen E, Sievers K, Tillikainen A. HLA-B27 in reactive arthritis following infection. Ann Rheum Dis. 1975;34 Suppl 1:29–30.

Boyum A. Separation of white blood cells. Nature. 1968;204:793–4.

Crowle AJ. Immunodiffusion. London: Academic; 1961.

Greenwood FC, Hunter WM, Glover JS. The preparation of ^{131}I-labelled human growth hormone of high specific radioactivity. Biochem J. 1963;89:114–23.

Staub AM. Preparation of cell wall antigens from Gram-negative bacteria. In: Williams CA, Chase MW, editors. Methods in immunology and immunochemistry, vol. I. London and New York: Academic; 1967. p. 28.

Welsh J, Avakian H, Cowling P, Ebringer A, Wooley P, Panayi G, Ebringer R. Ankylosing spondylitis, HLA-B27 and *Klebsiella*. I. Cross-reactivity studies with rabbit antisera. Br J Exp Pathol. 1980;61:85–91.

Westphal O, Luderitz O, Bister F. Über die Extraktion von Bakterien mit Phenol/Wasser. Z Naturforsch. 1952;7b:148.

Chapter 5
Molecular Mimicry Between HLA-B27 and *Klebsiella* Bacteria Investigated by Using Human Tissue Typing Sera

5.1 Introduction: Molecular Mimicry and Tissue Typing Sera

Rabbits immunised with human HLA-B27 lymphocytes have been shown to react against antigens obtained from several Gram-negative microorganisms. Xenoantigens are widely distributed throughout nature and induce the formation of cross-reactive antibodies which may be involved in the pathogenesis of various diseases (Whittingham and Mackay 1977).

Immunisation with xenogeneic lymphocytes however stimulates the production of antibodies which are directed predominantly against non-specific membrane components, thereby diluting the antigenic effects of HLA antigens. A possible way to avoid such limitations is to study sera obtained after immunisation with allogeneic lymphocytes.

Human tissue typing sera are usually obtained from pregnant women who have been immunised by fetal lymphocytes carrying paternal HLA antigens not shared with the mother.

Antibodies against HLA-A, HLA-B and HLA-C specificities are commonly found in sera of women who have had several pregnancies (Festenstein and Démant 1978).

Cross-reactions between Gram-negative bacteria and antigens of vertebrate cells have been demonstrated for *Escherichia coli*, *Salmonella typhimurium* (Rowley and Jenkin 1962) and *Klebsiella pneumoniae* (Asherson and Holborow 1966).

HLA antigens have been shown to cross-react with bacterial antigens obtained from *Escherichia coli* and *Salmonella* strains of microorganisms (Hirata et al. 1973).

In this study, monospecific HLA-B27 tissue typing sera have been compared with non-B27 tissue typing for their capacity to bind *Klebsiella* antigens. The majority of the anti-HLA-B27 tissue typing sera came from Bristol.

A. Ebringer, *Ankylosing Spondylitis and Klebsiella*,
DOI 10.1007/978-1-4471-4300-0_5, © Springer-Verlag London 2013

5.2 Bristol

Bristol is a famous seaport and university town in the west of England, on the River Avon and has a population of approximately half a million.

The name means in Old English, 'the place of the bridge'. The city obtained a royal charter in 1155.

The 'Clifton Suspension Bridge' spans the Avon Gorge, was designed by Isambard Kingdom Brunel and completed in 1864.

Bristol merchants sponsored many nautical explorations, especially by Italian and English sailors.

The 'Cabot Tower' was erected in 1867, to commemorate the 400th anniversary of John Cabot's discovery of North America.

5.3 HLA Tissue Typing Sera

Human tissue typing sera were obtained from the 'National Tissue Typing Reference Centre', in Southmead, a suburb of Bristol and supplied by Dr. C.C. Entwistle. Some 10 out of the 13 anti-HLA-B27 tissue typing sera came from Bristol.

Other tissue typing sera were obtained commercially from Searle (High Wycombe).

Typing sera from both sources were supplied neat and had been obtained from women who had been pregnant.

There were altogether 30 non-B27 and 13 B27 typing sera involved in this study.

5.4 Haemagglutination Method

Sheep erythrocytes coated with *Klebsiella* lipopolysaccharide (LPS) were prepared and assay carried out as previously described.

The titre of each typing serum was expressed as the $\log_2$ difference between the titre achieved with coated cells compared to the titre obtained with uncoated cells.

5.5 Labelling of *Klebsiella* Sonicate Preparation (KSP)

Klebsiella pneumoniae microorganisms, obtained from ankylosing spondylitis patient 100 attending the 'Ankylosing Spondylitis Research Clinic of the Middlesex Hospital', were grown on MacConkey plates, harvested, washed twice with cold PBS (4 °C), resuspended (20 ml; 1.3×10^{13} microorganisms), ultrasonicated and centrifuged.

Supernatant was filtered through Sephadex G-25 and ^{125}I-labelling of *Klebsiella* sonicate preparation, carried out as previously described.

5.6 Radio-Binding Assay for ^{125}I-*Klebsiella* Sonicate Preparation

The ability of various tissue typing sera to bind a fixed quantity of ^{125}I-*Klebsiella* sonicate preparation was tested by a radio-binding assay and carried out in LP3 plastic tubes (Luckhams).

Antigen and sera were diluted in 0.1 M phosphate buffer, pH 7.4, containing 0.015 M sodium azide, 0.1 M sodium chloride and 0.4 % w:v bovine serum albumin (BSA). To a 50 μl amount of assay buffer, 50 μl buffer containing 3 ng of ^{125}I-*Klebsiella* sonicate preparation was added and a 50 μl amount of serum dilution, incubated at 37 °C for 30 min, then co-precipitating rabbit anti-human (1:6) serum added, titrated to equivalence point and incubated overnight at 4 °C.

Unbound ^{125}I-*Klebsiella* sonicate preparation was removed by addition of 1 ml ice-cold phosphate buffer containing 0.01 M potassium iodide, centrifuged (MSE,Mistral) at 3,000 rpm for 30 min. Then, 1 ml amount from the supernatant discarded, and the washing procedure repeated.

Radioactivity was measured in a well-type gamma counter (Packard Model 578). Binding of ^{125}I-*Klebsiella* sonicate preparation was expressed as a percentage of the total remaining after correction for blank values, which contained labelled antigen with co-precipitating serum alone (Formula 5.1).

Each serum dilution was carried out in quadruplicate.

$$\text{Percentage bound } (\%\text{B}) = \frac{\text{Test cpm} - \text{Blank cpm}}{\text{Total cpm} - \text{Blank cpm}} \times 100 \tag{5.1}$$

5.7 Competition Assay for ^{12}I-*Klebsiella* Sonicate Preparation

Rabbit serum against *Klebsiella* sonicate preparation was able to bind ^{125}I-*Klebsiella* sonicate preparation in a radio-binding assay up to a dilution of 1/10,000 when compared to serum (control) obtained from the same rabbit before immunisation.

Previous studies had shown that maximum difference was obtained in the dilution range of 1/1,000 and 1/3,000.

Therefore, a dilution pf 1/2,000 of rabbit anti-*Klebsiella* sonicate preparation was selected for competition experiments with human tissue typing sera.

Since co-precipitating donkey anti-rabbit serum had no precipitating activity against human immunoglobulins, any binding of ^{125}I-*Klebsiella* sonicate preparation by human tissue typing sera would appear as a reduction in the radioactive counts of the precipitate and therefore could be expressed as a percentage inhibition by the tissue typing serum acting as a competitor.

Different tissue typing sera could thus be compared for their capacity to inhibit the ^{125}I-*Klebsiella* sonicate preparation radio-binding assay.

The method used was a modification of the radio-binding assay: Briefly, to 50 µl aliquots of human HLA typing sera diluted to 1/5 or 1/55 with buffer were added 50 µl of rabbit anti-*Klebsiella* serum at a dilution of 1/2,000 and a 50 µl solution containing 3 ng of ^{125}I-*Klebsiella* sonicate preparation as antigen. After incubation, the rabbit IgG was precipitated by donkey anti-rabbit IgG serum (Wellcome Reagents) and assay carried out as before.

The reduction in the binding of ^{125}I-*Klebsiella* sonicate preparation by rabbit anti-*Klebsiella* in the presence of HLA typing serum acting as competitor (%B) was compared to control assays containing no HLA typing serum but an equivalent volume of buffer (%B_0) and results expressed as percentage inhibition (% I; Formula 5.2).

Assays containing HLA-typing serum alone had very low binding activity (3–4 %) compared to control assays containing rabbit *Klebsiella* antiserum (19–20 % binding), and the inhibition values were corrected for these readings. Thus, Formula 5.2 becomes:

$$\text{Percentage inhibition } (\%\text{I}) = \left(1 - \frac{\%\text{B (with competitor)}}{\%\text{B}_0\text{ (without competitor)}}\right) \times 100 \qquad (5.2)$$

5.8 Results of Haemagglutination Studies with HLA Typing Sera

The results of the haemagglutination studies using HLA typing sera are summarised in Table 5.1.

In the HLA-A series, there were only two out of 15 sera which gave a positive response with *Klebsiella* LPS-coated sheep red cells (Table 5.1, group A).

The HLA-B series of typing sera were divided into two groups: a B27 group which consisted of sera with B27 specificity and a non-B27 group containing the remaining B-specific tissue typing sera.

Typing sera having specificities for HLA antigens cross-reacting with HLA-B27, such as B7, BW22 and BW42, were excluded from this study.

There were 4 out of 15 sera in the non-B27 group and 10 out of 13 in the B27 group that reacted with *Klebsiella*-coated sheep red cells, and this difference is statistically significant ($\chi^2 = 7.03$, $p < 0.01$).

When the B27 group is compared to all A and B tissue typing sera, the difference becomes more pronounced: 6 out of 30 sera reacted in the non-B27 group compared to 10 out of 13 sera in the B27 group, and this difference is statistically significant ($\chi^2 = 10.26$, $p < 0.001$).

5.9 Results of Radio-Binding Assay for ^{125}I-*Klebsiella* Sonicate Preparation by HLA Typing Sera

Twelve monospecific HLA-typing sera provided by the 'National Tissue Typing Reference Centre' in Southmead; Bristol (Table 5.2), were compared for their capacity to bind ^{125}I-*Klebsiella* sonicate preparation.

Table 5.1 Agglutination titres of *Klebsiella* LPS-coated sheep red cells by HLA typing sera

HLA-A series	Assigned specificity	Titre
(A) *Group A, non-B27 tissue typing sera*:		
1022	A1+11	1
83	A1+11	0
420	A1+B8 0	
54/60/3	A2	0
230	A2	0
35	A2+W17+W38	0
57/73/6	A3	0
257	A9	0
Fer/14	A9	0
M8/47	A9	1
204	A10	0
1093	A11	0
M6/18	W29+weak B12	0
72/39/6	W31+W30	0
73/57/7	W32+A10	0
(B) *Group B, non-B27 tissue typing sera*:		
M8/43	B5	0
3893 (Bristol)	B5	0
294	W5+B5	0
M8/38	W5+B5 0	
515	B8	0
5200 (Bristol)	B8	0
3572 (Bristol)	B8	0
3560 (Bristol)	B8	0
L18/670	B12	0
840	B12	1
63/33/5	B12	0
4609 (Bristol)	B12	2
5336 (Bristol)	B12	0
5/14/7	W14	0
21	W18+B5	0
(C) *Group C, B27 tissue typing sera*:		
837	W27	2
1018	W27	2
1058	W27	2
307 (Bristol)	B27	1
753 (Bristol)	B27	3
2503 (Bristol)	B27	0
3041 (Bristol)	B27	2
3086 (Bristol)	B27	1
3209 (Bristol)	B27	2
3356 (Bristol)	B27	0
3469 (Bristol)	B27	1
4480 (Bristol)	B27	1
5185 (Bristol)	B27	0

Results are expressed as the number of doubling dilutions greater than for uncoated cells (Titre = $\log_2$ coated titre – $\log_2$ uncoated titre)

NTTRC sera from Bristol are indicated; the remaining sera were obtained from Searle (High Wycombe)

Table 5.2 Cytotoxic specificity of 12 HLA typing sera supplied by the 'National Tissue Typing Reference Centre' (Bristol) used in radio-binding assays

U.K. number	Assigned HLA specificity	Lymphocyte cytotoxicity ++	+−	−+	−−
3086	B27	5	1	1	80
3209	B27	12	0	2	128
3469	B27	6	2	0	76
2503	B27	7	0	1	72
5185	B27	8	0	1	67
4480	B27	10	0	0	70
3560	B8	17	0	0	60
3572	B8	17	0	0	60
5200	B8	12	0	0	64
3893	B5	7	0	2	70
4609	B12	14	0	2	64
5336	B12	17	2	1	51

+ + Number of different lymphocytes carrying HLA antigen of assigned specificity detected by typing serum. +− Number of different lymphocytes carrying HLA antigen of assigned specificity not detected by typing serum. −+ Number of different lymphocytes not carrying HLA antigen of assigned detected by typing serum. − − Number of different lymphocytes not carrying HLA antigen of assigned specificity not detected by typing serum

The six B27 tissue typing sera bound more ^{125}I-*Klebsiella* sonicate preparation than the six non-B27 typing sera (Fig. 5.1) at each of the five dilutions tested (At 1/200 dilution, $t=2.45$, $p<0.025$).

5.10 Results of Competition Binding Assays

Competition studies using the HLA typing sera at two separate dilutions showed that HLA-B27 typing sera were acting as a better competitor than non-B27 tissue typing sera (Fig. 5.2). Monospecific anti-B27 tissue typing sera competed more strongly in the binding for ^{125}I-*Klebsiella* sonicate preparation by a rabbit anti-*Klebsiella* serum than did non-B27 typing sera, and these differences were statistically significant at both typing serum dilution tested: at 1/5 dilution ($t=2.73$; $p<0.02$) and at 1/55 dilution ($t=2.31$, $p<0.05$).

5.11 Discussion and Conclusions

The experiments reported here indicate that pregnant women immunised with HLA-B27 lymphocytes produce allogeneic sera that show increased binding for *Klebsiella* antigens compared to sera produced against non-HLA-B27 antigens (Avakian et al. 1980).

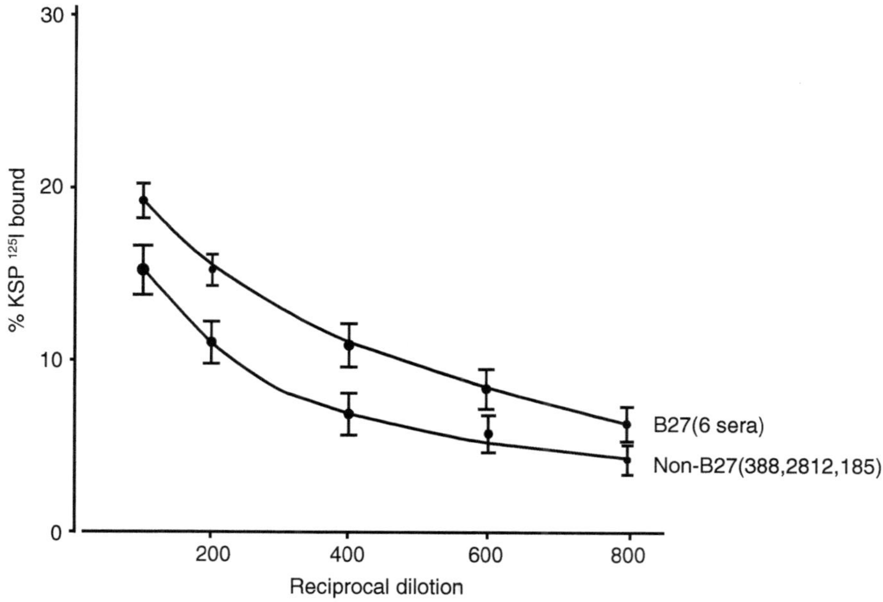

Fig. 5.1 Radio-binding assay using [125]I-*Klebsiella* sonicate preparation of monospecific HLA typing sera. Each point is a mean (± standard error) of estimations with six different typing sera. Each serum was tested in quadruplicate

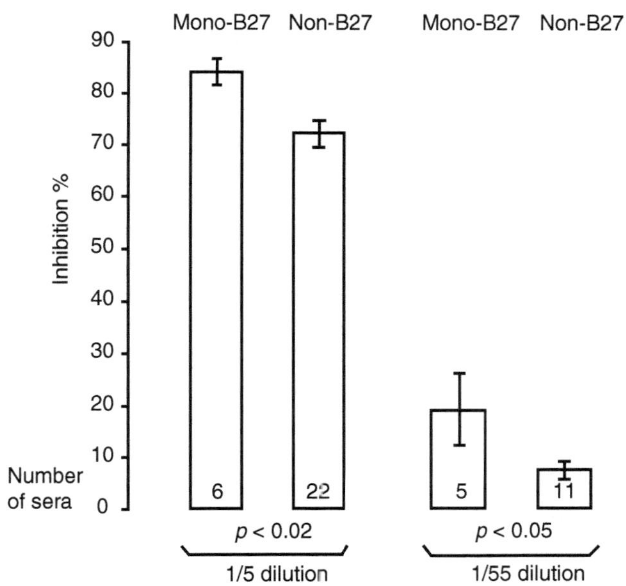

Fig. 5.2 Competition assay between HLA typing sera and rabbit anti-*Klebsiella* serum for [125]I-*Klebsiella* sonicate preparation. *Histograms* indicate mean (± standard error) of sera tested, and each serum estimation was done in quadruplicate

These investigations were started after the demonstration of an association between HLA-B27 and ankylosing spondylitis patients (Caffrey and James 1973).

Two main theories have been proposed to explain this association.

The first is the two-gene theory or linkage disequilibrium hypothesis which states that there is a separate susceptibility gene, closely linked to HLA-B27, whose gene product is somehow associated with the development of the disease.

The second is the one-gene theory or cross-tolerance hypothesis which states that the HLA-B27 gene codes codes for an HLA molecule that stereochemically resembles antigens found in environmental agents such as microorganisms (Ebringer 1978).

Infections by such microorganisms might lead to the production of cross-reactive autoantibodies which could be responsible for the tissue damage occurring in ankylosing spondylitis patients. A similar mechanism is thought to operate in rheumatic fever (Kaplan and Meyeserian 1962).

It has been suggested that such 'molecular mimicry' may be a general phenomenon of biological adaptation by the parasite to the host (Damian 1964).

In an endeavour to examine this second hypothesis, rabbits were immunised with HLA-B27 lymphocytes and tested against a number of microorganisms. Antigens obtained from the Gram-negative microorganisms *Enterobacter aerogenes*, *Klebsiella pneumoniae*, *Shigella sonnei* and *Yersinia enterocolitica* were found to react with such antisera. Examination of faecal cultures in patients with ankylosing spondylitis showed that *Klebsiella pneumoniae* microorganisms were found frequently in active cases, but the other microorganisms were rarely isolated from patients or control subjects. Therefore, further studies were confined to *Klebsiella* microorganisms.

The immunological activity of the rabbit lymphocyte antisera could have been due to non-specific factors, such as immunisation with xenogeneic cells or the effect of adjuvant.

Therefore, allogeneic, monospecific tissue typing sera were tested for their capacity to bind *Klebsiella* antigens. Studies with tissue typing sera obtained from two separate centres indicate that B27 antisera react to a greater extent with *Klebsiella* antigens than non-B27 sera by three separate techniques: haemagglutination, radio-binding assay and competition radioimmunoassay. Although these differences are small, they are readily reproducible and would appear to be compatible with the chronic nature of the pathogenesis of ankylosing spondylitis. More pronounced cross-reactions between host and microorganisms would evoke more acute pathological phenomena such as those observed during graft rejections or blood transfusion reactions.

A possible explanation for the results obtained from the studies with rabbit and human tissue typing sera is that there is partial cross-reactivity between some antigens present in HLA-B27 lymphocytes, including HLA-B27 itself and antigenic components of several Gram-negative bacteria such as *Klebsiella* or *Yersinia.*

These cross-reactions may be relevant in the pathogenesis of ankylosing spondylitis or 'reactive arthritis' following *Yersinia* or *Shigella* infections. Further studies are required to identify the parameters which control the pathogenesis of these diseases.

References

Asherson GL, Holborow EJ. Autoantibody production in rabbits. VII. Autoantibodies to gut produced by injection of bacteria. Immunology. 1966;10:161–7.

Avakian H, Welsh J, Ebringer A, Entwistle CC. Ankylosing spondylitis, HLA-B27 and *Klebsiella*. II. Cross-reactivity studies with human tissue typing sera. Br J Exp Pathol. 1980;61:92–6.

Caffrey MFP, James DCO. Human lymphocyte antigen association in ankylosing spondylitis. Nature. 1973;242:121.

Damian RT. Molecular mimicry: antigen sharing by parasite and host and its consequences. Am Nat. 1964;98:129–49.

Ebringer A. The link between genes and disease. New Sci. 1978;79:865–7.

Festenstein H, Démant P. HLA and H-2. London: Edward Arnold; 1978.

Hirata AA, McIntire FC, Terasaki PI, Mittal KK. Crossreactions between human transplantation antigens and bacterial lipopolysaccharides. Transplantation. 1973;15:441–5.

Kaplan MH, Meyeserian M. An immunological crossreaction between Group A *Streptococcal* cells and human heart. Lancet. 1962;1:706–10.

Rowley D, Jenkin CR. Antigenic crossreaction between host and parasite as a possible cause of pathogenicity. Nature. 1962;193:151–4.

Whittingham S, Mackay IR. Tissue antigens: autoantigens, alloantigens xenoantigens and neoantigens. Aust N Z J Med. 1977;7:172–94.

Chapter 6
Muscle Changes in Ankylosing Spondylitis

6.1 Introduction: Involvement of Muscle Pathology in Ankylosing Spondylitis

Ankylosing spondylitis patients attending the 'Ankylosing Spondylitis Research Clinic of the Middlesex Hospital' complained frequently of muscle stiffness and pain. Some even mentioned that there was never any day that they felt to be free of pain or stiffness.

Lumbar pain in ankylosing spondylitis patients strongly suggests that pathology of paraspinal muscles is involved in this disease. This could involve specific pathological damage as well as atrophic changes due to disuse and may occur in many muscles (Cooper et al. 1991).

6.2 Muscle Stiffness, Muscle Pain and the Enthesis

Muscle stiffness and often accompanied by tenderness is a well-recognised feature of ankylosing spondylitis. The source of these characteristic symptoms has long been attributed to joint inflammation and more recently to inflammation at the site of attachment of ligaments or tendons to bone, to the enthesis (Ball 1971).

The dramatic relief obtained by exercise, as compared to the slower less pronounced relief, produced in other inflammatory arthropathies, could indicate the involvement of the muscle itself.

A higher serum creatine phosphokinase level was found in a group of ankylosing spondylitis patients when compared to healthy subjects, and isoenzyme studies confirmed that muscle was the source of the enzyme (Calin 1975).

Significant histological changes in the muscle tissues of ankylosing spondylitis patients have been described in several studies. In a total of 23 ankylosing spondylitis patients with biopsies from paraspinal muscles, 6 showed neurogenic features, and

A. Ebringer, *Ankylosing Spondylitis and Klebsiella*,
DOI 10.1007/978-1-4471-4300-0_6, © Springer-Verlag London 2013

the remainder had a variety of non-specific atrophic changes with 4 exhibiting a mild degree of interstitial fibrosis (Pohl and Sievers 1974).

In a study of five quadriceps muscle biopsies, two were considered myopathic, two had indeterminate changes and one was normal (Roux et al. 1975).

To try to extend these studies, we have investigated the histological, surface electromyographic and plasma enzyme changes together with muscle strength measurements in a further group of ankylosing spondylitis patients with proven disease, attending the 'Ankylosing Spondylitis Research Clinic of the Middlesex Hospital'.

6.3 Patients and Controls

Patients with ankylosing spondylitis, as defined by the New York criteria (Gofton 1968), were studied: 18 were male and 2 were female with an age range of 21–59 years (mean 38.9 years). The male/female ratio was 9.0.

Six were considered to be definitely active at the time of the biopsy due to the presence of peripheral disease such as iritis (one patient) or moderate to severe pain and stiffness, requiring regular anti-inflammatory therapy up to maximum dosage. Past involvement of hip or knee had occurred in 13 patients, although none had overt activity in these joints at the time of the biopsy. There was a past history of iritis in 10 patients.

Nineteen patients were positive for HLA-B27 (95 %), the other one being positive for HLA-B7.

Fifteen were on anti-inflammatory agents (phenylbutazone 9, naproxen 3, indomethacin 1, flurbiprofen 1 and fenoprofen 1). In addition, one patient was also on D-penicillamine and one was on acetazolamide and potassium chloride for glaucoma. Four were not taking any tablets.

Sera were also collected from 34 patients with active rheumatoid arthritis (8 male/26 female) attending the Rheumatology Department of the Lister Hospital in Stevenage, Hertfordshire, with a mean age of 59.0 years (range = 21–83 years) having a mean erythrocyte sedimentation rate (± standard error) of 49.6 ± 4.8 mm/h.

The female/male ratio in the rheumatoid arthritis patients from Hertfordshire was 3.3. Erythrocyte sedimentation rates were not measured in the controls.

6.4 Blood Samples, Muscle Biopsies and Histology

A 10-ml sample of blood was taken for measurement of plasma creatine kinase in 17 patients immediately prior to biopsy.

All patients were subjected to mid-thigh needle biopsy using the method of Edwards and co-workers (1980).

Samples for histology and biochemistry were first orientated under the dissecting microscope and then frozen in isopentane cooled by liquid nitrogen.

Cryostat sections were prepared and stained with haematoxylin and eosin, modified Gomori trichrome and Miller's Van Gieson.

Histochemical sections for NADH tetrazolium reductase (NADH-TR), myosin ATPase (pre-incubated at pH 9.4) using the method of Round et al. (1980) and also for acid phosphatase were also performed, with simultaneous staining of normal sections as controls.

In addition, biopsy specimens from five patients were randomly selected and examined for IgG, IgM, IgA, C1q and C3 by the previously described method of Isenberg and Snaith (1981).

Fluorescein-conjugated antisera to these immunoglobulins (Behring Diagnostic Reagents, Hounslow, Middlesex) were incubated with muscle sections for 30 min and, after washing in phosphate buffered saline, examined under ultraviolet light.

6.5 Muscle Strength and Electromyographic Studies

Sixteen patients attended at a later date for muscle strength measurement. The 'maximum voluntary contraction force' for the quadriceps muscles was measured by the technique of Edwards et al. (1977). The patient sits in a muscle testing chair with the pelvis stabilised by a lap strap and an inextensible loop around the ankle. Forces generated by maximal voluntary knee extension are detected by a force transducer attached to the inextensible loop, amplified and displayed on an ultraviolet paper recorder.

The forces produced were compared with those of a large group of normal subjects, matched for weight and expressed as a percentage of the expected normal.

Quantitative electromyography was also studied in this muscle. Patients were set a visual target which was 25 % of the maximum voluntary contraction force of the left quadriceps muscle. Surface electromyograms from six positions on the anterior surface of the thigh, along a line joining the greater trochanter and the mid-point of the patella, of duration 1.28 s and digitised at 1 kHz, were sequentially entered into the computer memory (CBM 3032).

Frequency analysis using the fast Fourier transform algorithm was performed, and power spectra of the electromyogram for each position were averaged over the ensemble. The 'mean power frequency' (MPF), which reflects the overall frequency content from the contracting muscle, was computed from the final averaged spectrum using the Mills et al. (1982) method.

6.6 Results of Histological and Biochemical Investigations

All specimens showed some histological changes to a varying degree and are summarised in Table 6.1. Normal sections stained with haematoxylin-eosin showed pink, densely packed, uniform fibres with peripheral nuclei. No more than 9 % of these fibres should show central migration of their nuclei. In 80 % of our ankylosing

Table 6.1 Summary of histological changes

	Number of patients		Percentage of patients showing changes
Internal nuclei	Many cells	2	10
	Few cells	14	70
Atrophic fibres	Type I	2	10
	Type II	6	30
Acid phosphatase reaction	Local	15	75
	Generalised	2	10
NADH-TR peripheral condensation reaction	11	55	

spondylitis patients, central migration of nuclei was seen indicating a non-specific myopathic change.

Myosin ATPase, when incubated at pH 9.4, selectively stains type II fibres giving rise to a characteristic chequerboard pattern. This allows for assessment of fibre type distribution which in our case was normal. However, scattered small type II fibres with occasional atrophy were seen in 40 % of the sections.

A diffuse reaction with the acid phosphatase stain indicates lysosomal activity and muscle cell damage. This feature was seen in 10 % of our ankylosing spondylitis patients, but in 75 % of the patients there were scattered areas of local reaction not seen in normal control samples stained at the same time.

NADH-TR is an oxidative stain which selects type I fibres again giving rise to the characteristic chequerboard pattern. There was a peripheral condensing reaction product in 55 % of our samples. No abnormal fibrosis was demonstrated with the Miller's Van Gieson stain nor did the modified Gomori trichrome detect any evidence of mitochondrial damage. The fluorescent tests for immunoglobulins were negative in all five specimens.

The plasma creatine kinase was elevated above the laboratory normal in only 2 of the 17 ankylosing spondylitis patients studied.

6.7 Muscle Strength Measurements and Surface Electromyography

The 'maximum voluntary contraction force' was taken as the highest of three maximal voluntary quadriceps contractions, and the results were expressed as a percentage of predicted values obtained from healthy subjects of equivalent weight. Only 2 of the 16 ankylosing spondylitis patients exceeded the norm of 100 %. Less than 80 % was scored in both legs in four patients and in one leg in five patients. A value of less than 40 % was scored by two patients in both legs. These two patients also had the most internal nuclei on histological examination.

In 10 male patients (age range: 29–46 years) the mean power frequency (± standard deviation) was 70.2 ± 7.7 Hz as compared to 74.3 ± 6.1 Hz for the 16 controls (8 male, 8 female) (age range 22–35 years) indicating that there was some muscle impairment. Similar electromyographic changes in ankylosing spondylitis have been reported by others (Sadowska-Wroblewska 1968).

6.8 Pathological and Clinical Implications

Ankylosing spondylitis is a multi-system disease with uveal, cardiac, pulmonary and gastrointestinal involvements. The muscle changes described in this study together with those from other groups suggest that muscle pathology occurs in ankylosing spondylitis.

Central migration of nuclei and diffuse fibre atrophy are well recognised as non-specific myopathic features and indicate that muscles are also damaged in ankylosing spondylitis patients.

A diffuse reaction with the acid phosphatase stain is an indication of muscle cell damage and usually correlates with lipofuscin deposition. However, a scattered localised reaction, although occasionally present in a few fibres in many biopsies, is never seen to the extent observed in our patients. A possible explanation is that this represents a lesser degree of damage to the cell itself, such as sarcomere disruption, or it may indicate the presence of breakdown products from previous inflammatory cell infiltrates. Electron microscopy studies could resolve some of these questions by providing a more definite identification of the residual organelles present in those sites.

Peripheral condensation of reaction product in type I fibres is an occasional finding in a variety of muscle disorders and a frequent finding in marathon runners who have a type I fibre preponderance.

Although fibre distribution in our patients was normal, the changes seen may indicate a real increase in mitochondrial enzymes in response to the exercise from which ankylosing spondylitis patients gain relief. We were unable to correlate the changes observed in our patients with age, sex, disease activity and distribution or duration of the disease process.

In relation to drug therapy, it is well known that corticosteroids can produce myopathic damage with central migration of nuclei and type II fibre atrophy (Afifi et al. 1968). Perhaps non-steroidal anti-inflammatory drugs could produce similar, though less severe damage.

The muscle changes seen were not those of a hereditary disorder, and it is possible that an environmental factor may be involved in the development of these abnormalities. The persistent absence of inflammatory cells and immunoglobulins would appear to exclude an ongoing inflammatory process, but blind needle biopsy could well miss the areas of maximum involvement.

We conclude therefore that histological and electromyographic changes together with muscle strength impairment occur in patients with ankylosing spondylitis and may account for some of their symptoms (Hopkins et al. 1983).

References

Afifi AK, Berman RA, Harvey JC. Steroid myopathy: clinical, histological and cytological observations. John Hopkins Med J. 1968;123:158–74.

Ball J. Enhesopathy of rheumatoid arthritis and ankylosing spondylitis. Ann Rheum Dis. 1971; 1971(30):213–23.

Calin A. Raised creatine phosphokinase in ankylosing spondylitis. Ann Rheum Dis. 1975; 34:244–7.

Cooper RG, Freemont AJ, Fitzmaurice A, Alani SM, Jayson MIV. Paraspinal fibrosis: a specific pathological component in ankylosing spondylitis. Ann Rheum Dis. 1991;50:755–9.

Edwards RHT, Young A, Hoskins GP, Jones DA. Human skeletal Muscle function: description of tests and normal values. Clin Sci Mol Med. 1977;52:283–90.

Edwards RHT, Young A, Wiles CM. Needle biopsy of skeletal muscle in the diagnosis of myopathy and the clinical study of muscle function and repair. N Engl J Med. 1980;302:261–71.

Gofton JP. Differential diagnosis of ankylosing spondylitis and rheumatoid arthritis. Med Clin North Am. 1968;52:517–26.

Hopkins GO, McDougald J, Mills K, Isenberg D, Ebringer A. Muscle changes in ankylosing spondylitis. Br J Rheumatol. 1983;22:151–7.

Isenberg DA, Snaith ML. Muscle disease in systemic lupus erythematosus: a study of its nature, frequency and cause. J Rheumatol. 1981;8:917–24.

Mills KR, Newham DJ, Edwards RH. Force, contraction frequency and energy metabolism as determinants of ischaemic muscle pain. Pain 1982;14:149–54.

Pohl W, Sievers BU. Veränderungen der Muskulatur bei Spondylitis Ankylopoietica. Z Rheumatol. 1974;33:249–53.

Round JM, Matthews Y, Jones DA. A quick, simple and reliable histochemical method for ATPase in human muscle preparations. Histochem J. 1980;12:707–10.

Roux H, Serratrice G, Maestracci D, Gambarelli D, De Bisschop G, Cartouzou G, Mante S, Recordier AM. Les atteintes musculaires au cours de la pelvispondylite ankylosante. Rev Rhum Mal Osteoartic. 1975;42:231–8.

Sadowska-Wroblewska M. Electromyographic investigations in ankylosing spondylitis. Reumatologia. 1968;6:265–74.

Chapter 7
Raised Serum IgA Is Present in Ankylosing Spondylitis Patients

7.1 Introduction: Immunoglobulin Levels and Disease Activity in Ankylosing Spondylitis

There is evidence that gastrointestinal infection may be an important factor in the development and onset of ankylosing spondylitis.

Sacroiliitis and ankylosing spondylitis are common sequelae in persons who develop arthritis or Reiter's disease after dysenteric infection with *Salmonella*, *Shigella* or *Yersinia enterocolitica.*

Investigation by lymphangiography has shown that pelvic and paraspinal lymphadenopathy precedes the radiological changes of ankylosing spondylitis (Fournier et al. 1969).

Raised levels of serum IgA in ankylosing spondylitis patients have been reported from Belgium (Veys and Van Laere 1973). Polish workers reported that increased levels of β-2 macroglobulins were present in ankylosing spondylitis patients (Mackiewicz and Fenrych 1961).

Plasma cells in the 'gut associated lymphoid tissue' are the major source of serum IgA (Lamm 1976).

Investigations in animals raised in germ-free conditions have shown that after oral immunisation the main specific plasma cell response is IgA in character, and nearly all the circulating specific antibody is IgA (Crabbé et al. 1969).

Clearly if the aetiological factor in ankylosing spondylitis is acting in the gut, then this possibility should be reflected in the levels of circulating immunoglobulins, especially those of the IgA type.

Serum immunoglobulin levels were measured in ankylosing spondylitis patients attending the 'Ankylosing Spondylitis Research Clinic of the Middlesex Hospital' in London.

A. Ebringer, *Ankylosing Spondylitis and Klebsiella*,
DOI 10.1007/978-1-4471-4300-0_7, © Springer-Verlag London 2013

7.2 Ankylosing Spondylitis Patients and Controls

Blood was obtained from 122 ankylosing spondylitis patients during varying phases of disease activity. A total of 221 patient sera were randomly selected from a bank of stored sera, each patient being selected on average twice (range 1–5). Each patient visit was considered as a separate event, the shortest interval between visits being 1 month.

The New York criteria were used for the diagnosis of ankylosing spondylitis (Bennet and Wood 1968).

Patients with inflammatory bowel disease were excluded from the study.

The mean age of all patients was 34.5 years (range 11–68 years) and 29 were women.

Of 117 patients tested, 110 were HLA-B27 positive (94 %).

Single serum samples were obtained from 58 healthy subjects corresponding in age and sex distribution to the ankylosing spondylitis patients and who had no history of arthritis or backache.

7.3 Methods Used in Estimating Serum Immunoglobulins

Serum IgA, IgG and IgM estimations were determined by the radial immunodiffusion technique with commercially prepared immunodiffusion plates and protein standards (Behringwerke, Marburg/Lahn).

Blood for the erythrocyte sedimentation rate (ESR) was taken at each patient visit and measured by the Westergren method.

Serum C-reactive protein (CRP) estimations were determined by the radial immunodiffusion technique with commercial antisera (Hoechst), and each estimation was the mean of at least two separate measurements.

All measurements were carried out in code and without knowledge of the patient's clinical status.

7.4 Results of Serum IgA Estimations

The results of the serum immunoglobulin estimations are shown in Table 7.1.

The mean serum IgA in ankylosing spondylitis patients was 307 mg/dl compared to a mean serum IgA of 223 mg/dl in the healthy, control subjects. This is an increase of 38 % and is statistically significant ($t=3.14$, $p<0.005$).

There was a slight rise in the mean serum IgG and IgM estimations when compared to control subjects, but this was not statistically significant.

In an endeavour to study further the distribution pattern of the serum IgA, the ankylosing spondylitis patients were divided into two groups according to their

Table 7.1 The mean (± standard error) serum immunoglobulin levels in healthy controls and ankylosing spondylitis patients (SE = standard error)

	Controls		Ankylosing spondylitis patients	
	Mean (± SE) (mg/dl)	Number of estimations	Mean (± SE) (mg/dl)	Number of estimations
Serum IgA	223 ± 11	58	307 ± 13	221
Serum IgG	1,263 ± 36	58	1,361 ± 30	195
Serum IgM	140 ± 6	58	149 ± 6	185

'erythrocyte sedimentation rate': one group consisting of patients with an 'erythrocyte sedimentation rate' below 15 mm/h ('Normal ESR') and the other group consisting of ankylosing spondylitis patients having an 'erythrocyte sedimentation rate' of 15 mm/h or more ('Elevated ESR').

The mean serum IgA in ankylosing spondylitis patients having an 'elevated ESR' was 369 mg/dl, while in ankylosing spondylitis having a 'normal ESR', it was 236 mg/dl, and this difference is statistically significant ($t = 5.64$, $p < 0.001$) (Fig. 7.1).

The mean serum IgA in ankylosing spondylitis patients with an 'elevated ESR' was 65 % higher than the mean serum IgA in healthy, control subjects. Furthermore, there was no significant difference between the mean serum IgA in ankylosing spondylitis patients with a 'normal ESR' and the mean serum IgA in healthy, control subjects (Fig. 7.1).

Samples for 'C-reactive protein' estimations were selected randomly from the pool of sera available. The ankylosing spondylitis sera were divided into two groups: one group consisting of ankylosing spondylitis patients with a serum C-reactive protein level below 15 μg/ml and the second group having a serum C-reactive protein level of 15 μg/ml (15 mg/l) or more (Fig. 7.1).

It was considered that patients having the higher level of C-reactive protein were more likely as a group to be in an active inflammatory phase of the disease. The mean serum IgA in ankylosing spondylitis patients having an elevated C-reactive protein level was 387.8 mg/dl, while in patients having the lower C-reactive protein level, it was 236.5 mg/dl, and this difference is statistically significant ($t = 3.68$, $p < 0.001$) (Fig. 7.1).

The mean serum IgA in ankylosing spondylitis patients with an elevated serum C-reactive protein value was 74 % higher than in healthy control subjects. Again, as in the previous 'erythrocyte sedimentation rate' comparison, there was no significant difference between the mean serum IgA of the low 'C-reactive protein' group and the healthy control subjects (Cowling et al. 1980).

7.5 Results of Serum IgG Estimations

The mean serum IgG in ankylosing spondylitis patients was 1,361 mg/dl, which is a rise of 8 % compared with the mean serum IgG obtained for healthy, control subjects, but this difference is not statistically significant.

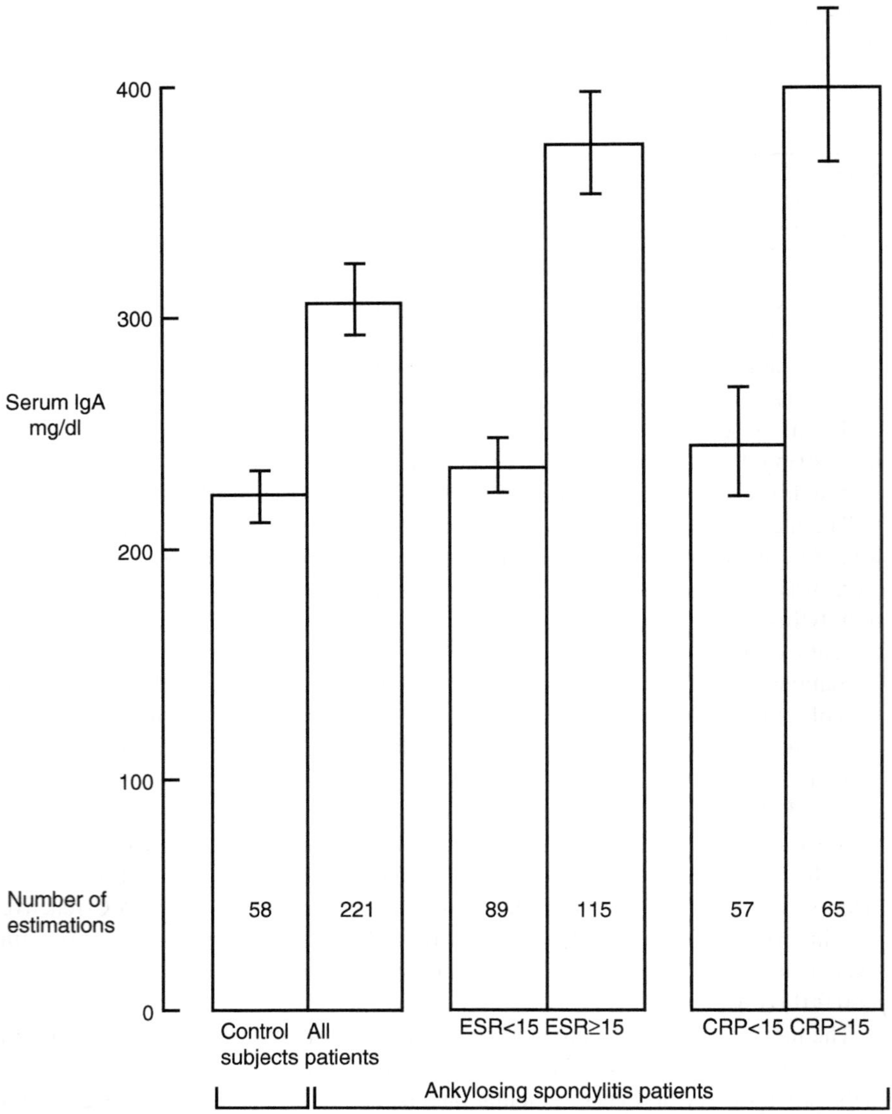

Fig. 7.1 Serum IgA (mean ± standard error) measured in healthy, control subjects and ankylosing spondylitis patients. Mean serum immunoglobulin levels in patients with elevated erythrocyte sedimentation rate (ESR ≥ 15 mm/h) and elevated C-reactive protein levels (CRP ≥ 15 μg/ml) were also compared to sera from patients having normal (ESR < 15 mm/h) or low C-reactive protein (CRP < 15 μg/ml) values

However, when the ankylosing spondylitis patients were divided into groups with increased inflammatory activity, either an erythrocyte sedimentation rate ≥15 mm/h or a C-reactive protein level ≥15 ug/ml, again there was a rise in the mean serum IgG level when compared to the level in healthy, control subjects (Fig. 7.2). The mean serum IgG level in ankylosing spondylitis with an 'elevated ESR' was

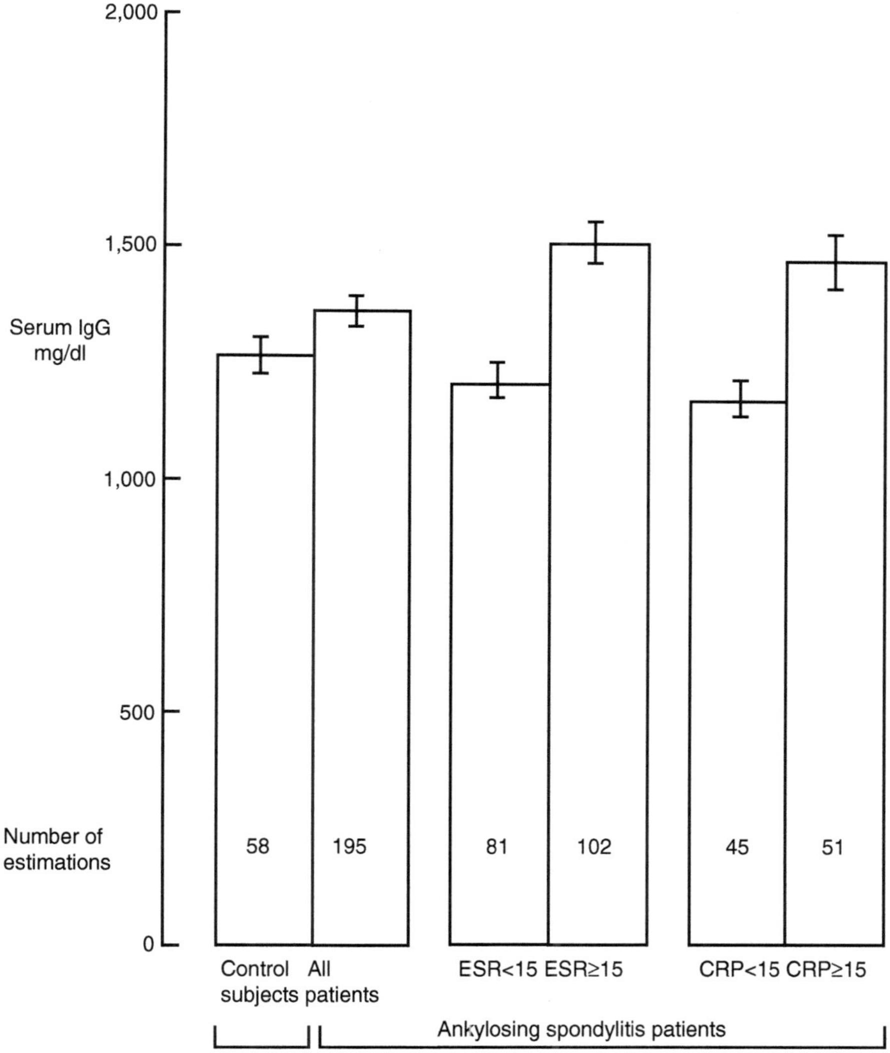

Fig. 7.2 Serum IgG (mean ± standard error) measured in healthy control subjects and ankylosing spondylitis patients. Mean serum immunoglobulin levels in patients with elevated erythrocyte sedimentation rate (ESR ≥ 15 mm/h) and elevated C-reactive protein levels (CRP ≥ 15 μg/ml) were also compared to sera from patients having normal (ESR < 15 mm/h) or low C-reactive protein (CRP < 15 μg/ml) values

1,508 mg/dl, and this 20 % rise, when compared to healthy control subjects, was statistically significant ($t = 9.85$, $p < 0.001$).

The mean serum IgG in ankylosing spondylitis patients with an "elevated C-reactive protein level" was 1,468 mg/dl and this 16 % rise, when compared with the level in healthy control subjects, is also statistically significant ($t = 3.40$, $p < 0.001$).

There was no significant difference between mean serum IgG levels in patients with 'normal ESR' and 'low CRP' values when compared to healthy control subjects.

7.6 Results of Serum IgM Estimations

The mean serum IgM in ankylosing spondylitis was 149 mg/dl, which is a 6 % rise compared to the mean serum IgM obtained for healthy, control subjects, but this difference is not statistically significant (Fig. 7.3).

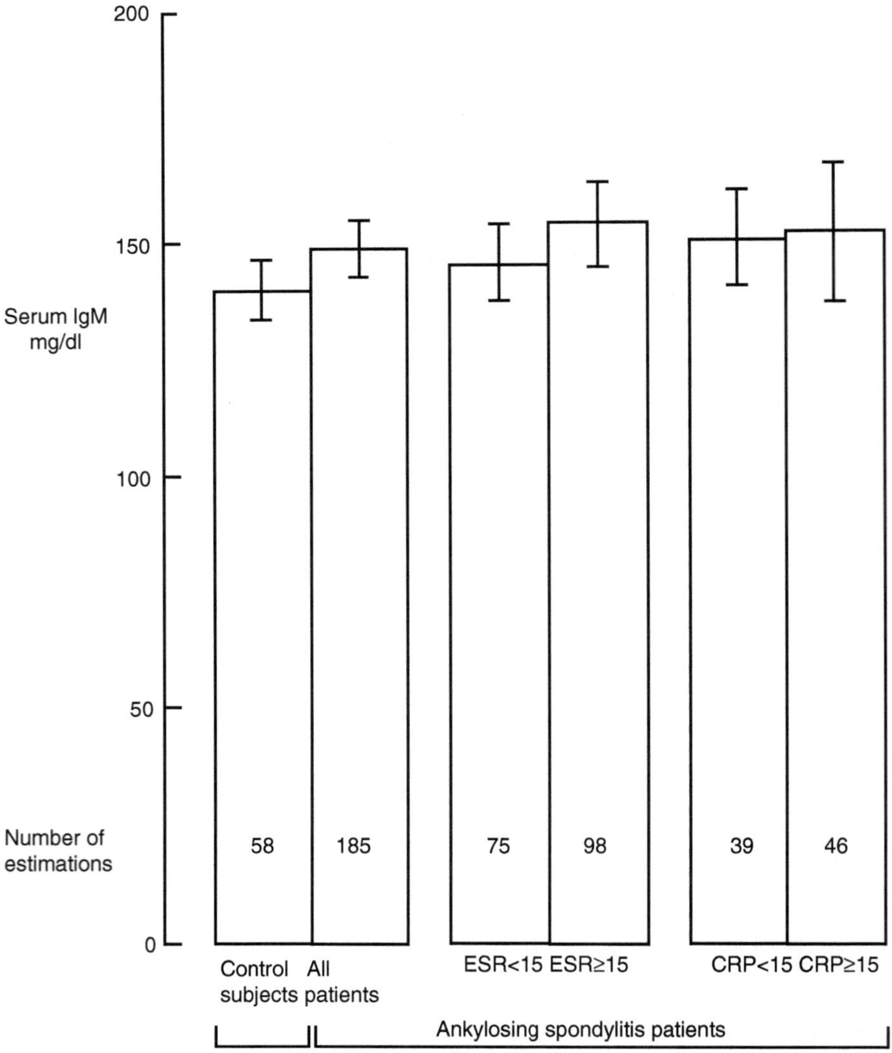

Fig. 7.3 Serum IgM (mean ± standard error) measured in healthy control subjects and ankylosing spondylitis patients. Mean serum immunoglobulin levels in patients with elevated erythrocyte sedimentation rate (ESR ≥ 15 mm/h) and elevated C-reactive protein levels (CRP ≥ 15 μg/ml) were also compared to sera from patients having normal (ESR < 15 mm/h) or low C-reactive protein (CRP < 15 μg/ml) values

Furthermore, when ankylosing spondylitis patients were divided into groups with increased inflammatory activity, again there was no statistically significant difference between serum IgM levels in patients with an elevated erythrocyte sedimentation rate or C-reactive protein level and control subjects or patients with 'normal' erythrocyte sedimentation rate or low C-reactive protein values.

7.7 Discussion

These studies have confirmed the findings of several previous investigators and shown that serum IgA is predominantly raised in patients with active, ankylosing spondylitis compared to serum IgG or serum IgM levels. The investigations have shown that these elevated serum IgA levels are most frequently associated with active phases of ankylosing spondylitis, as measured by erythrocyte sedimentation rates or C-reactive protein levels. These results clearly incriminate a pathological process involving the gastrointestinal tract in the development of ankylosing spondylitis.

A Belgian group from Ghent have emphasised that there is high prevalence, in over 50 % of samples, showing clinically silent inflammatory lesions in patients with spondyloarthropathies (Mielants et al. 1988).

A high frequency of endoscopic lesions in patients with spondyloarthropathy have also been reported from Finland (Leirisalo-Repo and Repo 1992).

There is also a comparatively smaller but definite rise in serum IgG during active phases of ankylosing spondylitis. If an immunoglobulin molecule were to be involved in the pathological processes of targeting lumbar tissues, muscle, uvea or entheses, then an IgG molecule being smaller than dimeric IgA would be a more likely pathogenic trigger.

Another striking observation from these studies is that there is no elevation in the mean serum IgA of ankylosing spondylitis patients when they are in inactive state of the disease, as measured by biochemical parameters, such as 'erythrocyte sedimentation rate' or C-reactive protein levels. It would appear that diagnostic or pathogenic immunoglobulins are unlikely to be found when there is no biochemical evidence of inflammation. Clinical criteria alone may not be sufficient to diagnose 'disease activity' when following ankylosing spondylitis patients in longitudinal studies.

Furthermore, this elevation in serum IgA indicates that it is not part of the clinical phenotype of ankylosing spondylitis but does correlate with the current level of inflammation in the patient. Thus, an ankylosing spondylitis with severe deformities due to long-standing disease but currently not inflamed will not have an elevation in serum IgA.

The elevation in total serum IgA strongly suggests that some external triggering factor is acting across the mucosal surface such as the lower gastrointestinal tract, thereby initiating the rise in serum IgA.

Lymphangiographic studies indicate that regional lymph nodes draining the pelvis, pelvic colon and rectum, namely, the pre-sacral and para-aortic lymph nodes become enlarged during active or progressive phases of ankylosing spondylitis and before the development of radiographic changes (Langness et al. 1971).

Inflammatory changes in the large bowel have been demonstrated in ankylosing spondylitis by rectal biopsy (Jayson et al. 1970). An association between inflammatory bowel disease and ankylosing spondylitis has been well established (Wright 1980).

Even if the large bowel does have an aetiological role in ankylosing spondylitis, it is still unclear why distal sites such as the spine, peripheral joints and the eye are affected. Although bacterial debris may be released from the gut, but that hypothesis alone cannot explain the strong predisposition in individuals with the tissue antigen HLA-B27.

One possible explanation is provided by the cross-reactivity or molecular mimicry theory which suggests that some microorganisms may carry surface antigens that have stereochemical similarity to self antigens of the host, such as HLA-B27.

Persistent infection may lead to production of cross-reacting antimicrobial antibodies which can act also as self-damaging autoantibodies. If these antimicrobial antibodies bind to self antigens, then tissue damage may follow complement activation with migration of leucocytes to inflamed regions and release of cytokines and lysosomal enzymes from inflammatory cells. The evoked generalised inflammation then leads to the clinical features observed in ankylosing spondylitis.

A similar mechanism may operate in the reactive arthritis of rheumatic fever or in the HLA-B27-positive reactive arthritis following infection with *Salmonella*, *Shigella* or *Yersinia enterocolitica* microorganisms.

7.8 Pathological and Clinical Implications

An increase in serum IgA immunoglobulin in patients during active phases of the disease would appear to be consistent with the hypothesis that microbial infection in the gut could act as an initiating agent or trigger factor in the development of ankylosing spondylitis.

References

Bennet PH, Wood PHN. In: Bennet PH, Wood PHN, editors. Population studies of the rheumatic diseases. Amsterdam: Excerpta Medica Foundation; 1968. p. 456.

Cowling P, Ebringer R, Ebringer A. Association of inflammation with raised serum IgA in ankylosing spondylitis. Ann Rheum Dis. 1980;39:545–9.

Crabbé PA, Nash DR, Bazin M, Eyssen H, Heremans JF. Antibodies of the IgA type in intestinal plasma cells of germ free mice after oral or parenteral immunisation with ferritin. J Exp Med. 1969;130:723–44.

Fournier AM, Denizet D, Delagrange A. La lymphographie dans la spondylarthrite ankylosante. J Radiol Electrol Med Nucl. 1969;50:773–84.

Jayson MIV, Salmon PR, Harrison WJ. Inflammatory bowel disease in ankylosing spondylitis. Gut. 1970;11:506–11.

Lamm ME. Cellular aspects of immunoglobulin A. Adv Immunol. 1976;22:223–90.

Langness U, Banavsky D, Alexopoulos J, Kriegel W, Burger R. Differentiation of inflammation and ossification in spondylitis ankylopoietica. Acta Rheumatol Scand. 1971;17:15–22.

Leirisalo-Repo M, Repo H. Gut and spondyloarthropathies. Rheum Dis Clin North Am. 1992;18:23–35.

Mackiewicz S, Fenrych W. Immuno-electrophoretic analysis of proteins in serum and synovial fluid in rheumatoid arthritis and ankylosing spondylitis. Ann Rheum Dis. 1961;20:265–73.

Mielants H, Veys EM, Cuvelier C, de Vos M. Ileocolonoscopic findings in seronegative spondyloarthropathies. Br J Rheumatol. 1988;27(Suppl II):95–105.

Veys EM, Van Laere M. Serum IgG, IgM and IgA levels in ankylosing spondylitis. Ann Rheum Dis. 1973;32:493–6.

Wright V. Seronegative polyarthritis: a unified concept. Arthritis Rheum. 1980;21:619–33.

Chapter 8
Faecal Cultures in Ankylosing Spondylitis and Uveitis

8.1 Introduction: The Origin of Ankylosing Spondylitis

An infective aetiology for ankylosing spondylitis has been postulated for many years (Romanus 1953). A high incidence of prostatitis has been reported in patients with ankylosing spondylitis (Mason et al. 1958), but no definite agent has been positively implicated or identified. Acute anterior uveitis is also frequently associated with ankylosing spondylitis, although it may manifest itself before the onset of the rheumatological disease.

A remarkable association between ankylosing spondylitis and HLA-B27 has been reported from the Westminster Hospital in London (Brewerton et al. 1973) and also from Los Angeles in the USA (Morris et al. 1974).

Most patients with ankylosing spondylitis possess HLA-B27, whilst its frequency in the general UK or US population is about 8 %.

Several hypotheses have been proposed to explain this remarkable association. The 'linked gene' theory suggests that an 'immune response gene', responsible for causing the disease, is situated close and on the same chromosome as the gene coding for HLA-B27. Therefore, on division and recombination of the chromosomes, these genes would travel together.

All other theories propose some form of interaction between the HLA-B27 molecule itself and external, infectious agents. The presence of an HLA-B27-like antigen on a microorganism would suggest that the individual is less able to mount an adequate immune response against that particular microorganism because it is recognised partially as a self-structure.

We have reported preliminary evidence of immunological cross-reactivity between HLA-B27-positive lymphocytes and *Klebsiella-Enterobacter* species and *Yersinia enterocolitica.*

Following these results, it was decided to determine the frequency of *Klebsiella-Enterobacter* species and *Yersinia enterocolitica* in the faeces and urine of ankylosing spondylitis patients and also in a control group of healthy subjects having a

A. Ebringer, *Ankylosing Spondylitis and Klebsiella*,
DOI 10.1007/978-1-4471-4300-0_8, © Springer-Verlag London 2013

similar age and sex distribution. It was also decided to correlate these findings with a simultaneous assessment of disease activity and to determine whether it was linked to acute, anterior uveitis.

8.2 Ankylosing Spondylitis Patients and Controls

There were 63 ankylosing spondylitis patients attending the 'Ankylosing Spondylitis Research Clinic of the Middlesex Hospital' and 124 healthy controls. The patients selected had been diagnosed as having ankylosing spondylitis and were aged under 40 years at the commencement of the study. The age and sex distribution of patients and controls is summarised in Table 8.1. Three of the 63 ankylosing spondylitis patients did not have HLA-B27.

The control group consisted of members of staff, students and ambulant, convalescent patients without arthritic disease. No patient or control subject had taken antibiotics for at least 6 weeks.

On examination they were assessed for current disease activity, and this was based on the following criteria:

1. Patient self-rated visual analogue scale of pain or discomfort
2. Evidence of active peripheral manifestation such as an acute arthritis, effusions or uveitis
3. Duration of 'early morning stiffness'
4. Range of lumbar spine flexion
5. Erythrocyte sedimentation rate
6. Anti-inflammatory and analgesic drug requirement

These criteria were used as the basis for classifying the ankylosing spondylitis patients into three grades of disease activity: 'active disease', 'probably active disease' and 'inactive disease'. The following guidelines were used to assess the ankylosing spondylitis patients.

8.2.1 *Active Disease*

The presence of peripheral manifestations appeared to be the most important feature. If these were present, then other criteria were nearly always strongly positive.

The other important consideration was recent worsening of symptoms especially increased 'early morning stiffness' and failure to control symptoms with current drug therapy. If this had occurred in the previous 4 weeks, it was considered to indicate 'active disease'.

Mild fluctuations in these criteria were not considered sufficient to classify 'active disease', and the patient was included in the next grade.

Table 8.1 Comparison of positive and negative faecal cultures for *Klebsiella/Enterobacter* microorganisms in ankylosing spondylitis patients with and without acute anterior uveitis (AAU), hospital controls, rheumatoid arthritis (RA) patients and female physiotherapy students

	Ankylosing spondylitis patients				
	With AAU	Without AAU	Hospital controls	RA	Students
Positive cultures	13	229	51	49	5
Negative cultures	4	536	106	201	45

8.2.2 *Probably Active Disease*

If only some of the above criteria showed recent worsening or if most of the criteria were positive but stable, in the absence of peripheral manifestations, then the patient was assessed as having 'probably active disease'.

8.2.3 *Inactive Disease*

This group of ankylosing spondylitis patients considered their symptoms to be well controlled and often volunteered that their disease was quiescent. Many used drugs infrequently or not at all.

The duration of 'early morning stiffness' was often short or had not changed for a long period. A raised 'erythrocyte sedimentation rate' did not preclude an assessment of 'inactive disease'.

8.3 Collection and Investigations of Urinary and Faecal Specimens

Midstream urine and faecal samples were obtained at the same visit as the time of the clinical assessment. Both urine and faecal specimens were examined for the presence of *Klebsiella-Enterobacter* species and also for *Yersinia enterocolitica.*

Faecal specimens were cultured on a differential medium containing inositol and incubated at 37 °C for 18 h before examination for inositol-fermenting colonies.

Isolation of *Yersinia enterocolitica* was facilitated by incubation at 37 °C for 48 h followed by enrichment culture using peptone water, pH 7.0, at 4 °C for 3 weeks (Bejot et al. 1975). Pure isolates of suspect colonies were identified by the API 20E system.

All cultures and identifications were performed under code by one person (D.R.C.) (Ebringer et al. 1977).

Fig. 8.1 Frequency of *Klebsiella* microorganisms in faecal cultures

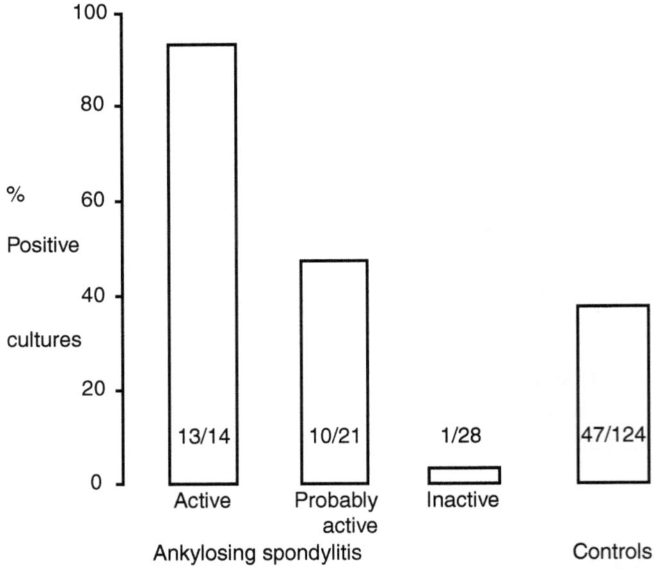

8.4 Results of Urine Investigations

No urine specimen was positive for *Enterobacter*, *Klebsiella* or *Yersinia enterocolitica* microorganisms.

Three specimens from control subjects were positive, but all three individuals were symptomless.

Subsequently, urine cultures were not collected or investigated in ankylosing spondylitis patients.

8.5 Results of Faecal Investigations

The results of the 'disease activity' classification and faecal cultures are summarised in Fig. 8.1.

Fourteen patients were assessed as having 'active disease', 21 as 'probably active disease' and 28 as having 'inactive disease'. Positive cultures for *Klebsiella* species were obtained in 13 (93 %) of the 'active group', 10 (48 %) of the 'probably active group' and in only 1 (4 %) of the 'inactive group'.

The difference in the prevalence of bacteria between the 'active' and 'inactive groups' ($\chi^2 = 29.58$, with Yates correction; $p < 0.001$) and between the 'active' and the 'control groups' ($\chi^2 = 13.30$, with Yates correction; $p < 0.001$) was highly significant.

Bacteriological analysis showed that *Enterobacter aerogenes* was isolated only three times, twice from control subjects and once from a patient with ankylosing spondylitis. The patient was in an 'active group', and *Klebsiella pneumoniae* microorganisms were also isolated from the same subject.

No *Yersinia enterocolitica* was isolated from either ankylosing spondylitis patients or healthy, control subjects.

All the remaining positive cultures were identified as *Klebsiella pneumoniae* by the API 20E system. With the inclusion of repeat faecal samples, 99 positive cultures were subjected to additional biochemical tests and 49 identified as *Klebsiella aerogenes* by the classification of Cowan (1974).

8.6 Acute Anterior Uveitis and Faecal Cultures

Acute anterior uveitis occurs not only in ankylosing spondylitis but also in Reiter's disease, ulcerative colitis and Crohn's disease. When sacroiliitis is present, all of these conditions are strongly associated with HLA-B27.

The incidence of HLA-B27 in all individuals presenting to eye clinics with uveitis is around 60 %. Although infective agents are known to cause some forms of acute anterior uveitis, most cases are idiopathic or associated with diseases whose aetiology is unknown.

Although we have reported evidence that there is cross-reactivity between three Gram-negative microorganisms *Enterobacter aerogenes*, *Klebsiella pneumoniae* and *Yersinia enterocolitica* with HLA-B27 in studying faecal cultures in ankylosing spondylitis patients, only one microbe from these three, namely, *Klebsiella pneumoniae*, was regularly isolated, especially during phases of active disease.

We have studied acute anterior uveitis in our group of patients with ankylosing spondylitis attending the 'Ankylosing Spondylitis Research Clinic of the Middlesex Hospital'.

We have examined 190 ankylosing spondylitis patients involving 782 separate outpatient visits. All patients fulfilled the New York criteria for ankylosing spondylitis. Patients with 'early' or 'possible' ankylosing spondylitis were excluded from the study. Some 155 patients were tissue typed, and 139 were positive for HLA-B27 (90 %).

All patients with acute anterior uveitis were seen, the diagnosis confirmed and treatment instituted by their ophthalmic physician.

Faecal cultures were carried out as previously described. All episodes where patients were taking antibiotics were excluded from the study.

A total of 159 healthy, hospital-associated controls provided one faecal sample each, and 93 rheumatoid arthritis patients attending another research clinic provided a faecal sample involving altogether 250 outpatient visits. The minimum interval between visits was 3 months. Fifty female physiotherapy students, on their first day of contact with a hospital environment, also provided a faecal sample.

8.7 Results of Faecal Cultures in Patients with Uveitis

The results of the studies on faecal cultures in ankylosing spondylitis patients with and without acute anterior uveitis are shown in Table 8.1. Positive cultures were found in 13 out of 17 outpatient visits when the ankylosing spondylitis patient also had acute anterior uveitis, and this was significant when compared to ankylosing spondylitis without uveitis ($\chi^2 = 14.75$ with Yates correction, $p < 0.001$), to hospital controls ($\chi^2 = 10.94$, $p < 0.001$), to rheumatoid arthritis patients ($\chi^2 = 25.77$ with Yates correction, $p < 0.001$) and to female physiotherapy students ($\chi^2 = 23.18$ with Yates correction, $p < 0.001$). Three patients had two episodes of acute anterior uveitis during the study, and each was counted separately.

Klebsiella/Enterobacter species were identified on 229 out of 763 outpatient visits in ankylosing spondylitis patients, at which acute anterior uveitis was not present. The incidence of *Klebsiella/Enterobacter* species in hospital controls, outpatients with rheumatoid arthritis and female physiotherapy students was 33, 20 and 10 %, respectively (Ebringer et al. 1979).

Many of the patients with acute anterior uveitis had positive cultures for *Klebsiella* for some months before the development of acute anterior uveitis at the time of the assessment. Two cases were excluded because no cultures were available at the onset of acute anterior uveitis, although a culture result was positive when tested 4 weeks later when mild signs of uveitis were still present.

8.8 Discussion

These studies have shown that *Klebsiella* microorganisms can be isolated from faecal cultures of patients with ankylosing spondylitis and also from ankylosing spondylitis having at the same time acute anterior uveitis. Only patients aged 40 years or under were selected for study with the intention of observing a greater proportion of patients with early, active inflammatory disease. The active phase of ankylosing spondylitis usually occurs in the second and third decade of life, after which the inflammatory process becomes often quiescent. It was considered that a study of patients with predominantly 'burnt out' disease would produce no conclusive result, in the same way that examination of patients with chronic rheumatic heart disease would produce little information about *Streptococcal* infections which initiated the illness.

There are many controversies in assessing 'disease activity' in ankylosing spondylitis patients. In assessing 'disease activity', it is not only important to consider peripheral manifestations of the condition and limitations of spinal flexion but also the presence of elevated levels of biochemical parameters such as 'erythrocyte sedimentation rate' and 'C-reactive protein' levels.

The taxonomy and classification of *Klebsiella* species is still under debate. Some authorities classify *Klebsiella pneumoniae* and *Klebsiella aerogenes* separately. Our results show that the presence of *Klebsiella pneumoniae* or *Klebsiella aerogenes* correlates positively with disease activity. These observations lend support to the hypothesis that *Klebsiella* species by latent infection or colonisation of the bowel may be the initiating factor in the onset of ankylosing spondylitis.

It is possible that most of the *Enterobacteriaceae* under favourable conditions may initiate inflammatory joint disease. "The enteric pathogens *Salmonellae*, *Shigellae* and *Yersinia enterocolitica* have been implicated in the post-dysenteric form of Reiter's disease or 'reactive arthritis', and this affects predominantly HLA-B27-positive individuals (Calin and Fries 1976)".

Autoantibodies have been reported in the serum of patients with ankylosing spondylitis (Howell et al. 1972). It is possible that cross-reactivity may restrict antibody production only to low-affinity, poorly specific antibodies which could persist and lead to the development of immune complex disease (Soothill and Steward 1971).

The cause of the joint and eye inflammation in HLA-B27-positive individuals is to some extent unknown. However, an infective agent has been suspected, particularly in view of the evidence that reactive arthritis can occur after dysentery.

The microbe *Klebsiella pneumoniae* is only conditionally pathogenic and is commonly found in the gastrointestinal tract. Our findings that this microorganism is frequently associated with and often precedes acute anterior uveitis support the hypothesis that many of the acute inflammatory episodes in HLA-B27-positive patients, whether acute peripheral arthritis, spinal disease or eye inflammation, are all responses to a common environmental aetiological factor. It remains to be seen whether *Klebsiella pneumoniae* is this environmental factor.

Increased recovery of *Klebsiella* microorganisms in patients with ankylosing spondylitis has been reported from Leeds in England (Eastmond et al. 1980), from Canada (Hunter et al. 1981) and from the USA (Kuberski et al. 1983). However, other workers found no correlation between faecal carriage of *Klebsiella* and disease activity in ankylosing spondylitis patients (Warren and Brewerton 1980).

8.9 Pathological and Clinical Implications

If the initiating factor in ankylosing spondylitis is a bacterial antigen due to *Klebsiella pneumoniae*, then it may be possible to modify the disease by elimination of the bacteria. Antibiotics or removal of the bacteria by substrate modification may result in a decrease of the inflammatory process or even complete prevention or recurrence of relapses.

References

Bejot J, Alonso JM, Mollaret HH. Bacteriological diagnosis of human yersinioses. Med Mal Infect. 1975;5:233–6.

Brewerton DA, Caffrey M, Hart FD, James DCO, Nicholls A, Sturrock RD. Ankylosing spondylitis and HLA-B27. Lancet. 1973;i:904–7.

Calin A, Fries JF. Epidemic Reiter's syndrome: follow-up evidence on genetic and environmental factors. Ann Intern Med. 1976;84:564–6.

Cowan ST. Cowan and Steel's manual for the identification of medical bacteria. 2nd ed. Cambridge: Cambridge University Press; 1974.

Eastmond CJ, Willshaw HE, Burgess SEP, Shinebaum R, Cooke F, Wright W. Frequency of *Klebsiella aerogenes* in patients with ankylosing spondylitis and controls with respect to the individual features of the disease. Ann Rheum Dis. 1980;39:118–23.

Ebringer R, Cooke D, Cawdell DR, Cowling P, Ebringer A. Ankylosing spondylitis: *Klebsiella* and HLA-B27. Rheumatol Rehabil. 1977;16:190–6.

Ebringer R, Cawdell D, Ebringer A. Klebsiella pneumoniae and acute anterior uveitis in ankylosing spondylitis. Br Med J. 1979;1:383.

Howell FA, Chamberlain MA, Perry RA, Torrigiani G, Roitt IM. IgG antiglobulin levels in patients with psoriatic arthropathy, ankylosing spondylitis and gout. Ann Rheum Dis. 1972;31:129–31.

Hunter T, Harding GKM, Kaprove RE, Schroeder M. Fecal carriage of *Klebsiella* and *Enterobacter* species in patients with active ankylosing spondylitis. Arthritis Rheum. 1981;24:106.

Kuberski TT, Morse HDG, Rate RG, Bonnell MD. Increased recovery of *Klebsiella* from the gastrointestinal tract of Reiter's syndrome and ankylosing spondylitis patients. Br J Rheumatol. 1983;22 Suppl 2:85–90.

Mason RM, Murray RS, Oates JK, Young AC. Prostatitis and ankylosing spondylitis. Br Med J. 1958;1:748–51.

Morris RI, Metzger AL, Bluestone R, Terasaki PI. HLA-W27. A useful discriminator in the arthropathies of inflammatory bowel disease. New Engl J Med. 1974;290:1117–9.

Romanus R. Pelvo-spondylitis ossificans and genito-urinary infection. Acta Med Scand. 1953;145 Suppl 280:172–8.

Soothill JF, Steward MW. The immunological significance of the heterogeneity of antibody affinity. Clin Exp Immunol. 1971;9:193–9.

Warren RE, Brewerton DA. Faecal carriage of *Klebsiella* by patients with ankylosing spondylitis and rheumatoid arthritis. Ann Rheum Dis. 1980;39:37–44.

Chapter 9
Biochemical Parameters and *Klebsiella* in Ankylosing Spondylitis

9.1 Introduction: The Use of Biochemical Parameters in Ankylosing Spondylitis

An association between clinically active inflammatory disease in ankylosing spondylitis and the presence in faecal cultures of the Gram-negative microorganism *Klebsiella pneumoniae* has been reported by our group.

Disease activity in those studies was assessed for each individual visit on the basis of the patient's assessment and the clinical findings.

The biochemical parameters of inflammation, namely, 'erythrocyte sedimentation rate' and 'C-reactive protein' levels have been shown to be useful indicators of disease activity in other rheumatic diseases such as rheumatoid arthritis (Amos et al. 1977).

C-reactive protein is produced in the liver, and only low levels are found in normal human serum. Elevated levels of C-reactive protein are found during acute infections, tissue injury or inflammatory disease (Mortensen et al. 1976). C-reactive protein is an acute phase reactant, and its physiological role is to bind phosphocholine found on the surface of dead and dying cells.

The molecule is capable of activating the complement cascade and initiating both the opsonic (Siegel et al. 1975) and lytic components of the system (Osmand et al. 1975).

It is a member of the pentraxin family of proteins, and its gene is located on chromosome 1. It is an annular pentameric disc consisting of 224 amino acid residues.

Elevated levels of C-reactive protein have been found in several rheumatic diseases during active inflammatory phases (Glynn and Irving 1959).

In this study, we set out to determine if 'erythrocyte sedimentation rate' and 'C-reactive protein' levels correlated or contributed to our understanding of the pathology in ankylosing spondylitis when compared to clinically assessed disease activity and the presence of positive faecal cultures.

A. Ebringer, *Ankylosing Spondylitis and Klebsiella*,
DOI 10.1007/978-1-4471-4300-0_9, © Springer-Verlag London 2013

9.2 Selection of Ankylosing Spondylitis Patients and Controls

Serum samples were obtained from 149 patients attending the 'Ankylosing Spondylitis Research Clinic of the Middlesex Hospital' on 469 outpatient visits.

Each patient had an average of 3 visits (range 1–10).

The patients' samples were selected randomly from a bank of serum samples obtained over a period of 2 years.

The diagnosis of ankylosing spondylitis was made by the New York criteria.

Five patients with psoriatic spondylitis and six who had inflammatory bowel disease with spondylitis were also included. Of 125 patients who had been tissue typed, 117 carried the HLA-B27 antigen (94 %).

Two patients with colitic spondylitis and two with psoriatic spondylitis did not possess the HLA-B27 antigen.

Six patients were included who had normal or suspicious sacroiliac X-ray changes with low back pain. All six were HLA-B27 positive, and most had a positive family history, a positive sacroiliac scintiscan or peripheral joint involvement.

The mean age of all patients was 34.5 years (range 13–72) with a mode of 26 years. There were 33 female patients.

Sixty healthy control subjects having no previous history of arthritis or back pain and not in a hospital environment were bled for estimations of C-reactive protein.

9.3 Assessment of Disease Activity

Assessment was done during the time of the patient's outpatient visit and before the results of the 'erythrocyte sedimentation rate', the C-reactive protein level and the faecal culture were available.

Three grades of disease activity were considered: 'active disease', 'probably active disease' and 'inactive disease'. The following guidelines were used to assess the ankylosing spondylitis patients:

9.3.1 Active Disease

The presence of peripheral manifestations such as active synovitis, dactylitis, joint or spinal tenderness or acute anterior uveitis appeared to be the most important features.

Assessment of active disease was also made on the basis of recent, within the last 4 weeks, exacerbation of peripheral or spinal symptoms.

Anti-inflammatory drug intake had usually increased, or the maintained dose had failed to control symptoms. There was nearly always worsening of the patient's self-rated visual analogue scale of pain.

Mild fluctuations in these criteria were not considered sufficient to classify 'active disease', and the patient was included in the next grade.

9.3.2 *Probably Active Disease*

Patients with probably active disease usually had symptoms which were stable or constant and well controlled with anti-inflammatory therapy.

Alternatively, they may have had more severe symptoms and signs in the previous months and now appeared to be improving. Short fluctuations in symptoms were usually disregarded. If a patient had an effusion which was not tender or inflamed, this was more likely to be assessed as 'probably active disease'.

9.3.3 *Inactive Disease*

This group of ankylosing spondylitis patients considered their symptoms to be well controlled or had only occasional mild or short-lived symptoms. They usually did not require medication, or if they did, the dose was regular and effective. Many used drugs infrequently or not at all.

9.4 Methods Used in These Studies

9.4.1 *C-Reactive Protein Estimation*

The Mancini radial immunodiffusion technique with commercial antisera (Hoechst) was used.

Each estimation was the mean of at least two separate measurements.

All estimations were carried out without knowledge of the patient's clinical status.

9.4.2 *Erythrocyte Sedimentation Rate Measurement*

Blood for estimation of 'erythrocyte sedimentation rate' was taken on the day of the outpatient visit and measured by the Westergren method.

The normal hospital service was used, and there was no special identification for the 'erythrocyte sedimentation rate' samples being measured.

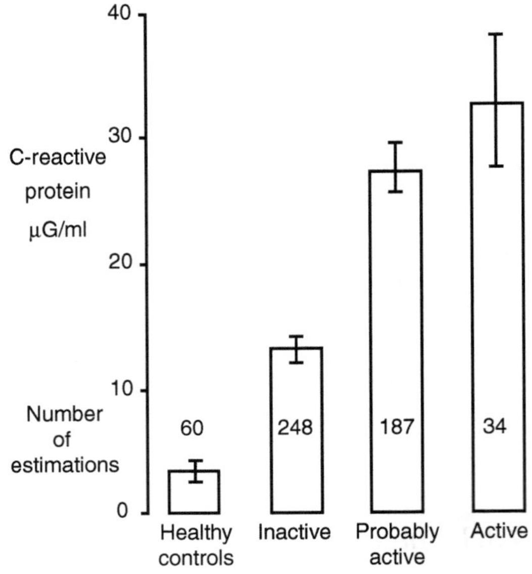

Fig. 9.1 Mean serum 'C-reactive protein' levels in healthy control subjects and patients with ankylosing spondylitis during different phases of disease activity. *Bars* indicate standard errors of the mean

9.4.3 Faecal Cultures

Faecal specimens were collected and cultured as described previously.

Faecal cultures were read without knowledge of the patient's clinical status. Some patients were also on an antibiotic co-trimoxazole at the time of assessment. These results were analysed separately when disease activity was assessed.

9.5 C-Reactive Protein and Disease Activity

The mean serum C-reactive protein level in active ankylosing spondylitis patients was 32.78 ± 5.33 μg/ml (mean ± standard error); in probably active patients, it was 27.64 ± 1.99 μg/ml, and in inactive patients, it was 13.22 ± 0.82 μg/ml (Fig. 9.1). The difference in mean levels between active and inactive patients ($t = 6.62$, $p < 0.001$), as well as between probably active patients and inactive patients ($t = 7.33$, $p < 0.001$), was statistically significant.

The mean serum C-reactive protein level in healthy control subjects was 3.57 ± 0.61 μg/ml. Of the 60 control subjects, 31 (52 %) had zero values for their C-reactive protein level.

The difference in mean serum C-reactive protein levels between the two different disease activity groups in ankylosing spondylitis compared to healthy control subjects was statistically significant: active patients ($t = 7.17$, $p < 0.001$), probably active patients ($t = 6.82$, $p < 0.001$) and inactive patients ($t = 5.68$, $p < 0.001$).

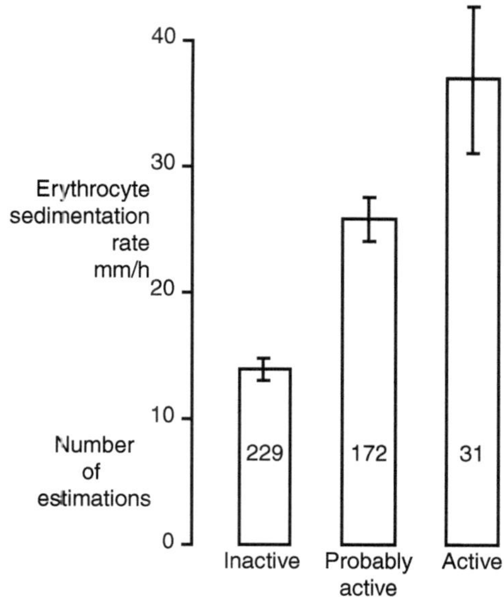

Fig. 9.2 Mean 'erythrocyte sedimentation rate' levels in patients with ankylosing spondylitis during different phases of disease activity. *Bars* indicate standard errors of the mean

9.6 Erythrocyte Sedimentation Rate and Disease Activity

The mean 'erythrocyte sedimentation rate' in active ankylosing spondylitis patients was 37.10 ± 5.99 mm/h Westergren (mean ± standard error); in probably active patients, it was 25. 99 ± 99 mm/h, and in inactive patients, it was 14.28 ± 0.90 mm/h (Fig. 9.2).

The differences in mean erythrocyte sedimentation rate between the active and inactive patients ($t = 6.96$, $p < 0.001$) and probably active and inactive patients ($t = 6.62$, $p < 0.001$) were statistically significant.

Not only was there a correlation between mean C-reactive protein values and mean erythrocyte sedimentation rates in various phases of disease activity, but individual values of high or low erythrocyte sedimentation rates were closely correlated with high or low values in serum C-reactive protein levels, irrespective of disease activity ($r = +0.6947$, $p < 0.001$).

9.7 Isolation of *Klebsiella* and Disease Activity

The results of culture investigations in ankylosing spondylitis patients with active, probably active and inactive phases of disease activity are summarised in Table 9.1.

Klebsiella species of microorganisms were isolated more frequently from ankylosing spondylitis patients during active and probably active phases than during

Table 9.1 Frequency of isolation of *Klebsiella/Enterobacter* microorganisms in ankylosing spondylitis patients with active, probably active and inactive disease

	Active	Probably active	Inactive
Culture positive	11 (0)	45 (6)	42 (4)
Culture negative	14 (6)	104 (34)	154 (24)
% of positive cultures in all patients	44 %	30 %	21 %
% of positive cultures in patients not taking antibiotics	58 %	36 %	23 %

Numbers in brackets indicate number of episodes where patients were on antibiotics

inactive phases. The difference between isolation rate of *Klebsiella* in active patients compared to inactive patients was statistically significant ($\chi^2=5.02$, $p<0.025$, Yates correction), but not significant when probably active patients were compared to inactive patients.

This study included some patients who were taking antibiotics. If the episodes where taking antibiotics are excluded (Table 9.1), the frequency of isolation of *Klebsiella* microorganisms increases in all three categories of disease activity.

The difference between the isolation of *Klebsiella* microorganisms in both active ($\chi^2=9.18$, $p<0.005$, Yates correction) and probably active ($\chi^2=5.07$, $p<0.025$, Yates correction) not taking antibiotics is statistically significant when compared to a similar group of inactive ankylosing spondylitis patients.

9.8 C-Reactive Protein and Erythrocyte Sedimentation Rate in Ankylosing Spondylitis Patients with and Without *Klebsiella*

All the outpatient visits in ankylosing spondylitis patients where *Klebsiella* microorganisms were isolated from faecal cultures were grouped together irrespective of disease activity and compared to all the visits where no *Klebsiella* microbes had been isolated.

The mean serum C-reactive protein level in ankylosing spondylitis patients having a positive *Klebsiella* culture was 21.17 ± 2.91 μg/ml (mean ± standard error), whilst in patients not having *Klebsiella* was 18.57 ± 1.21 μg/ml (Fig. 9.3), and this difference is statistically significant ($t=2.48$, $p<0.01$).

The mean erythrocyte sedimentation rate in ankylosing spondylitis patients having a positive faecal *Klebsiella* culture was 24.15 ± 2.56 mm/h, whilst in patients not having *Klebsiella* in their faecal culture was 18.78 ± 1.13 mm/h (Fig. 9.4), and this difference is statistically significant ($t=2.21$, $p<0.025$).

The presence of faecal cultures positive for *Klebsiella pneumoniae* would appear to correlate with biochemical parameters of inflammation (Cowling et al. 1980).

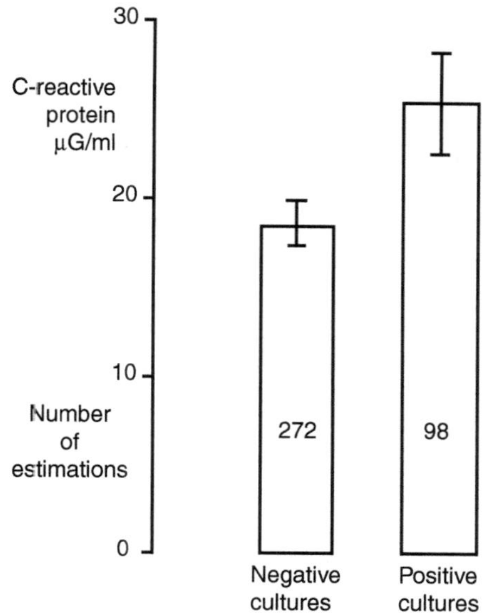

Fig. 9.3 Mean 'C-reactive protein' levels in patients with positive or negative faecal cultures for *Klebsiella/Enterobacter* microorganisms. *Bars* indicate standard errors of the mean

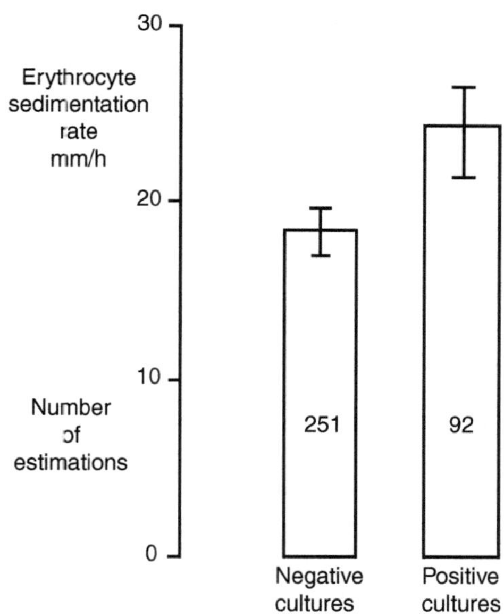

Fig. 9.4 Mean 'erythrocyte sedimentation rate' levels in patients with positive or negative faecal cultures for *Klebsiella/Enterobacter* microorganisms. *Bars* indicate standard errors of the mean

9.9 Discussion

These results show that ankylosing spondylitis patients have elevated levels of C-reactive protein and erythrocyte sedimentation rates similar to those observed in active rheumatoid arthritis patients (Amos et al. 1977). Moreover, the elevations in

C-reactive protein levels and erythrocyte sedimentation rates correlate with clinically assessed states of increased disease activity.

Furthermore, the presence of *Klebsiella/Enterobacter* species of microorganisms in faecal cultures is associated with a higher mean C-reactive protein level and elevated erythrocyte sedimentation rate, irrespective of the clinically assessed state of diseased activity.

Thus, there is an association between the presence of *Klebsiella* in ankylosing spondylitis and active disease as assessed independently by clinical and laboratory criteria.

The assessment of disease activity was deliberately aimed at patients with acute inflammatory disease whether these were episodes of acute anterior uveitis, peripheral arthritis, spinal disease or a combination of all these three clinical states. It is more difficult to assess such active episodes when the symptoms relate to pelvic or spinal disease alone, and it is for this reason that recent worsening of symptoms played a major role in guiding the grading of disease activity.

Clinical observation suggests that ankylosing spondylitis is not an inexorable progressive disease and that it follows a pattern of exacerbations and remissions.

The sacroiliitis and spinal disease as evidenced by limitation of movement and radiographic changes would, under this hypothesis, more probably reflect the gradual accumulation of partially irreversible, chronic secondary changes due to the initial inflammatory episodes. It is possible that each major flare-up of disease in the ankylosing spondylitis patients, whether acute anterior uveitis, peripheral arthritis or spinal inflammation, may be due to reinfection or rechallenge by the agent or agents responsible for triggering the inflammation.

This hypothesis therefore suggests that ankylosing spondylitis and the episodes of acute anterior uveitis associated with HLA-B27 are due to a form of reactive arthritis or reactive inflammation, mediated immunologically by exposure to *Klebsiella pneumoniae* microorganisms.

It is possible that *Klebsiella pneumoniae* is the main microbe triggering such exacerbations of inflammatory spinal, joint and eye disease.

In this sense, ankylosing spondylitis closely resembles the 'reactive arthritis' occurring following dysenteric episodes by *Shigella*, *Salmonella* and *Yersinia enterocolitica* microorganisms. However, ankylosing spondylitis patients living in London do not appear to have been infected by *Salmonella*, *Shigella* or *Yersinia enterocolitica* microorganisms but have been exposed to episodes of *Klebsiella pneumoniae* located in the bowel by a microorganism showing some 'molecular mimicry' to HLA-B27.

The best model of 'reactive arthritis' is acute rheumatic fever. In this disease, there is a clear difference between the acute rheumatic symptoms occurring several weeks after a *Streptococcal* throat infection and the complications and functional limitations due to incompetent or stenosed cardiac valves of chronic rheumatic heart disease. Here, there is an analogy between the inflammatory episodes of acute rheumatic fever and the chronically diseased cardiac valves and the acute inflammatory episodes of ankylosing spondylitis and the sacroiliitis and spondylitis of established disease. The search for an aetiological agent in rheumatic fever would have been unrewarding if only patients with established rheumatic heart disease had been studied. Similarly we anticipated that the 'active disease' or acute inflammatory episodes of ankylosing spondylitis were the times to search for potential aetiological agents.

In rheumatic fever, the infection is located in the upper respiratory tract and inflammatory damage is mediated by cross-reacting anti-*Streptococcal* antibodies which affect the brain and endomyocardium, producing chorea and rheumatic heart disease.

In ankylosing spondylitis, the infection might be located in the lower gastrointestinal tract and inflammatory damage is triggered by cross-reacting antimicrobial antibodies affecting the spine, entheses, joint and eyeball, producing sacroiliitis and uveitis. Such antibodies remain to be demonstrated in ankylosing spondylitis.

These studies on C-reactive protein and erythrocyte sedimentation rates were made on the assumption that each outpatient visit could be considered as an independent event to see if there was a trend between clinical disease activity and elevated levels of markers of biochemical inflammation. This meant that the same patient was investigated over several outpatient visits. It appeared that *Klebsiella* bacterial isolation occurred more frequently during states of increased disease activity, whether assessed clinically or measured biochemically by erythrocyte sedimentation rate or C-reactive protein. For subsequent investigations, when specific anti-*Klebsiella* antibodies were measured, it was considered that each ankylosing spondylitis patient should have an elevated erythrocyte sedimentation rate and a raised C-reactive protein level.

9.10 Pathological and Clinical Implications

It would appear that active phases of ankylosing spondylitis, either assessed clinically or by biochemical parameters such as C-reactive protein or erythrocyte sedimentation rates, are associated with the presence of *Klebsiella pneumoniae* microbes in the gut.

References

Amos RS, Constable TJ, Crockson RA, Crockson AP, McConkey B. Rheumatoid arthritis: relation of C-reactive protein and erythrocyte rates to radiographic changes. Br Med J. 1977;1:195–7.

Cowling P, Ebringer R, Cawdell D, Ishii M, Ebringer A. C-reactive protein, ESR and *Klebsiella* in ankylosing spondylitis. Ann Rheum Dis. 1980;39:45–9.

Glynn JH, Irving M. Laboratory investigations in the diagnosis of Rheumatic diseases. Ann Phys Med. 1959;5:1–9.

Mortensen RF, Osmand AP, Lint TF, Gewurz H. Interaction of C-reactive protein with lymphocytes and monocytes, complement dependent adherence and phagocytosis. J Immunol. 1976; 117:774–81.

Osmand AP, Mortensen RF, Siegel J, Gewurz H. Interaction of C-reactive protein with the complement system. III Complement dependent passive haemolysis initiated v by CRP. J Exp Med. 1975;142:1065–77.
Siegel J, Osmand AP, Wilson MF, Gewurz H. Interactions of C-reactive protein with the complement system. C-reactive protein mediated consumption of complement by poly-L-lysine polymers and other polycations. J Exp Med. 1975;142:709–21.

Chapter 10
Binding of *Klebsiella* Antisera to HLA-B27 Cells

10.1 Introduction: The Problem of HLA-B27 in Ankylosing and Its Link to *Klebsiella*

Ankylosing spondylitis is a chronic inflammatory arthritis primarily affecting the axial skeleton and sacroiliac joints. Some studies have suggested an association between clinically active inflammatory disease in ankylosing spondylitis and the presence in faecal cultures of the Gram-negative microorganism *Klebsiella pneumoniae.*

Approximately 96 % of patients with ankylosing spondylitis possess HLA-B27, whereas its frequency in the general population is only 8 %. The two-gene theory suggests that an ankylosing spondylitis gene is in linkage disequilibrium with HLA-B27.

The one-gene theory suggests that the HLA-B27 molecule is directly involved in the disease. There are two variants of the one-gene theory: (a) the molecular mimicry theory and (b) the plasmid theory.

The molecular mimicry proposes that there is cross-reactivity or similarity between HLA-B27 and the external putative pathogen, probably the *Klebsiella* microbe (Ebringer 1983).

The plasmid theory proposes that a plasmid in *Klebsiella* microbes somehow modifies the HLA-B27 molecule so that cells from ankylosing spondylitis patients will express bacterial antigens but not cells obtained from healthy HLA-B27 individuals (Seager et al. 1979).

The molecular mimicry or cross-tolerance hypothesis predicts that an anti-*Klebsiella* serum would bind equally well to HLA-B27-positive lymphocytes obtained from ankylosing spondylitis patients or from healthy HLA-B27-positive individuals but would bind less to cells obtained from HLA-B27-negative individuals.

The plasmid theory predicts that an anti-*Klebsiella* serum would bind more to HLA-B27 cells obtained from ankylosing spondylitis patients when compared with either HLA-B27 cells obtained from healthy donors or HLA-B27-negative cells.

The following study was undertaken to test the mutually exclusive predictions of these two competing one-gene theories.

A. Ebringer, *Ankylosing Spondylitis and Klebsiella*,
DOI 10.1007/978-1-4471-4300-0_10, © Springer-Verlag London 2013

10.2 Patients and Control Subjects

The study was carried out on peripheral blood lymphocytes from 84 tissue-typed subjects.

There were 30 ankylosing spondylitis patients satisfying the New York criteria attending the 'Ankylosing Spondylitis Research Clinic of the Middlesex Hospital', all of whom were HLA-B27 positive. Erythrocyte sedimentation rate (Westergren) was carried out by the hospital service.

Control subjects were healthy bone marrow donors attending the Anthony Nolan Research Laboratories: 21 of them were HLA-B27 positive and the remaining 33 were HLA-B27 negative.

There were only four ankylosing spondylitis patients attending the 'Ankylosing Spondylitis Research Clinic of the Middlesex Hospital' who were HLA-B27 negative. All four were 'clinically inactive', and because of the small number of subjects, they were excluded from the study.

10.3 Rabbit Antisera

All antisera were raised in New Zealand white rabbits.

Two antisera to *Klebsiella* sonicate preparation (KSP) were obtained from the same rabbit after 18 and 24 immunisations and denoted serum A and serum B, respectively.

A third antiserum to *Klebsiella* sonicate preparation was obtained from a different rabbit after 28 immunisations (serum E).

Two rabbit anti-myoglobin sera were obtained from another rabbit after five and eight immunisations and designated serum M1 and serum M2, respectively.

Non-immune sera were obtained from two unimmunised rabbits, pooled and designated serum C.

Finally, serum A was absorbed with *Klebsiella* microorganisms and designated serum D.

Klebsiella microorganisms were grown overnight in nutrient broth, harvested, washed in sterile PBS and then resuspended in a minimum volume of distilled water. Samples were frozen at −20 °C and freeze-dried overnight.

In the absorption procedure, 1 ml of serum A was mixed with 20 mg of freeze-dried *Klebsiella* microorganisms, vortexed and mixed at 4 °C for 2 h by rotation. The mixture was then centrifuged at 10,000 rpm for 15 min at 4 °C, the supernatant decanted and absorbed twice more, as described. After final absorption, the supernatant was centrifuged at 10,000 rpm for 30 min at 4 °C, aliquoted and stored.

Donkey anti-rabbit IgG serum (DAR-IgG) was obtained from Wellcome Reagents. Horseradish peroxidase-conjugated swine anti-rabbit serum was obtained from Dako Immunoglobulins Ltd.

10.4 Specificity Tests on Antisera

The binding values (B_o and B) of anti-*Klebsiella* sonicate preparation sera A and B were determined in radio-binding experiments.

Sera A to D were diluted in radioimmunoassay buffer (PBS containing 0.015 M sodium azide and 0.4 % w/v bovine serum albumin) over the serial dilution range 10^{-3} to 10^{-8} inclusive. Fifty microliter aliquots of each serum dilution were incubated with 50 µl of radio-iodinated *Klebsiella* sonicate preparation (KSP) and 50 µl radioimmunoassay buffer at 37 °C for 30 min in duplicate. Fifty microliter of co-precipitating donkey anti-rabbit IgG, containing rabbit serum at 1:100 as carrier, was added to each tube at 1:25 dilution and incubated overnight at 4 °C.

The precipitates were washed 2 × 1 ml in PBS containing 0.01 M potassium iodide by centrifugation for 30 min at 4 °C.

Residual radioactivity was counted, and the percentage of ^{125}I-*Klebsiella* sonicate preparation (KSP) bound, calculated according to the formula:

$$\text{Percentage bound }(\%\text{B}) = \frac{\text{Test cpm} - \text{Blank cpm}}{\text{Total cpm} - \text{Blank cpm}} \times 100 \tag{10.1}$$

where:
Total = total radioactivity added
Blank = radioactivity of precipitation mixture alone
Test = radioactivity of precipitation mixture + test serum

Anti-*Klebsiella* sonicate preparation sera A and B were tested for specificity by liquid-phase radioimmunoassay. *Klebsiella* sonicate preparation (KSP) competitor was diluted in radioimmunoassay buffer over the dilution range 0.1 g/ml–0.1 mg/ml inclusive. Similarly, sonicate preparations of *Escherichia coli*, *Yersinia enterocolitica* and *Shigella sonnei* prepared by the same method as for *Klebsiella* sonicate were diluted in radioimmunoassay buffer over the range 0.5–5 mg/ml inclusive.

Fifty microliter each of serum A and serum B, at dilution B_o, were incubated separately, with 50 µl of ^{125}I-*Klebsiella* sonicate preparation (KSP) and 50 µl of each competitor over the concentration range at 37 °C for 30 min. Fifty microliter of co-precipitating donkey anti-rabbit IgG, containing non-immune rabbit at 1:100 as carrier, was added to each tube at 1:25 dilution and incubated overnight at 4 °C. The precipitates were then washed 2 × 1 ml in PBS containing 0.01 M potassium iodide by centrifugation for 30 min at 4 °C.

Residual activity was counted, and the percentage inhibition calculated according to the formula:

$$\text{Percentage inhibition }(\%\text{I}) = \left(1 - \frac{\%\text{B (with competitor)}}{\%\text{B}_o\text{ (without competitor)}}\right) \times 100$$

where:
%B = percentage binding with competitor
%B_0 = percentage binding without competitor

10.5 Enzyme Immunoassay to Investigate the Binding of Anti-*Klebsiella* Sonicate Preparation to HLA-B27 Lymphocytes

Human peripheral blood lymphocytes were obtained from three groups according to tissue type and clinical status:

(i) Ankylosing spondylitis patients who were HLA-B27 positive
(ii) Healthy HLA-B27-positive individuals
(iii) Healthy HLA-B27-negative individuals

Peripheral blood lymphocytes were separated from whole blood by density gradient centrifugation, washed and resuspended in PBS at a cell density 20×10^6 cells/ml. Fifty microliter of cell suspensions in triplicate were incubated with 50 μl of either serum A, serum B or one of the three different non-immune sera, 1:100 PBS at 37 °C for 1 h. The cells were washed 2×1 ml in PBS by centrifugation, and 50 μl of horseradish peroxidase swine anti-rabbit serum, 1:10 from stock in PBS, was added to each sample and incubated at 37 °C for 1 h.

Cells were washed 3×1 ml in PBS and placed on ice. One ml of the electron donor 5-aminosalicylic acid, 1.3 mM in PBS containing 0.08 mM H_2O_2, was added to all samples and incubated at 37 °C for 1 h (Van Weemen and Schuurs 1971).

The reaction was stopped on ice, and 500 μl para-amino-benz-hydroxamic acid, 0.9 mM in PBS, was used to competitively inhibit the oxidation of 5-aminosalicylic acid by hydrogen peroxide (Schonbaum 1973).

Samples were centrifuged at 800 g for 5 min, and 1 ml of supernatant buffer containing enzyme reaction product was removed and the absorbance determined at 450 nm.

The enzyme immunoassays were performed over a period of several months, ensuring that on each occasion the assays included cells from at least one from each of the three groups: ankylosing spondylitis HLA-B27-positive, healthy HLA-B27-positive and healthy HLA-B27-negative individuals.

All cells provided were coded and the code broken on completion of the assay. Cells from each individual were tested in triplicate for binding with a non-immune serum and either anti-*Klebsiella* sonicate preparation (anti-KSP) serum A or anti--*Klebsiella* sonicate preparation (anti-KSP) serum B.

The mean absorbance value for the binding of non-immune control was calculated and subtracted from each absorbance value obtained for binding of the test sera (A or B) to give a mean absorbance value for the binding of that serum to human peripheral blood lymphocytes obtained from one individual.

The enzyme immunoassay was also used to test human peripheral blood lymphocytes for their ability to bind anti-myoglobin antibodies. The experimental protocol was as described previously, except that sera A and B were replaced by one of the anti-myoglobin sera M1 or M2 at 1:100 dilution in PBS.

The binding of the anti-myoglobin sera was compared with non-immune serum binding and the results calculated in the same way. Cells from ten healthy controls who were HLA-B27 positive compared to ten healthy individuals who were HLA-B27 negative were tested for binding by sera M1 or M2.

10.6 Absorption Experiments

Anti-*Klebsiella* sonicate preparation (anti-KSP) serum E was diluted 1:10 in PBS. Two hundred microliter of diluted serum was absorbed with either a pellet of 40×10^6 pooled peripheral blood lymphocytes obtained from 3 ankylosing spondylitis patients who were HLA-B27 positive or a pellet of 40×10^6 pooled peripheral blood lymphocytes obtained from three healthy controls who were HLA-B27 negative.

In each case, the peripheral blood lymphocytes were resuspended in the diluted serum and mixed thoroughly overnight at 4 °C by rotation.

The absorbed samples were centrifuged at 3,000 rpm at 4 °C for 30 min, and a 150 μl aliquot of serum was removed in a single-point radio-binding assay. Anti-*Klebsiella* sonicate preparation (anti-KSP) serum E, 1:10 in PBS, and absorbed serum E were then compared for their ability to bind tritiated *Klebsiella* sonicate preparation (KSP).

^{3}H-*Klebsiella* sonicate preparation (KSP) was radiolabelled by reductive alkylation using tritiated formaldehyde obtained from New England Nuclear (Rice and Means 1971).

Fifty microliter of absorbed or unabsorbed serum E was incubated with 50 μl of ^{3}H-*Klebsiella* sonicate preparation (KSP) (10,000 cpm) and 50 μl of radioimmunoassay buffer at 37 °C for 30 min. Fifty microliter of co-precipitating donkey anti-rabbit IgG, containing non-immune rabbit serum at 1:100 as carrier, was added to each tube at 1:25 dilution and incubated overnight at 4 °C.

The precipitates were washed 2×1 ml in PBS by centrifugation at 4 °C for 30 min. The precipitated were then dissolved in 500 μl of 10 % potassium hydroxide containing 10 % methanol and the mixture neutralised using an equivalent volume of 1 M hydrochloric acid. One milliliter of the neutralised mixture was placed in 6 ml of cocktail T scintillant and counted in a scintillation counter.

Altogether 200 μl aliquots of anti-*Klebsiella* sonicate preparation (anti-KSP) serum E were absorbed on three separate occasions with ankylosing spondylitis HLA-B27-positive cells and four separate occasions with healthy, HLA-B27-negative cells. The tests were carried out under code.

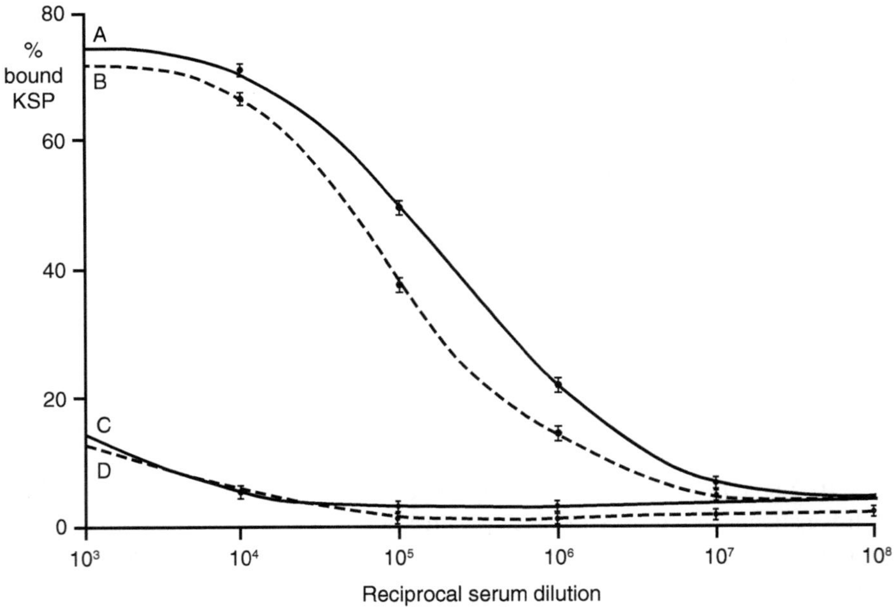

Fig. 10.1 Dilution response of rabbit anti-*Klebsiella* sonicate preparation (anti-KSP) sera A and B, compared with non-immune rabbit serum C and serum D (three times absorbed serum A). Results are expressed as percentage bound (mean ± standard error)

10.7 Results of Antisera Specificity

Anti-*Klebsiella* sonicate preparation (anti-KSP) sera A and B bound significant amounts of ^{125}I-*Klebsiella* sonicate preparation at 10^{-7} dilution above non-immune serum C and absorbed serum D ($p<0.001$) (Fig. 10.1).

B_0 values for serum A and serum B were 40 % (dilution 10^{-6}) and 36 % (dilution 1:400,000), respectively.

In the liquid-phase radioimmunoassay using serum A, inhibition by *Klebsiella* sonicate preparation (KSP) at 0.1 mg/ml was 100 %, whereas *Escherichia* sonicate preparation, *Yersinia* sonicate preparation and *Shigella* sonicate preparation did not exceed 15 % at 5 mg/ml (Fig. 10.2).

A similar curve was obtained for serum B.

There was no significant difference between serum A and serum B.

The liquid-phase radioimmunoassay results define the specificity of *Klebsiella* sonicate preparation (KSP) sera A and B under the conditions used in these experiments.

Serum E gave similar results with ^{125}I-*Klebsiella* sonicate preparation (KSP)-binding studies as sera A and B but was not tested in inhibition studies.

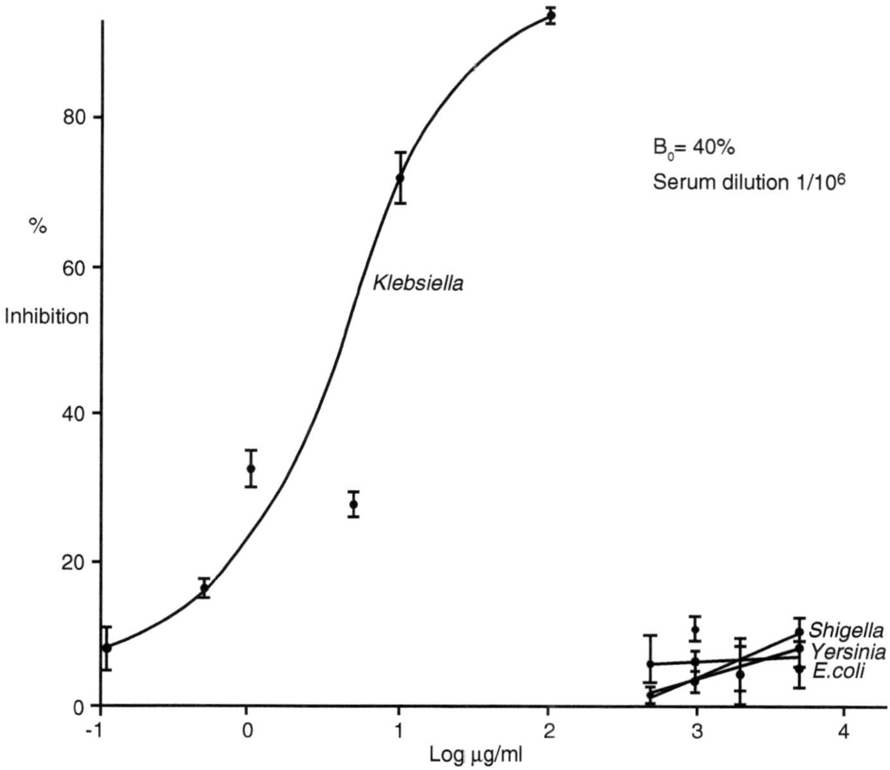

Fig. 10.2 Competitive radioimmunoassay of anti-*Klebsiella* sonicate preparation (anti-KSP) serum A using *Klebsiella* sonicate preparation (KSP) as standard competitor, compared with sonicates from *Escherichia coli*, *Yersinia enterocolitica* and *Shigella sonnei* microorganisms. Results are expressed as percentage inhibition (mean ± standard error)

10.8 Results of Enzyme Immunoassay and Absorption Experiments

The mean absorbance values for the actual binding of anti-*Klebsiella* sonicate preparation (anti-KSP) sera A or B to peripheral blood lymphocytes obtained from 33 healthy, HLA-B27-negative individuals was 5.79 ± 0.48 (mean ± standard error); from 21 healthy, HLA-B27-positive individuals, it was 9.10 ± 0.82, and from 30 ankylosing spondylitis patients who were all HLA-B27 positive, it was 9.16 ± 0.83 optical density (O.D.) units (Fig. 10.3).

The results show that ankylosing spondylitis patients who are HLA-B27 positive ($t = 3.60$, $p < 0.001$) and healthy individuals who are also HLA-B27 positive ($t = 3.77$, $p < 0.001$) bind more anti-*Klebsiella* sonicate preparation (anti-KSP) serum than do healthy, HLA-B27-negative cells (Baines et al. 1990).

There was no significant difference in the amount of anti-*Klebsiella* sonicate preparation (anti-KSP) serum bound by HLA-B27-positive lymphocytes obtained from either ankylosing spondylitis patients or healthy bone marrow donors.

In ankylosing spondylitis patients, the binding of the rabbit anti-*Klebsiella* sonicate preparation (anti-KSP) to peripheral blood lymphocytes was not associated with disease activity when this was assessed clinically or by measuring erythrocyte sedimentation rate.

Anti-myoglobin sera (M1 and M2) were tested in the same enzyme immunoassay as the anti-*Klebsiella* sonicate preparation (anti-KSP) sera. There was no significant difference in the amount of anti-myoglobin serum bound by cells from healthy HLA-B27-positive individuals and cells from healthy HLA-B27-negative individuals.

In a single-point radio-binding assay, there was no significant difference in the binding of ^{3}H-*Klebsiella* sonicate preparation (KSP) by unabsorbed serum E compared with serum E absorbed with healthy, HLA-B27-negative peripheral blood lymphocytes.

Serum E absorbed with ankylosing spondylitis peripheral blood lymphocytes bound significantly less ^{3}H-*Klebsiella* sonicate preparation (KSP) than unabsorbed serum E (paired t-test, $t=9.04$, $p<0.02$).

The mean absorption by ankylosing spondylitis HLA-B27-positive lymphocytes in three different assays was significantly greater than the mean absorption obtained with cells obtained from healthy, HLA-B27-negative individuals carried out in four separate absorption experiments ($t=6.76$, degrees of freedom $=5$, $p<0.005$).

10.9 Pathological and Clinical Implications

A complement-independent enzyme immunoassay was used to investigate the binding of anti-*Klebsiella* sonicate preparation (anti-KSP) sera to peripheral blood lymphocytes obtained from three different groups of individuals according to tissue type and clinical status.

A total of 84 individuals were investigated in these experiments: 33 healthy HLA-B27-negative individuals, 21 healthy HLA-B27-positive individuals and 30 patients who had ankylosing spondylitis and were also HLA-B27 positive.

Peripheral blood lymphocytes obtained from HLA-B27-positive ankylosing spondylitis patients and from HLA-B27-positive healthy individuals were found to bind significantly more anti-*Klebsiella* sonicate preparation (anti-KSP) than cells obtained from healthy bone marrow donors who were HLA-B27 negative.

The important observation is that there is no difference in the binding of anti-*Klebsiella* antibodies by HLA-B27-positive cells obtained from ankylosing spondylitis patients or from healthy, HLA-B27-positive individuals.

If *Klebsiella* antigens or fragments were present on the cells of ankylosing spondylitis patients who are HLA-B27 positive but absent from HLA-B27-positive

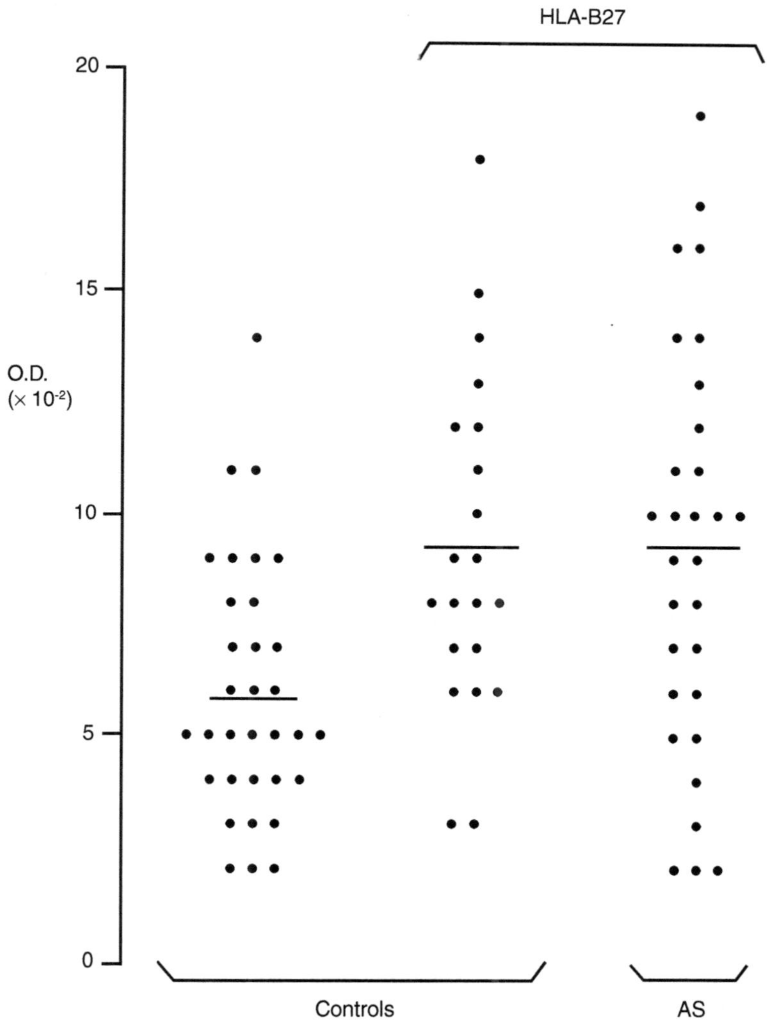

Fig. 10.3 The mean absorbance values (1 O.D. = A_{450} × 100) obtained from the binding of anti-*Klebsiella* sonicate preparation (anti-KSP) sera to lymphocytes from HLA-B27-positive ankylosing spondylitis (AS) patients, HLA-B27-positive healthy controls and HLA-B27-negative healthy controls. Each point represents the mean of triplicate experiments from one individual after subtraction for binding of non-immune control serum. All assays were carried out under code

healthy individuals, as suggested by the plasmid theory (Geczy et al. 1980), then anti-*Klebsiella* antibodies would have bound to a greater extent to cells obtained from ankylosing spondylitis patients.

The observation that there was no difference in the binding of anti-*Klebsiella* antibodies to HLA-B27-positive lymphocytes, irrespective of the clinical status of the donor, and that there was more binding of these antibodies by all HLA-B27-positive cells than by HLA-B27-negative cells suggests a degree of direct antigen recognition by anti-*Klebsiella* sera of some moiety on HLA-B27 lymphocytes.

Further evidence of a direct stereochemical relationship of HLA-B27 to *Klebsiella* has been provided by studies with anti-HLA-B27 monoclonal antibodies which suggested that there was no difference in the HLA-B27 molecule present on cells from patients with ankylosing spondylitis and from healthy HLA-B27-positive individuals (Grumet et al. 1981).

These various results indicate that the fine specificity of HLA-B27 cannot be subdivided into normal and disease variants.

Further studies with monoclonal antibodies to HLA-B27 have demonstrated direct cross-reactivity with antigens found on *Yersinia*, *Klebsiella* and *Shigella* microorganisms (Van Bohemen et al. 1984).

Similarly, an anti-*Yersinia* monoclonal antibody was shown to preferentially cross-react with HLA-B27 lymphoblastoid cell lines. When one of these cell lines was modified so that it no longer expressed HLA-B27, the anti-*Yersinia* monoclonal antibody failed to react with it (Kono et al. 1985).

Furthermore, sera from HLA-B27-positive patients with ankylosing spondylitis or Reiter's disease have antibodies directed against a peptide sequence of *Klebsiella pneumoniae* nitrogenase. The sequence is shared with a sequence present in HLA-B27 and appears to be expressed on the molecule's outer surface (Schwimmbeck et al. 1987).

Immunoperoxidase studies were carried out on synovial tissues obtained from patients with ankylosing spondylitis or reactive arthritis, using antisera to synthetic peptides shared between HLA-B27.1 and *Klebsiella pneumoniae* nitrogenase. All HLA-B27-positive patients with synovial inflammation showed strong immunoperoxidase in synovial lining cells, vascular endothelium and infiltrating inflammatory cells (Husby et al. 1989).

Thus, cross-reactive epitopes are present in the tissues of ankylosing spondylitis patients which can be targeted by anti-*Yersinia*, anti-*Shigella* but especially by anti-*Klebsiella* antibodies. The role of such antibodies in the pathogenesis of the disease remains to be evaluated.

References

Baines M, Ebringer A, Avakian H, Samuel D, James DCO. The use of enzyme immunoassay (EIA) and radiobinding assay to investigate the crossreactivity of *Klebsiella* antigens in ankylosing spondylitis patients and healthy controls. Scand J Rheumatol. 1990;19:341–9.

Ebringer A. The crosstolerance hypothesis, HLA-B27 and ankylosing spondylitis. Br J Rheumatol. 1983;22 Suppl 2:63–6.

Geczy AF, Alexander K, Bashir HV, Edmonds J. A factor (s) in *Klebsiella* culture filtrates specifically modifies an HLA-B27 associated cell surface component. Nature. 1980;283:782–4.

Grumet FC, Fendly BM, Engleman EG. Monoclonal anti-HLA-B27 antibody (B27M): production and lack of detectable typing difference between patients with ankylosing spondylitis, Reiter's syndrome and normal controls. Lancet. 1981;ii:174–6.

Husby G, Tsuchiya N, Schwimmbeck PL, Keat A, Pahle JA, Oldstone MBA, Williams Jr RC. Crossreactive epitope with Klebsiella pneumoniae nitrogenase in articular tissue of HLA-B27 positive patients with ankylosing spondylitis. Arthr Rheum. 1989;32:437–45.

Kono DH, Ogasawara M, Effros RB, Park MS, Wallford RL, Yu DTY. Ye-1: a monoclonal antibody that crossreacts with HLA-B27 lymphoblastoid cell lines and an arthritis causing bacteria. Clin Exp Imm. 1985;61:503–8.

Rice RH, Means GE. Radioactive labelling of proteins in vitro. J Biol Chem. 1971;246:831–2.

Schonbaum GR. New complexes of peroxidases with hydroxamic acids, hydrazides and amides. J Biol Chem. 1973;248:502–11.

Schwimmbeck PL, Yu DTY, Oldstone MBA. Autoantibodies to HLA-B27 in the sera of HLA-B27 patients with ankylosing spondylitis and Reiter's syndrome. J Exp Med. 1987;166:173–81.

Seager K, Bashir HV, Geczy AF, Edmonds J, De Vere Tyndall A. Evidence for a specific B27 associated cell marker on lymphocytes of patients with ankylosing spondylitis. Nature. 1979;277:68–70.

Van Bohemen CG, Grumet FC, Van Zanen HC. Identification of HLA-B27 M1 and M2 cross-reactive antigens in *Klebsiella*, *Shigella* and *Yersinia*. Immunology. 1984;52:607–10.

Van Weemen BK, Schuurs AHWM. Immunoassay using antigen-enzyme conjugates. FEBS Lett. 1971;15:232–6.

Chapter 11
IgA Antibodies to *Klebsiella* and Other Gram-Negative Bacteria in Ankylosing Spondylitis

11.1 Introduction: The Problem of Elevated Serum IgA in Ankylosing Spondylitis and Its Link to *Klebsiella*

In 'reactive arthritis', enteric infection by certain well-characterised Gram-negative bacteria is linked with the subsequent development of arthritis, especially in individuals carrying HLA-B27.

HLA-B27 is found in 90–96 % of patients with ankylosing spondylitis. The question arises as to whether this genetic predisposition reflects a common aetiology, especially whether the pathological processes associated with ankylosing spondylitis are triggered by Gram-negative infection of the gastrointestinal tract.

Several studies have shown that *Klebsiella* bacteria can be isolated from the faecal cultures of patients with active ankylosing spondylitis, not only in the UK, but also in the USA and Canada (Hunter et al. 1981).

In patients with *Yersinia* reactive arthritis, high titres of serum IgA antibodies to *Yersinia* serotype 03 correlate directly with disease severity in the presence of HLA-B27 (Granfors et al. 1980).

In view of the elevated levels of total serum IgA in active ankylosing spondylitis, it was decided to investigate the possibility that this increase might be due to an IgA immune response to bacteria, especially *Klebsiella*, present in the gastrointestinal tract. The methods used in these investigations were enzyme-linked immunosorbent assay (ELISA) (Trull et al. 1983).

In a second study, specific antibodies to several Gram-negative microorganisms were carried out against *Klebsiella pneumoniae*, *Salmonella typhimurium*, *Yersinia enterocolitica* and *Pseudomonas aeruginosa*.

A. Ebringer, *Ankylosing Spondylitis and Klebsiella*,
DOI 10.1007/978-1-4471-4300-0_11,

11.2 Selection of Serum Samples from Ankylosing Spondylitis Rheumatoid Arthritis, Psoriasis Patients and Healthy Controls

Blood was obtained from 65 patients attending the 'Ankylosing Spondylitis Research Clinic of the Middlesex Hospital': 50 patients were seen once, 13 patients twice and 2 patients were bled on 3 separate outpatient visits, making a total of 82 sera available for studies. The sera were selected at random from a stored collection. The shortest interval between visits was 1 month.

The patients were diagnosed according to the New York criteria for ankylosing spondylitis. Of 55 patients tested for HLA-B27, 53 were found to be HLA-B27 positive (96 %).

Patients with inflammatory bowel disease were excluded from the study.

Control sera were obtained from 57 healthy subjects: 34 being female from the Anthony Nolan Laboratories at St Mary Abbots Hospital.

Blood collected from the Rheumatology Clinic at Guy's Hospital provided 53 serum samples from 43 rheumatoid arthritis and 35 serum samples from 21 psoriatic arthritis patients. Definite or classical rheumatoid arthritis was diagnosed according to the ARA criteria. The mean age of the rheumatoid arthritis was 54.8 years, and 28 (64 %) were female. The diagnosis of psoriatic arthritis was based upon the presence of a seronegative anodular arthritis and psoriasis. The mean age of the psoriatic patients was 45.8 years, and 7 (30 %) were female. All sera were stored at −20 °C prior to assay.

Estimations of C-reactive protein and IgA were carried out by the single radial immunodiffusion technique, as previously described.

Faecal specimens passed within the 24 h prior to clinical assessment were cultured on a differential medium containing inositol and incubated at 37 °C for 18 h before examination for inositol-fermenting colonies. Pure isolates of suspect colonies were identified by the API 20E system.

Clinical assessment of disease activity was carried out, as previously described.

11.3 Enzyme-Linked Immunosorbent Assay (ELISA)

The microorganisms *Klebsiella pneumoniae* (Department of Bacteriology, Middlesex Hospital), *Escherichia coli*, *Pseudomonas aeruginosa* (Department of Clinical Bacteriology, Guy's Hospital) and *Candida albicans* (Department of Immunology, St Mary's Hospital) were cultured for 24 h at 37 °C in a minimal salts medium supplemented with 2 mg/ml glucose (Clowes and Hayes 1980).

The cultures were centrifuged at 1,000 g (MSE-6 L) for 30 min, and the supernatant decanted. It was then Millipore filtered (0.45 μm) and freeze-dried before reconstitution in PBS to a final concentration of 0.05 mg/ml protein, using purified IgG as standard.

Aliquots of 100-μl freeze-dried reconstituted culture supernatant were absorbed for 24 h at 37 °C onto polystyrene, 96-well flat-bottom Microelisa plates (Dynatech

Microelisa systems). Plates were washed once with PBS and any remaining non-specific binding sites blocked with human serum albumin (HAS, Sigma Chemical Co.) at a concentration of 20 mg/ml PBS for 2 h at 37 °C. Excess human serum albumin was flicked off, and duplicate 100-μl aliquots of test or control sera were added to the wells at 1/100 dilution in PBS, supplemented with 2 mg/ml human serum albumin, 0.05 % w/v Tween 20 (Sigma Chemical Co.) and sodium azide at 0.5 mg/ml (assay buffer), and the plates incubated for 1 h at 37 °C.

The wells were washed three times in PBS containing Tween 20. Then 100 μl of rabbit anti-human IgA (Dako Immunoglobulins) at 1/100 in assay buffer was added to each well, followed by 1-h incubation at 37 °C.

The plates were then washed in Tris buffer, pH 8.0 (BDH, Chemical Ltd.) supplemented with Tween 20, and 100 μl of goat anti-rabbit IgG conjugated with alkaline phosphatase (Miles Yeda Ltd.), added at 1/2,000 dilution in Tris/Tween 20. The plates were incubated for 45 min at 37 °C, washed three times in Tris buffer and 100 μl of phosphatase substrate (Sigma 104) added at a concentration of 1 mg/ml in diethanolamine buffer, pH 9.8 (BDH Chemicals Ltd.).

After developing for 30 min at 37 °C, the reaction was stopped with 100-μl 9 M sodium hydroxide and the optical absorbance measured spectrophotometrically with a Microelisa minireader (MR590, Dynatech Instruments) at 410 nm. The results are expressed as O.D. units × 100.

Comparison of ELISA results between groups was analysed using Student's *t*-test.

11.4 Absorption Studies

Cultures of *Klebsiella pneumoniae* and *Pseudomonas aeruginosa* were sedimented by centrifugation at 1,000 g (MSE-6L centrifuge) for 30 min. The bacteria were resuspended in distilled water, sub-aliquoted into four equal volumes and freeze-dried immediately. Serum samples from four ankylosing spondylitis patients containing different quantities of IgA antibody to *Klebsiella* were diluted 1/10 in PBS and 1-ml volumes absorbed with either the *Klebsiella* or *Pseudomonas* freeze-dried preparation.

A control serum sample was prepared without the addition of bacteria. The sera were incubated overnight at 4 °C on a Rolamix (Luckham Ltd.). The bacteria were removed by centrifugation and the sera retested by ELISA.

11.5 C-Reactive Protein Results

Ankylosing spondylitis patients with an erythrocyte sedimentation rate greater than or equal to 15 mm/h had a mean serum C-reactive protein level of 45.2 μg/ml, and this was significantly higher than the level of 14.0 μg/ml found in ankylosing spondylitis patients with an erythrocyte sedimentation rate less than 15 mm/h ($t=4.28$, $p<0.001$).

The psoriatic arthritis and rheumatoid arthritis patients had a mean serum C-reactive protein levels of 40.0 and 92.1 μg/ml, respectively.

The mean C-reactive protein concentration in 54 healthy control subjects was 2.7 μg/ml, of whom 38 (70 %) had zero values.

11.6 Total Serum IgA Values

The mean total serum IgA in ankylosing spondylitis patients with an erythrocyte sedimentation rate equal to or greater than 15 mm/h was 3.93 mg/ml, whereas in ankylosing spondylitis patients with an erythrocyte sedimentation rate less than 15 mm/h, it was 2.60 mg/ml, and this difference is statistically significant ($t = 3.93$, $p < 0.001$).

The mean total serum IgA in psoriatic patients was 2.16 mg/ml; in rheumatoid arthritis patients, it was 2.33 mg/ml, and in healthy controls, it was 2.07 mg/ml.

There was a significant difference in total serum IgA levels between ankylosing spondylitis patients with an elevated erythrocyte sedimentation rate and the mean total serum IgA in psoriatic patients ($t = 4.19$, $p < 0.001$), in rheumatoid arthritis patients ($t = 9.95$, $p < 0.001$) and in healthy controls ($t = 6.55$, $p < 0.001$).

There was a positive correlation both between erythrocyte sedimentation rate and total serum IgA ($r = +0.4086$, $p < 0.001$) and between serum C-reactive protein level and total serum IgA concentrations ($r = +0.411$, $p < 0.001$) in patients with ankylosing spondylitis.

11.7 IgA Antibodies to *Klebsiella*

The mean serum IgA antibody to *Klebsiella* antigen in 43 sera from ankylosing spondylitis patients with an erythrocyte sedimentation rate equal to or greater than 15 mm/h was 14.00 ± 1.16 ELISA units (mean ± standard error) (Fig. 11.1), whereas in 39 sera from ankylosing spondylitis patients with an erythrocyte sedimentation rate less than 15 mm/h, it was 10.67 ± 0.73, and this difference is statistically significant ($t = 2.38$, $p < 0.02$).

Although there was no direct correlation between serum anti-*Klebsiella* IgA and erythrocyte sedimentation rate, antibody levels tended to rise concurrently with erythrocyte sedimentation rate (Fig. 11.2).

The mean serum IgA anti-*Klebsiella* level of 14.24 ± 1.54 (mean ± standard error) in ankylosing spondylitis patients with an erythrocyte sedimentation rate greater than 30 mm/h was significantly higher ($p < 0.025$) when compared with the mean antibody level of 10.79 ± 0.80 in ankylosing spondylitis patients with an erythrocyte sedimentation rate between 0 and 10 mm/h, whilst in patients with an intermediate erythrocyte sedimentation rate had intermediate values in *Klebsiella* antibody levels (Fig. 11.2).

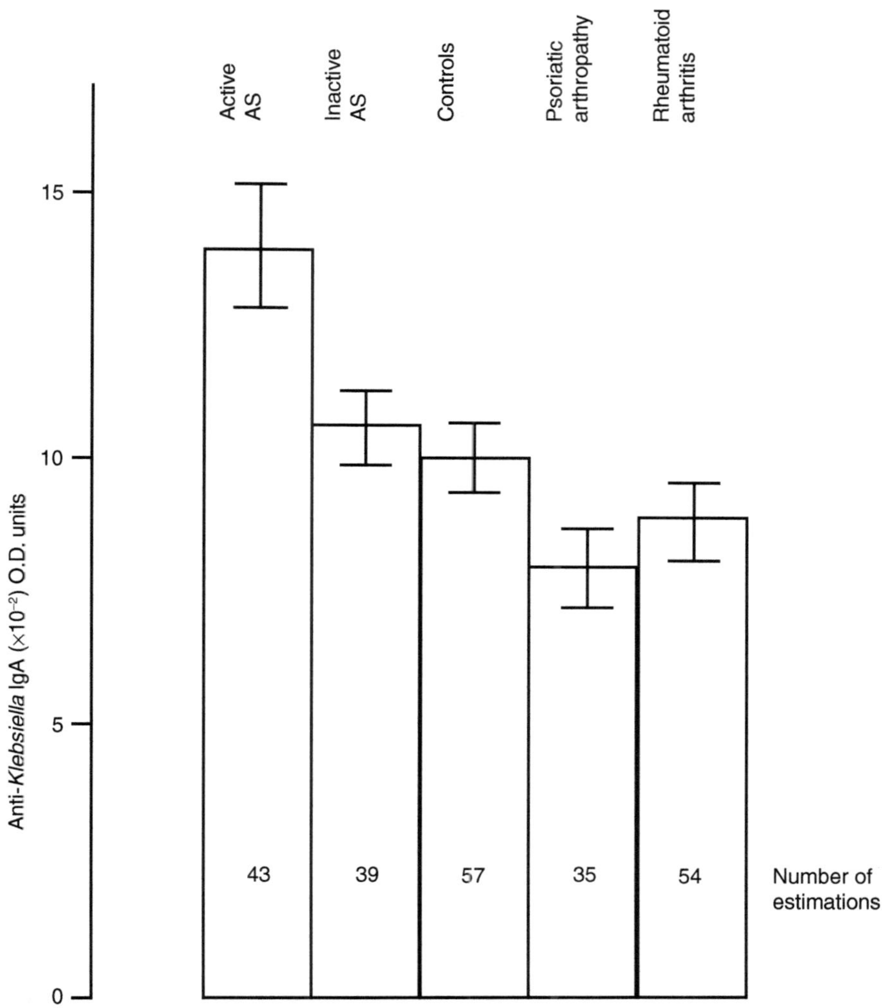

Fig. 11.1 Specific serum IgA antibody to *Klebsiella pneumoniae* (mean ± standard error) measured in ankylosing spondylitis patients with active and inactive disease, healthy controls and patients with psoriatic arthropathy and rheumatoid arthritis

The mean anti-*Klebsiella* antibody level in 35 psoriatic patients was 7.97 ± 0.72; in 54 rheumatoid arthritis patients, it was 8.84 ± 0.64, and in 57 normal control sera, it was 10.00 ± 0.64.

There was a significant elevation in anti-*Klebsiella* antibody levels in ankylosing spondylitis patients with an elevated erythrocyte sedimentation rate compared to psoriatic patients ($t=4.19$, $p<0.001$), rheumatoid arthritis patients ($t=4.12$, $p<0.001$) and healthy controls ($t=3.21$, $p<0.005$).

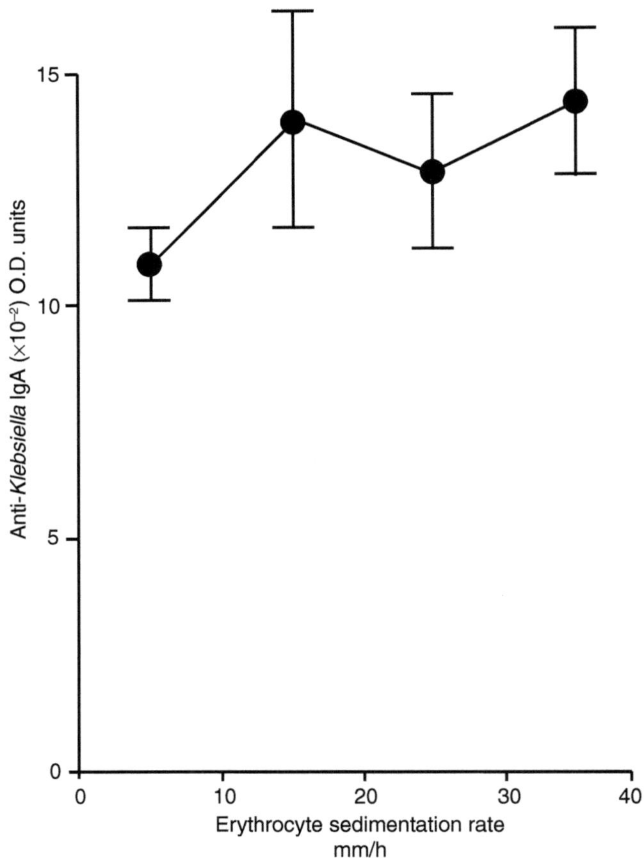

Fig. 11.2 Specific serum IgA antibody (mean ± standard error) to *Klebsiella pneumoniae* and erythrocyte sedimentation rate in ankylosing spondylitis patients

There was no significant difference between healthy controls and patients with rheumatoid arthritis, psoriatic arthritis or ankylosing spondylitis having a low erythrocyte sedimentation rate.

Psoriatic and rheumatoid arthritis patients having an erythrocyte sedimentation rate greater than 15 mm/h were found to have similar *Klebsiella* IgA antibody levels when compared to controls.

Mean IgA antibody levels to *Candida albicans* or *Escherichia coli* did not differ in patients when compared to control subjects.

The absorption of four sera containing differing titres of IgA antibodies to soluble *Klebsiella* antigens with whole inactivated *Klebsiella pneumoniae* microorganisms reduced the level of antibody, but absorption with *Pseudomonas aeruginosa* microorganisms had no effect upon the concentration of IgA antibody to *Klebsiella* as measured by ELISA (Table 11.1).

Table 11.1 Anti-*Klebsiella* antibody activity after absorption. IgA antibodies to *Klebsiella* measured by ELISA before and after a single absorption with inactivated *Pseudomonas aeruginosa* and *Klebsiella pneumoniae* 1 mg/ml (mean ± standard error)

		After absorption with	
Serum sample	Pre-absorption	*Pseudomonas*	*Klebsiella*
1.	30.5 ± 0.7	34.5 ± 0.7	12.0 ± 1.4
2.	27.5 ± 0.7	28.0 ± 0.0	11.5 ± 0.7
3.	15.5 ± 0.7	14.5 ± 0.7	8.5 ± 0.7
4.	9.0 ± 1.4	7.0 ± 0.0	6.0 ± 1.4

11.8 Faecal Cultures and Anti-*Klebsiella* Antibodies

The mean serum anti-*Klebsiella* IgA antibody was found to be higher in ankylosing spondylitis with positive faecal cultures for *Klebsiella* compared to patients with negative cultures, but this difference was not statistically significant.

Furthermore, the mean anti-*Klebsiella* IgA antibody was found to be higher in patients with active or probably active disease when compared to inactive patients, but again this difference was not statistically significant.

However, when faecal culture and disease activity were examined together, an additive effect was observed such that patients having either a positive culture or diagnosed as being clinically active or both had a significantly higher serum anti-*Klebsiella* IgA level when compared with patients with negative cultures who were clinically inactive ($t = 6.27$, $p < 0.001$) (Fig. 11.3).

11.9 Second Study Against the Gram-Negative Microorganisms: *Klebsiella, Salmonella, Yersinia* and *Pseudomonas*

In a second study, blood was obtained from 107 patients attending the 'Ankylosing Spondylitis Research Clinic of the Middlesex Hospital': 75 patients were seen once, 26 patients were seen twice, 5 patients were seen three times and 1 patient was bled on four separate occasions, making a total of 146 sera available for study (Trull et al. 1984).

Control sera were obtained from 110 healthy tissue-typed bone marrow donors attending the Anthony Nolan Laboratories at St Mary Abbots hospital. The sera were selected at random, stored at −20 °C and coded prior to analysis.

Total serum immunoglobulins IgA, IgG and IgM, serum C-reactive protein and erythrocyte sedimentation rate were determined, as previously described.

For statistical analysis, the sera were divided into three grades of disease activity as assessed by the level of C-reactive protein: Sixty patients with a serum C-reactive protein concentration greater than or equal to 30 μg/ml were considered to have

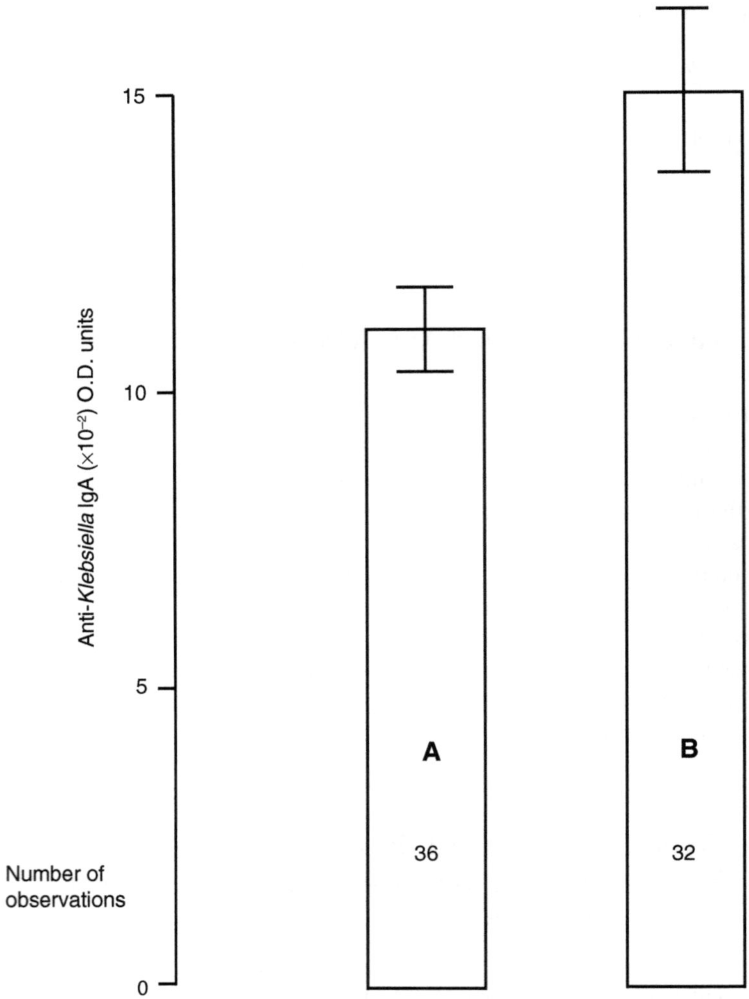

Fig. 11.3 Specific serum IgA antibody (mean ± standard error) to *Klebsiella pneumoniae* in ankylosing spondylitis patients with inactive disease and negative culture (*column A*) compared to patients having either active disease or positive culture or both (*column B*)

'active disease', 56 patients with a C-reactive protein level 10–30 μg/ml were considered to have 'moderately active disease' and, in 30 patients, a C-reactive protein level of less than 10 μg/ml was considered to indicate 'inactive disease'.

Bacterial antigens to *Klebsiella pneumoniae* and *Yersinia enterocolitica* (Department of Rheumatology, Middlesex Hospital), *Salmonella typhimurium* and *Pseudomonas aeruginosa* (Department of Clinical Bacteriology, Guy's Hospital) were prepared as previously described.

The ELISAs were also carried out as previously described. In brief, the assay employs a double antibody technique: The bacterial antigen in microtitre plate is treated first with human or test control serum, then with class-specific rabbit anti-human serum and developed with goat anti-rabbit immunoglobulin alkaline phosphatase conjugate and substrate.

The results were expressed as O.D. units × 100. The results of the absorption studies indicate that specific antibody was absorbed predominantly by the homologous bacteria.

11.9.1 Serum C-Reactive Protein Level

The mean serum C-reactive level in ankylosing spondylitis patients was 37.31 ± 9.17 mg/l (mean ± standard error), and in healthy controls, it was 4.19 ± .06 mg/l. Healthy HLA-B27-positive individuals had a mean C-reactive protein level of 3.39 ± 0.75 mg/l, and this was comparable with the level of 4.65 ± 0.92 mg/l in non-HLA-B27 healthy subjects. Thirty-seven out of 110 (34 %) normals had zero values for C-reactive protein.

11.9.2 Serum IgA

The mean serum concentration of IgA in ankylosing spondylitis patients was 2.72 ± 0.11 g/l, and this was significantly higher than the levels of 2.00 ± 0.09 in healthy controls ($t = 4.65$, $p < 0.001$).

The level of serum IgA in patients with 'active disease' was 3.13 ± 0.20 g/l and this was significantly than the level of 2.00 ± 0.16 g/l in 'inactive patients' ($t = 3.70$, $p < 0.001$) or the level in healthy controls ($t = 5.78$, $p < 0.001$) (Fig. 11.4).

The serum IgA concentration in patients with 'moderately active' disease was 2.66 ± 0.15 mg/l, and this was also significantly elevated when compared with patients with 'inactive disease' ($t = 2.77$, $p < 0.01$) and healthy controls ($t = 9.92$, $p < 0.001$).

The level of serum IgA in 40 healthy HLA-B27-positive subjects was 2.13 ± 0.13 g/l, and this did not differ significantly from the level of 1.93 ± 0.13 g/l found in 67 healthy HLA-B27-negative subjects.

There was a statistically significant positive correlation between the serum IgA concentration and both erythrocyte sedimentation rate ($r = +\,0.278$, $p < 0.001$) and serum C-reactive protein level ($r = +0.189$, $p < 0.05$).

11.9.3 Serum IgG

The mean serum IgG in ankylosing spondylitis patients was 12.15 ± 0.35 g/l, and this was significantly higher than the level of 11.01 ± 0.32 g/l in healthy controls ($t = 2.22$, $p < 0.05$).

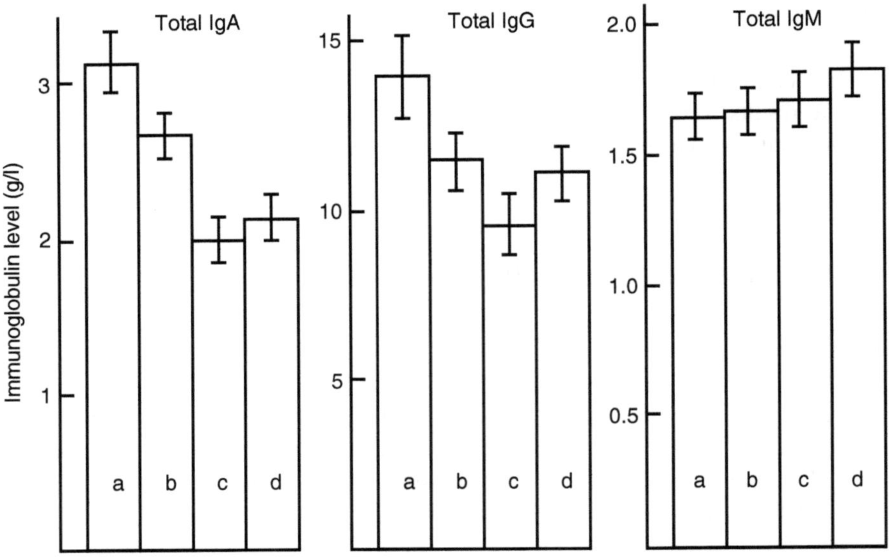

Fig. 11.4 Total serum immunoglobulin A, G and M levels (mean ± standard error) in active (*a*), moderately active (*b*) and inactive (*c*) ankylosing spondylitis patients and healthy controls (*d*)

The level of serum IgG in active patients was 14.01 ± 0.63 g/l, and this was significantly greater than the level of 9.57 ± 0.47 g/l in inactive patients ($t = 4.64$, $p < 0.001$) and the level in healthy controls ($t = 4.56$, $p < 0.001$).

There was again a significant correlation between the serum IgG concentration and both erythrocyte sedimentation rate ($r = +0.370$, $p < 0.001$) and C-reactive protein level ($r = +0.528$, $p < 0.001$).

11.9.4 Serum IgM

The mean serum IgM concentration in ankylosing spondylitis patients was 1.67 ± 0.05 g/l, and this was comparable with the level of 1.70 ± 0.05 g/l found in healthy controls. There was also no association between serum IgM levels and either with erythrocyte sedimentation rate or C-reactive protein.

11.9.5 ELISA IgA Antibodies

The serum *Klebsiella pneumoniae* IgA in ankylosing spondylitis patients was 12.02 ± 0.59 ELISA units (± standard error), and this was significantly greater when compared with the level of 9.97 ± 0.57 found in healthy controls ($t = 2.42$, $p < 0.02$).

IgA antibodies to other Gram-negative bacteria were similar in patients and controls.

Ankylosing spondylitis patients with 'active disease' had a mean *Klebsiella pneumoniae* IgA level of 12.85 ± 0.97, and this was significantly higher than the level of 9.52 ± 0.86 found in patients with 'inactive disease' ($t = 2.22$, $p < 0.025$) and healthy controls ($t = 2.32$, $p < 0.025$), although it did not differ significantly from the *Klebsiella pneumoniae* IgA level in the 'inactive disease' group. There was no difference between *Klebsiella pneumoniae* IgA antibody levels in 'inactive patients' and healthy controls.

IgA antibody levels to *Salmonella typhimurium*, *Yersinia enterocolitica* and *Pseudomonas aeruginosa* were similar in patients and controls, irrespective of disease activity.

In order to illustrate the relationship between the raised total serum IgA in ankylosing spondylitis patients and specific IgA antibodies to Gram-negative bacteria, 12 patients with a total serum IgA concentration exceeding the normal mean serum IgA + 2 standard deviations (equivalent to 4.6 g/l) were compared with the healthy controls. Ankylosing spondylitis patients with elevated serum IgA had a mean *Klebsiella pneumoniae* IgA level of 18.65 ± 2.32, and this was significantly elevated when compared with HLA-B27-positive healthy controls ($t = 3.21$, $p < 0.005$), healthy HLA-B22/B7-positive controls ($t = 9.16$, $p < 0.005$) and B7CREG-negative controls ($t = 6.05$, $p < 0.001$) (Fig. 11.5).

Antibodies to other Gram-negative bacteria were not increased in ankylosing spondylitis patients with high total serum IgA.

11.9.6 ELISA IgG Antibodies

The mean level of IgG antibody to *Salmonella typhimurium* antigens in ankylosing spondylitis patients was 15.88 ± 0.76, and this was significantly greater than the level of 13.15 ± 0.86 in healthy controls ($t = 2.36$, $p < 0.02$).

When patients were divided according to disease activity, there was no difference in *Salmonella typhimurium* antibody levels between active and inactive patients.

However, there was a significant correlation between *Klebsiella pneumoniae* IgG and both erythrocyte sedimentation rate ($r = +0.193$, $p < 0.05$) and C-reactive protein ($r = +0.173$, $p < 0.05$).

Ankylosing spondylitis patients with 'active disease' had a mean serum *Klebsiella pneumoniae* IgG level 40.92 ± 3.03, and this was significantly higher than the level of 24.50 ± 2.52 in patients with 'inactive disease' ($t = 9.53$, $p < 0.001$).

Patients with 'moderately active' disease had an intermediate antibody level of 33.84 ± 9.38.

However, the level of *Klebsiella pneumoniae* IgG in ankylosing spondylitis patients with 'active' or 'moderately active' disease did not differ from the level of 38.05 ± 2.12 found in healthy controls.

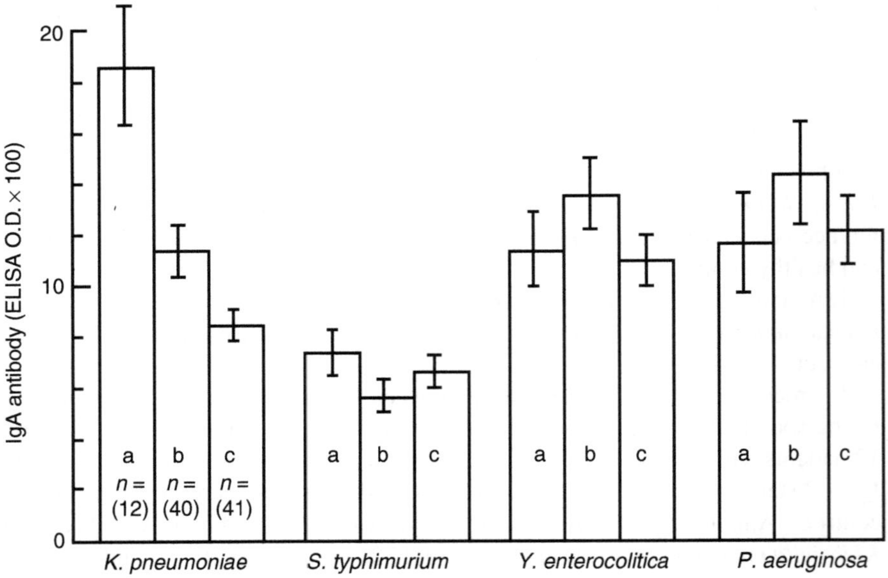

Fig. 11.5 Serum antibacterial IgA levels (mean ± standard error) in ankylosing spondylitis patients with an elevated total serum IgA (>4.6 G/L) (*a*) compared to the levels found in healthy HLA-B27-positive (*b*) and non-HLA-B27 control subjects (*c*)

IgG antibodies to other Gram-negative bacteria did not correlate with disease activity.

11.9.7 ELISA IgM Antibodies

There was no elevation of IgM antibodies to Gram-negative bacteria in ankylosing spondylitis patients when compared to healthy subjects.

11.10 Pathological and Clinical Implications

It would appear that during active phases of ankylosing spondylitis, either assessed clinically or by biochemical parameters such as C-reactive protein or erythrocyte sedimentation rates, elevated levels of specific antibodies to *Klebsiella pneumoniae* microbes can be detected in such patients.

The clear elevation of *Klebsiella pneumoniae* antibody titres compared to other Gram-negative microorganisms such as *Salmonella typhimurium*, *Yersinia enterocolitica* and *Pseudomonas aeruginosa* suggests that these specific microbes may be involved in the pathology of the disease.

It is thus possible that active inflammatory enthesopathy lesions occur during periods when elevations of specific anti-*Klebsiella* serum IgA antibodies can be detected in serum, suggesting that a gut microbial trigger event may have been responsible for the exacerbations or relapses that occur in ankylosing spondylitis.

Measurement of levels of secretory IgA antibodies in the saliva may provide more conclusive evidence of mucosal immunity to potentially arthritogenic bacteria in patients with ankylosing spondylitis (Calguneri et al. 1981).

The adherence of pathogenic bacteria to mucosal epithelium is an important step in colonization and invasion of the intestinal tract. The production of specific antibodies to *Klebsiella pneumoniae* may have been the starting trigger leading to pathology in the spine and peripheral joints which eventually produced the classical picture of ankylosing spondylitis. Although serum IgA antibodies were clearly identified, it is more likely that the smaller IgG anti-*Klebsiella* antibodies may have penetrated to the enthesopathic sites, peripheral joints and spinal sites where together with complement factors it may have started the inflammatory process leading to the established features of ankylosing spondylitis.

References

Calguneri M, Swinburne L, Shinebaum R, Cooke EM, Wright V. Secretory IgA: Immune defence pattern in ankylosing Spondylitis and *Klebsiella*. Ann Rheum Dis. 1981;40:600–4.

Clowes RC, Hayes W. Experiments in microbial genetics. New York: Wiley; 1980.

Granfors K, Viljanen M, Tiilikainen A, Toivanen A. Persistence of IgM. IgG and IgA antibodies to Yersinia in Yersinia arthritis. J Infect Dis. 1980;141:424.

Hunter T, Harding GKM, Kaprove RE, Schroeder ML. Fecal carriage of *Klebsiella* and *Enterobacter* species in patients with active ankylosing spondylitis. Arthritis Rheum. 1981;24:106.

Trull AK, Ebringer R, Panayi GS, Colthorpe D, James DCO, Ebringer A. IgA antibodies to *Klebsiella pneumoniae* in ankylosing spondylitis. Scand J Rheumatol. 1983;12:249–53.

Trull AK, Ebringer A, Panayi GS, Ebringer R, James DCO. HLA-B27 and the immune response to enterobacterial antigens in ankylosing spondylitis. Clin Exp Immunol. 1984;55:74–80.

Chapter 12
IgA Antibodies to *Klebsiella* Measured by Immunoblotting

12.1 Introduction: The Problem of Elevated Serum IgA in Ankylosing Spondylitis and Its Link to *Klebsiella*

Several studies have shown that *Klebsiella* bacteria can be isolated from the faecal cultures of patients with active ankylosing spondylitis. No such increased isolation is found for other Gram-negative microorganisms, such as *Salmonella*, *Shigella* or *Yersinia* species which are known to cause 'reactive arthritis'. All four species of Gram-negative microorganisms associated with 'reactive arthritis' *Salmonella*, *Shigella* and *Yersinia*, as well as *Klebsiella*, carry antigens cross-reacting with HLA-B27, but only serological studies can distinguish which of these bacteria is associated with ankylosing spondylitis in HLA-B27-positive patients. The concept of 'reactive arthritis' implies that there is a primary microbiological and clinical event characterised by diarrhoea and presence of a positive faecal culture with presence of antibacterial antibodies which is then followed several weeks or even months later by a secondary event involving 'reactive arthritis' of the large joints with no bacteria present in the synovial fluid. Whether ankylosing spondylitis falls into this group of diseases is unclear because the 'primary event' of a bacterial infection would appear to be 'clinically silent'.

In a survey of 39 different strains of *Klebsiella* isolated from faecal samples obtained from patients attending the 'Ankylosing Spondylitis Research Clinic of the Middlesex Hospital', 14 were *Klebsiella oxytoca*, (36 %), 24 were *Klebsiella aerogenes* (62 %) and 1 was *Klebsiella pneumoniae* (sensu stricto) (3 %) (Pease et al. 1982).

It has been suggested that after exposure to Gram-negative bacteria, ankylosing spondylitis is produced by bacteria binding to cross-reacting self-antigens such as HLA-B27, situated predominantly in the region of lymphatic drainage of the colon and rectum. To demonstrate the presence of such antibodies further, the following study was carried out with a western immunoblotting technique involving sodium dodecyl sulphate polyacrylamide gel electrophoresis (SDS-PAGE).

A. Ebringer, *Ankylosing Spondylitis and Klebsiella*,
DOI 10.1007/978-1-4471-4300-0_12,

Table 12.1 General characteristics of the 4 study groups

Tests	Controls	Inactive AS	Active AS	RA
Number subjects	51	38	28	31
Mean age (years)	35	48	44	63
Mean ESR (mm/h)	ND	5.8	38.9	28.4
Mean CRP (μg/ml)	3.5	4.9	35.9	21.1
Mean IgA (g/l)	1.82	2.04	4.50	2.73

AS ankylosing spondylitis, *RA* rheumatoid arthritis, *ESR* erythrocyte sedimentation rate, *CRP* C-reactive protein

12.2 Selection of Serum Samples from Ankylosing Spondylitis, Rheumatoid Arthritis Patients and Healthy Controls

Blood was obtained from patients attending the 'Ankylosing Spondylitis Research Clinic of the Middlesex Hospital' and rheumatoid arthritis patients attending the 'Gold Clinics' (Table 12.1).

The diagnosis of ankylosing spondylitis was made according to the New York criteria and that for rheumatoid arthritis according to the criteria of the American Rheumatism Association (Ropes et al. 1958).

The ankylosing spondylitis patients were classified into those with 'active' and 'inactive disease' according to the erythrocyte sedimentation rate and total serum IgA concentration at the time of the study. Patients with 'active disease' were defined as those with an erythrocyte sedimentation rate above 15 mm/h and a total serum IgA above 3 g/l, whereas patients with 'inactive disease' had an erythrocyte sedimentation rate below 15 mm/h and a total serum IgA below 3 g/l. Patients with only one of these variables elevated were deemed to be 'probably active' and excluded from the study. The sera from all subjects were coded and decoded after immunoblotting.

All patients were measured for erythrocyte sedimentation rate, C-reactive protein and total serum IgA, as previously described.

The Gram-negative bacteria *Klebsiella pneumoniae* var *oxytoca* (MX 100) and *Proteus mirabilis* (B17) were grown as previously described. Overnight cultures were centrifuged at 10,000 rpm for 20 min, washed three times in phosphate-buffered saline (pH 7.5), the pellet resuspended in 10-ml phosphate-buffered saline and ultrasonicated at an amplitude of 12 μm with 30-s bursts and 60-s rest periods (seven cycles).

12.3 Sodium Dodecyl Sulphate Polyacrylamide Gel Electrophoresis (SDS-PAGE)

The protein content of the sonicated sample was measured by Bradford's method (Bradford 1976).

The sample was then diluted in sample buffer (0.05 M TRIS.HCl pH 6.8, 2 mM EDTA, 2 % SDS, 50 mM dithiothreitol and 0.001 % bromophenol blue) to a protein concentration of 1 mg/ml and allowed to dissociate for 3 h at 37 °C. The samples were then subjected to SDS-PAGE.

Electrophoresis was performed in a discontinuous system with a 10 % polyacrylamide resolving gel and a 9.5 % stacking gel (Laemmli 1970).

A number of molecular weight markers (Sigma Chemical) were prepared at a concentration of 1 mg/ml in SDS sample buffer, and 100 μl was applied to the gel. The polypeptide markers, in order of decreasing molecular weight, were phosphorylase B (94,000), bovine serum albumin (67,000), ovalbumin (43,000), carbonic anhydrase (30,000), soybean trypsin inhibitor (20,100) and lactalbumin (14,400).

The treated sample of the microorganism was also applied to the gel, after which electrophoresis was performed at a constant current of 50 mA until the bromophenol blue had travelled 10 cm in the resolving gel.

The gels were stained either with Coomassie blue G-250 or immunoblotted, and molecular weights were estimated from a calibration curve obtained with standard proteins.

12.3.1 Immunoblot Analysis

The separated components of the bacterium were transferred electrophoretically from the gel onto a sheet of nitrocellulose (sartorius membrane, pore size 0.45 μm) (Towbin et al. 1979).

The transfer buffer was 25-mM TRIS.HCl, 192-mM glycine (pH 8.3) containing 29 % vol/vol methanol, and blotting was carried out for 1 h at 10 V/cm.

After transfer, the nitrocellulose sheet was cut into 3-mm strips, which were then shaken for 2 h at room temperature in a blocking buffer.

12.4 Characteristics of the Four Study Groups

The number of men and women in the control group was almost equal, whereas the ratio of men to women in the 'active ankylosing spondylitis' was 4:1, in the group with 'inactive ankylosing spondylitis', it was 2:1 and in the rheumatoid arthritis group, 1:2.

The mean erythrocyte sedimentation rate in the group with 'active disease' was significantly higher than that found in the group with 'inactive disease' ($t = 7.84$, $p < 0.001$) but not significantly different when compared to the group with rheumatoid arthritis.

The mean erythrocyte sedimentation rate in the group with rheumatoid arthritis was significantly raised in comparison with the 'inactive ankylosing spondylitis' group ($t = 6.07$, $p < 0.001$).

The mean C-reactive protein in the group with 'active ankylosing spondylitis' was significantly higher than that in groups with rheumatoid arthritis ($t = 2.69$, $p < 0.01$) and 'inactive ankylosing spondylitis' ($t = 7.58$, $p < 0.001$) and in the controls ($t = 9.27$, $p < 0.001$).

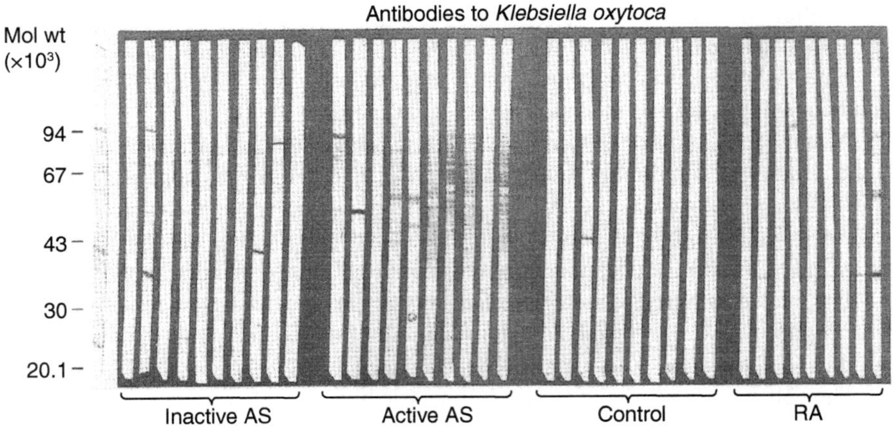

Fig. 12.1 Immunoblotting antigenic bands developed with serum samples from patients with 'inactive AS' and 'active AS', from controls and from patients with RA against sonicated *Klebsiella oxytoca*. The first strip on the left shows the protein profile of *Klebsiella oxytoca* after being separated by SDA-PAGE onto nitrocellulose paper and stained with amino black. Molecular weights markers ($\times 10^3$) are indicated (*AS* ankylosing spondylitis, *RA* rheumatoid arthritis)

The mean total serum IgA concentration in the group with 'active ankylosing spondylitis' was significantly raised compared with that in the groups with rheumatoid arthritis ($t=4.69$, $p<0.001$) and 'inactive ankylosing spondylitis' ($t=7.93$, $p<0.001$) and in the controls ($t=10.87$, $p<0.001$).

The mean total serum IgA of the group with rheumatoid arthritis was significantly higher than that of the group with 'inactive ankylosing spondylitis' ($t=3.29$, $p<0.005$) and the control group ($t=6.02$, $p<0.001$). The mean total serum IgA concentration of the group with 'inactive ankylosing spondylitis' was not significantly different from that found in the control group.

12.5 Analysis of the Results of the Immunoblotting Assay

The sera from 'active ankylosing spondylitis patients' showed many lines against *Klebsiella* homogenates compared to sera from 'inactive ankylosing spondylitis patients', rheumatoid arthritis patients and controls (Fig. 12.1).

The antigenic bands on each strip were counted, the origin of the serum samples decoded and the mean number of bands calculated (Table 12.2).

The mean number of bands in the group with 'active ankylosing spondylitis' was significantly higher than that in the 'inactive ankylosing spondylitis' group ($t=8.65$, $p<0.001$), rheumatoid arthritis group ($t=11.46$, $p<0.001$) and in controls ($t=15.10$, $p<0.001$).

The mean number of bands in the group with 'inactive ankylosing spondylitis' was also significantly higher than that in the control group ($t=2.76$, $p<0.01$), but not that in the group with rheumatoid arthritis. There was no significant difference

Table 12.2 Mean number of antigenic bands measured by immunoblotting against both *Klebsiella* and *Proteus* microorganisms in the 4 study groups

Tests	Controls	Inactive AS	Active AS	RA
Number subjects	51	38	28	31
Number of bands against *Klebsiella*	1.9	3.7	13.0	2.2
Number of bands against *Proteus*	0.7	1.3	3.0	1.4

AS ankylosing spondylitis, *RA* rheumatoid arthritis

in the mean number of bands between the group with rheumatoid arthritis and the control group (Shodjai-Moradi et al. 1992).

The mean number of antigenic bands against *Proteus* in patients with 'active ankylosing spondylitis' was significantly higher than that in the groups with 'inactive ankylosing spondylitis' (t =9.51, $p<0.001$), rheumatoid arthritis (t =2.96, $p<0.005$) and in the control group (t=5.04, $p<0.001$).

12.6 Comparison of Serum and Synovial Fluids

Paired samples of serum and synovial fluid from two patients with ankylosing spondylitis who also had knee effusions, one having 'active disease' and the other one 'inactive disease', were tested against a sonicated preparation of *Klebsiella* using a horseradish peroxidase-conjugated anti-human IgA, as previously described.

Each patient's synovial fluid and the corresponding serum sample showed exactly the same pattern of bands on the immunoblot (Fig. 12.2). The number and intensity of bands in the serum and synovial fluid obtained from the patient with 'inactive ankylosing spondylitis' (Patient A) was less than that of the bands in the fluids from the patient with 'active ankylosing spondylitis' (Patient B).

12.7 Pathological and Clinical Implications

Immunoblotting showed that sera from active ankylosing spondylitis patients have an increased number of IgA antibodies to different Gram-negative bacterial components of *Klebsiella* and to a lesser extent to *Proteus* microorganisms.

This is in agreement with earlier reports of raised antibodies to *Klebsiella* in patients with active ankylosing spondylitis when measured by enzyme-linked immunosorbent assay (ELISA), bacterial absorption (Ebringer et al. 1985) and indirect Coombs agglutination.

The increased levels of IgA antibodies indicate enterobacterial antigenic stimulation via the gut during active phases of the disease, and this is compatible with the increased levels of faecal isolation of *Klebsiella* found in such patients. Whether *Klebsiella* is the only Gram-negative microbe involved in such a pathogenic process remains to be established.

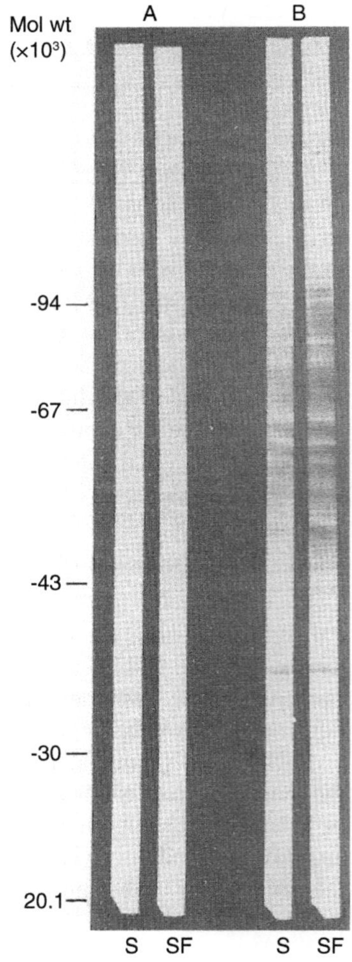

Fig. 12.2 Specific IgA antibodies to *Klebsiella* in serum (*S*) and synovial fluid (*SF*) in two patients with ankylosing spondylitis, one having 'inactive disease' (Patient A) and the other one having 'active disease' (Patient B), detected by immunoblotting

However, an immunoblotting assay performed under code with *Yersinia enterocolitica* showed antibodies to *Yersinia* in Finnish patients with *Yersinia* reactive arthritis, but no such antibodies were found in English patients with ankylosing spondylitis, thereby confirming similar studies carried out with ELISA (Toivanen et al. 1986).

Gram-negative bacteria share common antigens, and thus it is not surprising that some serum samples from patients with active ankylosing spondylitis detected three to four *Proteus* antigenic bands though the number detected against *Klebsiella* was much higher. In some patients with ankylosing spondylitis, up to 25 *Klebsiella* bands were detected.

Examination of the immunoblots showed that active ankylosing spondylitis patients had antibodies to a number of *Klebsiella* bacterial components with molecular weights ranging from 43,000 to 94,000. The common bands among the ankylosing spondylitis patients with active disease were to proteins with molecular weights 102,000 (22 %), 90,000 (30 %), 65,000 (37 %) and 48,000 (19 %). None of the control samples had antibodies against the 65,000 and 48,000 proteins.

Whether these proteins are involved in the pathogenesis of the disease remains to be determined.

An independent study was also carried out on two paired samples of serum and synovial fluid against a sonicated preparation of *Klebsiella* microorganisms, which showed a similar IgA antibody pattern in the serum and synovial fluid. This would appear to be consistent with the hypothesis that antibodies to *Klebsiella* found in the synovial fluid might have been derived from circulating immunoglobulins, probably produced in the lymph nodes draining the gastrointestinal tract and not produced locally in the inflamed joint.

Other workers have also carried out antibody investigations in ankylosing spondylitis and found raised titres against *Klebsiella* microorganisms. A group from Glasgow investigated 64 patients with ankylosing spondylitis, 25 with rheumatoid arthritis, 30 with Crohn's disease, 20 with ulcerative colitis and 35 controls using ELISA on *Klebsiella pneumoniae* as target antigen. The results of their studies showed that antibodies to *Klebsiella* were raised not only in ankylosing spondylitis but also in ulcerative colitis, Crohn's disease and rheumatoid arthritis when compared to controls (Cooper et al. 1988).

Their conclusion differs from ours as they suggest that patients with ankylosing spondylitis have a 'leaky' gut mucosa because of bowel inflammation which allows all gut bacteria to penetrate across the bowel. However, such a hypothesis implies that bacterial peritonitis should occur relatively frequently in patients with such diseases.

Clearly, further studies are required to resolve these differences, but there seems to be agreement that bacterial antigens, especially from *Klebsiella*, can be detected in ankylosing spondylitis patients with active disease. However, at this stage, it is not clear whether these antigens have a specific pathological role or only represent a non-specific immunological marker of a compromised bowel mucosa.

References

Bradford M. A rapid and sensitive method for the quantitation of microgram quantities of protein utilising the principle of protein dye binding. Anal Biochem. 1976;72:248–54.

Cooper R, Fraser SM, Sturrock RD, Gemmel CG. Raised titres of anti-*Klebsiella* IgA in ankylosing spondylitis, rheumatoid arthritis and inflammatory bowel disease. Br Med J. 1988; 296:1432–4.

Ebringer A, Baines M, Childerstone M, Ghuloom M, Ptaszynska T. Etiopathogenesis of ankylosing spondylitis and the cross-tolerance hypothesis. In: Ziff M, Cohen SB eds. Advances in Inflammation Research: The Spondyloarthropathies. New York Raven Press. 1985;9: 101–28.

Laemmli UK. Cleavage of structural proteins during the assembly of the head of bacteriophage T4. Nature. 1970;227:680–5.

Pease PE, Tyler RA, England JR, Colthorpe D, Ebringer A. An investigation into the properties of *Klebsiella* strains isolated from ankylosing spondylitis patients. J Hyg (Lond). 1982;89:119–23.

Ropes MW, Bennett GA, Cobb S, Jacox R, Jesar RA. Revision of diagnostic criteria for rheumatoid arthritis. Bull Rheum Dis. 1958;9:175–6.

Shodjai-Moradi F, Ebringer A, Abuljadayel I. IgA antibody response to *Klebsiella* in ankylosing spondylitis measured by immunoblotting. Ann Rheum Dis. 1992;51:233–7.

Toivanen A, Stahlberg TH, Granfors K, Ebringer A. Absence of antibodies to *Yersinia enterocolitica* in patients with ankylosing spondylitis in London. Lancet. 1986;ii:1400.

Towbin H, Stachelin T, Gordon J. Electrophoresis transfer of proteins from polyacrylamide gels to nitrocellulose sheets: procedure and some applications. Proc Natl Acad Sci USA. 1979;76:4350–7.

Chapter 13
Antibodies to *Klebsiella* in Ankylosing Spondylitis Measured by Bacterial Agglutination and ELISA Against Lipopolysaccharides

13.1 Introduction: Gram-Negative Bacteria in Ankylosing Spondylitis

The association between HLA-B27 and ankylosing spondylitis has been well established, and it has been suggested that *Klebsiella* bacteria may have a role to play in the pathogenesis of ankylosing spondylitis.

Several Gram-negative bacteria are known to be responsible for the development of 'reactive arthritis' especially in individuals who are HLA-B27 positive.

Agglutinating antibodies may be present in such patients or antibodies against bacterial lipopolysaccharides (LPS). Bacterial LPS is an important virulence factor for some members of the *Enterobacteriaceae* (Robbins et al. 1974). Elevated levels of serum LPS have been found in active ankylosing spondylitis patients (Wagener et al. 1988) although this has been disputed by others (Maki-Ikola et al. 1997).

It has been suggested that LPS plays a role in the pathogenesis of reactive arthritis caused by *Yersinia* (Granfors et al. 1989) and *Salmonella* (Maki-Ikola et al. 1991) microorganisms.

In this study, ankylosing spondylitis patients were compared to rheumatoid arthritis patients by two different techniques: bacterial agglutination and antibodies to bacterial LPS.

In the bacterial agglutination method, antibodies were measured against *Klebsiella* and *Proteus* microorganisms.

In the ELISA method, antibodies to LPS were measured against 4 different Gram-negative bacteria: *Klebsiella pneumoniae*, *Escherichia coli*, *Salmonella typhimurium* and *Salmonella enteritidis*.

A. Ebringer, *Ankylosing Spondylitis and Klebsiella*,
DOI 10.1007/978-1-4471-4300-0_13, © Springer-Verlag London 2013

13.2 First Study: Patients and Controls

13.2.1 Sera from Ankylosing Spondylitis Patients

Serum samples were obtained from 52 patients with ankylosing spondylitis, satisfying the New York criteria and attending the 'Ankylosing Spondylitis Research Clinic of the Middlesex Hospital'.

Ankylosing spondylitis patients with serum IgA greater or equal to 3 G/l were allocated to the active ankylosing spondylitis group, and those with serum IgA less than 3 G/l and erythrocyte sedimentation rate less than 15 mm/h were placed in the inactive group. Ankylosing spondylitis patients with a serum IgA less than 3 G/l but with an erythrocyte sedimentation rate above 15 mm/h were excluded from the study. Previous studies had shown that active ankylosing spondylitis patients had elevated levels of serum IgA (Table 13.1).

Control sera were samples obtained from 41 healthy blood donors.

13.2.2 Sera from Rheumatoid Arthritis Patients

Serum samples were obtained from 30 rheumatoid arthritis patients attending the weekly 'Gold Clinic' at the Middlesex Hospital.

It was considered that rheumatoid arthritis requiring second-line therapy represented a group with more active disease than rheumatoid arthritis patients being treated with non-steroidal anti-inflammatory drugs.

There were 14 men and 16 women. Their mean age was 59 years (range: 40–78 years), and the diagnosis was made according to the American Rheumatism Association criteria (Ropes et al. 1958).

All serum samples were investigated for C-reactive protein, IgG and IgA by the single radial immunodiffusion method of Mancini.

The hospital service measured the erythrocyte sedimentation rate (ESR) of all patients by the method of Westergren.

The mean (± standard error) erythrocyte sedimentation rate (ESR) in the rheumatoid arthritis was 28.2 ± 5.2 mm/h, and the mean (± standard error) C-reactive protein level was 22.7 ± 5.6 μg/ml (Table 13.1).

13.3 Statistical Analysis of Patient Groups and Controls

The mean (± standard error) erythrocyte sedimentation rate in the rheumatoid arthritis group was 28.2 ± 5.2 mm/h, and this was significantly higher ($p < 0.001$, $t = 4.17$) than the level of 5.7 ± 1.0 mm/h found in the inactive ankylosing spondylitis group.

Table 13.1 Characteristics of the first study groups

	Controls	Active AS	Inactive AS	RA
Number	41	24	28	30
M/F	23/18	20/4	21/7	14/16
Age range	20–50	28–62	24–69	40–78
Mean age	ND	41	44	59
ESR mm/h	ND	41.6±5.0	5.7±1.0	28.2±5.2
CRP μg/ml	1.6±0.6	35.9±5.8	3.8±0.8	22.7±5.6
IgG g/l	12.4±0.4	20.6±0.1	14.0±0.8	15.2±0.9
IgA g/l	1.96±0.1	4.74±0.2	1.74±0.1	2.55±0.2

AS ankylosing spondylitis, *RA* rheumatoid arthritis, *ESR* erythrocyte sedimentation rate, *CRP* C-reactive protein, *ND* not done, Mean ± standard error, *M/F* male/female, Mean age: years

The mean (± standard error) erythrocyte sedimentation rate in the active ankylosing spondylitis was 41.6±5.0 mm/h, and this was significantly higher ($p<0.001$, $t=7.67$) than the level of 5.7 ± 1.0 mm/h found in the inactive ankylosing spondylitis group.

For C-reactive protein levels, all three patient groups, active ankylosing spondylitis ($p<0.001$, $t=7.60$), inactive ankylosing spondylitis ($p<0.05$, $t=2.23$) and rheumatoid arthritis ($p<0.001$, $t=5.85$), had significantly higher levels than the one with 1.6±0.6 μg/ml measured in the controls.

Furthermore, the inactive ankylosing spondylitis group had significantly lower C-reactive protein level compared to the active ankylosing spondylitis group ($p<0.001$, $t=5.87$) and the rheumatoid arthritis group ($p<0.001$, $t=3.23$).

The mean (± standard error) serum IgG in active ankylosing spondylitis was 20.60±0.15 g/l, and this was significantly higher than the level of 14.04±0.82 g/l found in inactive ankylosing spondylitis ($p<0.001$, $t=3.93$), the level of 15.20±0.94 g/l found in the rheumatoid arthritis group ($p<0.005$, $t=3.15$) and the level of 12.44±0.44 g/l found in the controls ($p<0.001$, $t=6.28$).

The mean (± standard error) serum IgA of the active ankylosing spondylitis was 4.74±0.24 g/l, and this was significantly higher than the level of 2.55±0.21 g/l found in the rheumatoid arthritis group ($p<0.001$, $t=6.82$) or the level of 1.96±0.15 g/l found in the control group ($p<0.001$, $t=10.35$).

The mean (± standard error) serum IgA of the rheumatoid arthritis group was 2.55±0.21 g/l, and this was significantly higher than the level of 1.74±0.08 g/l found in the inactive ankylosing spondylitis group ($p<0.001$, $t=3.53$) or the level of 1.96±0.15 g/l found in the control group ($p<0.025$, $t=2.34$).

13.4 Coombs Agglutination Assay

Klebsiella pneumoniae var oxytoca (MX100) and *Proteus mirabilis* (B17) were obtained from the Department of Microbiology at Queen Elizabeth College. The cultures were maintained on nutrient agar slopes at room temperature.

Nutrient broth (Oxoid) 13 g/l of water was autoclaved at 121 °C, 1.05 kg/cm^2 for 15 min. A starter culture was prepared in 25 ml of autoclaved nutrient broth in a 250-ml conical flask and inoculated from the agar slope, incubated at 37 °C for 6 h and agitated at 250 rpm on an orbital shaker.

Shake flask cultures were prepared by inoculating 200 ml of nutrient broth, in a 2-l conical flask with 10-ml culture from the starter broth, incubated at 37 °C and shaken for 16 h at 250 rpm on an orbital shaker.

Overnight cultures were centrifuged at 2,500 × g for 15 min, washed three times with phosphate-buffered saline and the pellet resuspended in 25 ml phosphate-buffered saline.

The concentration of the bacteria was adjusted to give an optical density of 1.64 in a spectrophotometer 1,800 at 540 nm, since this had been found to give optimum agglutination. It was equivalent to 1.57 × 10^{12} cells/ml for *Klebsiella* and 2.05 × 10^{11} cells/ml for *Proteus* microorganisms, when measured in a Coulter counter (Model 2B1).

The agglutination assay was carried out as follows: 100 μl volumes of bacterial suspension were added to 100 μl doubling dilutions of test serum in Dreyer's tubes. The mixtures were incubated at 37 °C for 2 h, then 350 μl phosphate-buffered saline was added and the tubes were centrifuged for 20 min (1,500 × g, Mistral 6 L) at 4 °C.

The supernatant was decanted, the pellet resuspended in 350 μl fresh phosphate-buffered saline and the washing repeated twice. After the final wash, the pellet was resuspended in 100 μl one-tenth dilution in phosphate-buffered saline of Coombs rabbit anti-human immunoglobulin reagent. The tubes were incubated at 37 °C for 2 h, then at 4 °C overnight, and the agglutination end point determined.

All test serum samples were coded and end points read blind, in that the tester was unaware whether patient or control sera were being investigated.

13.5 Results of Coombs Agglutination Assay

Three separate agglutination studies were carried out against whole *Proteus mirabilis* and *Klebsiella pneumoniae var oxytoca* microorganisms. There were approximately 40 serum samples in each run, all tests were carried out blind and all samples came from different individuals. Therefore, each coded run was an independent investigation, and the pooled results are shown (Fig. 13.1) (Ebringer et al. 1985).

The mean (± standard error) *Klebsiella pneumoniae* agglutination titre in the active ankylosing spondylitis patients was 5.80 ± 0.20 $\log_2$ dilution units, and this was significantly higher than the level of 3.79 ± 0.21 $\log_2$ dilution units found in the inactive ankylosing spondylitis group ($p<0.001$, $t=6.26$), the titre of 3.67 ± 0.24 $\log_2$ dilution units in the rheumatoid arthritis patients ($p<0.001$, $t=7.22$) or the level of 3.85 ± 0.15 $\log_2$ dilution units in the healthy controls ($p<0.001$, $t=7.61$).

The mean (± standard error) *Proteus mirabilis* agglutination titre in the rheumatoid arthritis patients was 4.50 ± 0.18 $\log_2$ dilution units, and this was

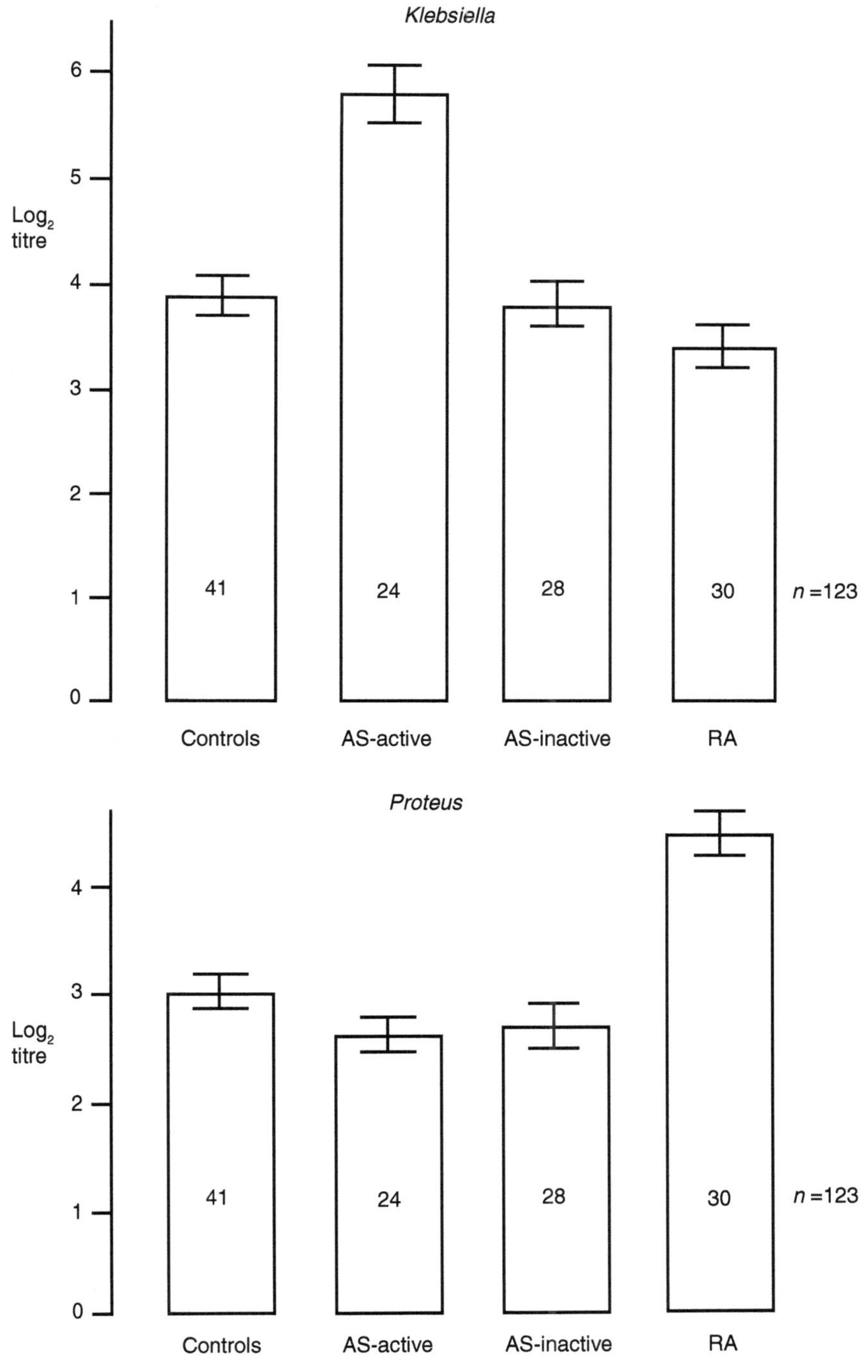

Fig. 13.1 Antibody agglutination titres (mean ± standard error) from three pooled runs. Number of subjects in each group is indicated

significantly higher than the level of 3.08 ± 0.17 $\log_2$ dilution units found in the active ankylosing spondylitis group ($p < 0.001$, $t = 5.69$), the titre of 2.68 ± 0.16 $\log_2$ dilution units found in the inactive ankylosing spondylitis patients ($p < 0.001$, $t = 7.60$) or the level of 2.63 ± 0.16 $\log_2$ dilution units found in the healthy controls ($p < 0.001$, $t = 9.27$).

13.6 Second Study: Patients and Controls

Ankylosing spondylitis sera were obtained from patients attending the 'Ankylosing Spondylitis Research Clinic of the Middlesex Hospital', and rheumatoid arthritis sera were obtained from patients attending the Rheumatology Department at the Lister Hospital, Stevenage.

Healthy control samples were supplied by the Blood Transfusion Service, London. Both ankylosing spondylitis and rheumatoid arthritis serum samples were randomly selected from our stock stored at −20 °C.

The groups examined in the second study were as follows: 100 patients with ankylosing spondylitis (81 males/19 females; mean age 47 years), 50 rheumatoid arthritis patients (15 males/35 females; mean age 57 years) and 50 healthy control subjects (30 males/20 females; mean age 44 years).

C-reactive protein levels were determined by the single radial immunodiffusion method, as previously described.

13.7 ELISA of Bacterial Lipopolysaccharide Samples

In the second study, IgG, IgA and IgM immunoglobulin antibodies to purified bacterial LPS from four different species of microorganisms were measured in 200 subjects.

LPS was isolated from *Klebsiella pneumoniae*, *Escherichia coli* serotype 055:B5, *Salmonella typhimurium* and *Salmonella enteritidis* (Sigma Ltd. UK). All LPS used had been purified by gel filtration.

The ELISA was carried out as follows: 96-well flat-bottomed, rigid polystyrene microtitre plates (Dynatech) were coated with 2.0 μg/well of bacterial LPS overnight at 4 °C.

After adsorption and washing with phosphate-buffered saline (PBS) containing 0.1 % (v/v) Tween 20 (Sigma), the plates were saturated with 2 % (w/v) casein (BDH) in PBS Tween 20, incubated for 1 h at 37 °C to block the non-specific binding, followed by washing with PBS Tween.

Serum samples diluted 1:200 in PBS Tween were added to the plates, incubated for 90 min at 37 °C, followed by washing and addition of peroxidase-conjugated rabbit anti-human class-specific IgG, IgA or IgM (Dako Ltd.) diluted in 1:500 in PBS Tween, and the plates incubated for 90 min at 37 °C.

After washing, the substrate solution, 0.5 mg/ml 2,2′-azinobis (3-ethylbenzthiazoline-6-sulphonic acid) (ABTS) (Sigma) in citrate/phosphate buffer (pH 4.1), containing 0.98 $H_2 O_2$ (Sigma), was added to each well, the plates were incubated at room temperature for 20 min, the reaction stopped with 2 mg/ml sodium fluoride (Sigma) and optical density (OD) measured at 630 nm with a microtitre plate reader (Dynatech, MR 600).

All assays were carried out under code, in that tester did not know which sera came from patients or controls.

13.8 Results of Study on Bacterial Lipopolysaccharides

The ankylosing spondylitis patients had significantly elevated antibody levels of the IgG class (mean ± standard error) (0.49 ± 0.01 OD units, $t=9.82$, $p<0.001$) and IgA class (0.75 ± 0.03 OD units, $t=7.63$, $p<0.001$) to *Klebsiella pneumoniae* LPS when compared to the healthy control group (Ahmadi et al. 1998).

The ankylosing spondylitis patients also had elevated IgA antibody levels to *Escherichia coli* LPS (0.23 ± 0.01 OD units, $t=208$, $p<0.05$) when compared with the healthy control group.

However, none of the study groups had elevated antibody levels to *Salmonella typhimurium* and *Salmonella enteritidis.*

Furthermore, there was no elevation of antibodies against *Klebsiella pneumoniae*, *Escherichia coli*, *Salmonella typhimurium* or *Salmonella enteritidis* in the rheumatoid arthritis patients.

The mean (± standard error) C-reactive protein level was 21.6 ± 2.4 mg/l in the ankylosing spondylitis patients, 39.1 ± 3.9 mg/l in the rheumatoid arthritis patients and 6.9 ± 1.7 mg/l in the healthy control group.

There was a significant correlation between serum IgG ($r=+0.466$, $p<0.001$) (Fig. 13.2) and serum IgA ($r=+0.558$, $p<0.001$) (Fig. 13.3) antibody levels against *Klebsiella pneumoniae* LPS and serum C-reactive protein levels, respectively.

There was no significant correlation between serum IgA anti-*Escherichia coli* LPS antibody and C-reactive protein levels.

13.9 Clinical Implications and Discussion

The data presented here show that there are specific and significant antibody elevations against the bowel microbe *Klebsiella pneumoniae* in active ankylosing spondylitis patients when compared to inactive ankylosing spondylitis patients, rheumatoid arthritis patients or healthy controls.

There are also specific and significant antibody elevations against the urinary microbe *Proteus mirabilis* in rheumatoid arthritis patients when compared to active or inactive ankylosing spondylitis patients or healthy controls.

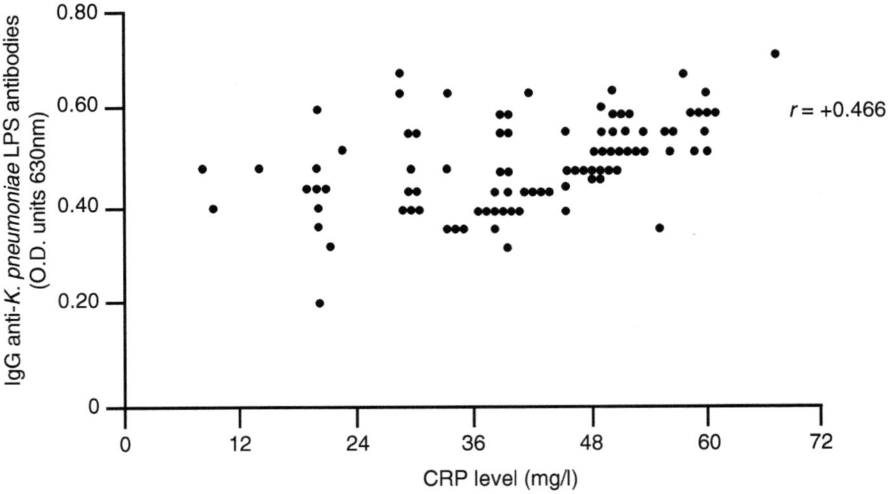

Fig. 13.2 Correlation between class-specific IgG anti-*Klebsiella pneumoniae* LPS and C-reactive protein levels in sera of ankylosing spondylitis patients

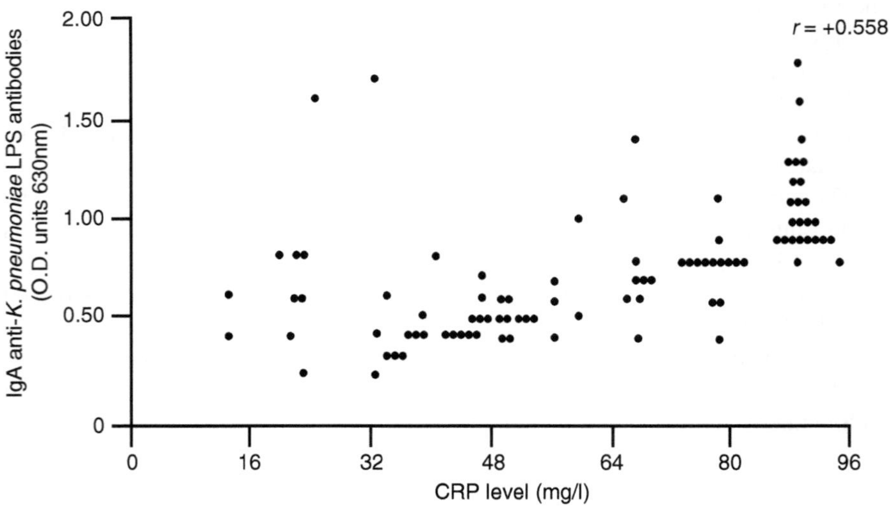

Fig. 13.3 Correlation between class-specific IgA anti-*Klebsiella pneumoniae* LPS and C-reactive protein levels in sera of ankylosing spondylitis patients

The high level of *Proteus* antibodies in rheumatoid arthritis was not due to non-specific effects of high immunoglobulin levels, since the patients with active ankylosing spondylitis had higher serum levels of IgG and IgA than the rheumatoid arthritis patients, yet their levels of *Proteus* antibodies were similar to those of inactive ankylosing spondylitis patients and healthy controls. To some extent, the two groups of patients with inflammatory arthritis acted as reciprocal controls to one another, in that ankylosing spondylitis patients had high antibody titres against *Klebsiella* microbes but not against *Proteus*, whilst rheumatoid arthritis patients had high levels of antibodies to *Proteus* but not against *Klebsiella*.

It is relevant to note that inactive ankylosing spondylitis did not have elevated levels of anti-*Klebsiella* antibodies despite having bony changes and sacroiliitis, features characteristic of the disease. The elevated antibody level to *Klebsiella* microbes is not associated with the phenotype of the disease but with the presence of inflammation.

Previous studies may have suggested that the bacteria or bacterial fragments may enter the joints and explain the pathology of 'reactive arthritis'.

One serious problem with these previous investigations is that an assumption is being made that the external microbiological agent would target the joint and could be isolated from the synovial cavity. However, the possibility that an autologous agent such as an antibody made by the ankylosing spondylitis patient being responsible for the joint and spinal inflammation was not considered as a possibility. Yet, this is exactly what happens in rheumatic fever: an infection by *Streptococcus pyogenes* located in the tonsils and upper respiratory tract evokes antibacterial antibodies which not only bind to the microbe wherever it is located but also to cross-reacting self-antigens found in the heart causing rheumatic fever and to the basal ganglia of the brain and giving rise to Sydenham's chorea.

In the second study, increased levels of IgG and IgA class-specific antibodies against *Klebsiella pneumoniae* LPS were found in ankylosing spondylitis patients compared to rheumatoid arthritis patients or healthy controls.

In addition, IgA class-specific antibodies against *Escherichia coli* LPS were found to be slightly elevated in ankylosing spondylitis patients.

However, there was no significant elevation of antibody levels against *Salmonella typhimurium* or *Salmonella enteritidis*.

There was a good correlation between IgG and IgA *Klebsiella* LPS antibodies and C-reactive protein in ankylosing spondylitis patients.

These observations are in agreement with previous findings that antibody elevations to *Klebsiella* but not to other Gram-negative bacteria such as *Escherichia coli*, *Proteus mirabilis*, *Pseudomonas aeruginosa*, *Salmonella*, *Shigella* and *Yersinia* are present in ankylosing spondylitis patients (Ebringer 1992).

In a study by another group, patients with a peripheral type of ankylosing spondylitis were reported to have increased levels of IgM and IgA class antibodies against *Klebsiella*, whereas patients with axial ankylosing spondylitis had IgG and IgA class antibodies against *Klebsiella*, as well as IgA antibodies against *Proteus mirabilis* and *Escherichia coli* (Maki-Ikola et al. 1994). In a related study, by the same group, ankylosing spondylitis patients were shown to have elevated IgM and IgA against *Klebsiella* LPS, as well as IgM antibodies to *Escherichia coli* LPS. They also observed a significant decrease in antibodies to *Klebsiella* LPS following treatment with sulphasalazine.

In a Japanese study, it was reported that patients with ankylosing spondylitis have increased levels of antibodies to *Klebsiella* LPS, as well antibodies to *Salmonella typhimurium* LPS and *Salmonella enteritidis* LPS (Tani et al. 1997).

However, our findings are not in agreement with others who reported increased levels of antibodies to *Salmonella* LPS in ankylosing spondylitis patients. A difference in methodology, the nature of the antigen preparation and cross-reactivity between the LPS of members of the *Enterobacteriaceae* may be responsible for the slightly elevated levels of anti-*Escherichia coli* antibodies found in our study as well as in the reports of other workers.

The elevated levels of IgA antibodies against *Klebsiella pneumoniae* bacteria in ankylosing spondylitis patients would tend to suggest that there is antigenic stimulation at a mucosal site, such as the gut.

The LPS molecule, especially the O-antigen polysaccharide chains, contributes to complement-mediated serum bactericidal activity of *Klebsiella* strains (Ciurana et al. 1987).

It is clear that antibodies to a variety of components of the gut microbe *Klebsiella pneumoniae* can be demonstrated in ankylosing spondylitis patients during active phases of the disease. It raises the therapeutic issue whether control of the bowel flora may be relevant in the treatment of this disease.

References

Ahmadi K, Wilson C, Tiwana H, Binder A, Ebringer A. Antibodies to *Klebsiella pneumoniae* lipopolysaccharide in patients with ankylosing spondylitis. Br J Rheumatol. 1998;37:1330–3.

Ciurana B, Thomas JM. Role of lipopolysaccharide and complement in susceptibility of Klebsiella pneumoniae to nonimmune serum. Infect Immun. 1987;55:2741–6.

Ebringer A. Ankylosing spondylitis is caused by *Klebsiella*. Rheum Dis Clin North Am. 1992; 18:105–21.

Ebringer A, Ptaszynska T, Corbett M, Wilson C, Macafee Y, Avakian H, Baron P, James DCO. Antibodies to *Proteus* in rheumatoid arthritis. Lancet. 1985;ii:305–7.

Granfors K, Ogasawara M, Hill JL, Lahesmaa-Rantala R, Toivanen A, Yu DTY. Analysis of IgA antibodies to lipopolysaccharide in *Yersinia*-triggered reactive arthritis. J Infect Dis. 1989; 159:1142–7.

Maki-Ikola O, Yli-Kerttula U, Saario R, Toivanen P. Granfors K. Antibodies to arthritis-associated microbes in inflammatory joint diseases. Rheumatol Int. 1991;10:231–4.

Maki-Ikola O, Lehtinen K, Nissila M, Granfors K. IgM, IgA and IgG class serum antibodies against *Klebsiella pneumoniae a*nd *Escherichia coli* lipopolysaccharides in patients with ankylosing spondylitis. Br J Rheumatol. 1994;33:1025–9.

Maki-Ikola O, Mertsola J, Granfors K. No endotoxin detected in the plasma in patients with ankylosing spondylitis. Ann Rheum Dis. 1997;56:279.

Robbins JB, McCracken GH, Gotschild EC, Orskov F, Orskov L, Hanson LA. *Escherichia coli* K1 capsular polysaccharide associated with neonatal meningitis. N Engl J Med. 1974;290:1216–20.

Ropes MW, Bennett GA, Cobb S, Jacox R, Jessar RA. Review of diagnostic criteria for rheumatoid arthritis. Bull Rheum Dis. 1958;3:175–6.

Tani Y, Sato H, Tanaka N, Mori K, Doida Y, Hukuda S. Serum IgA1 and IgA2 subclass antibodies against collagens in patients with ankylosing spondylitis. Scan J Rheum. 1997;26:380–2.

Wagener P, Bush J, Hammer M, Brunkhorst R. Endotoxin in the plasma of patients with inflammatory rheumatic diseases. Scand J Rheumatol. 1988;17:301–3.

Chapter 14
Dutch and German Patients with Ankylosing Spondylitis Have Antibodies to *Klebsiella*

14.1 The Netherlands Connection: An Introduction

In the early 1980s, the Immunology Unit of King's College had shown that there were elevated levels of antibodies to the Gram-negative bowel microbe *Klebsiella* in patients suffering from ankylosing spondylitis.

In 1992, I was attending a Rheumatology Congress in Barcelona when the late Professor Bert Feltkamp from Amsterdam approached me and said: 'Alan, we have done 3 studies in the Netherlands and we cannot find antibodies in our Dutch ankylosing spondylitis patients as you do in London. It must be the London water'. Clearly, here was a challenge as I knew there was nothing wrong with the London water.

I said: 'Bert, you code the Dutch ankylosing spondylitis and uveitis patients in Amsterdam and send them to us in London. We will send you the results back to Amsterdam and you can decode them'.

'For good measure, send us also sera from active, rheumatoid arthritis patients who have an erythrocyte sedimentation rate greater than 30 mm/hour (ESR>30 mm/hour) at the time the blood sample is taken, as we have also found the probable cause of this disease'.

'It is caused by a urinary tract infection by *Proteus* bacteria'. The sera were sent and the studies were carried out, using an immunofluorescence assay. For ankylosing spondylitis, we used an IgA anti-*Klebsiella* assay, whilst for rheumatoid arthritis, we used an IgG anti-*Proteus* assay.

14.2 Amsterdam: Location and History

Amsterdam is the capital and largest city of the Netherlands with a population of about two million. The city is in the province of North Holland, but the Ophthalmic Research Institute collects patients from the whole of the Netherlands.

A. Ebringer, *Ankylosing Spondylitis and Klebsiella*,
DOI 10.1007/978-1-4471-4300-0_14, © Springer-Verlag London 2013

Its name is derived from Amstellerdam, the city on the dam of the river Amstel. It started as a fishing village but in 1306 was granted city rights.

It is not as old as other Dutch cities such as Rotterdam, Utrecht and Nijmegen. However, it flourished in the Middle Ages because it traded with the Hanseatic League.

In the sixteenth century, the Dutch rebelled against Philip II of Spain which led to the 'Eighty Years' War' at the end of which the Netherlands gained its independence.

The seventeenth century is considered Amsterdam's 'Golden Age' when it traded all over the world.

The Amsterdam merchants founded the Dutch East India Company and opened the first stock exchange in the world.

During the Second World War, the Dutch people suffered a severe famine. It was noticed by Dutch doctors that patients with coeliac disease improved when there was a shortage of wheat. It led eventually to the discovery that gliadin, a component of wheat, was involved in this disease.

14.3 Patients and Controls

The incidence of 'acute anterior uveitis' in HLA-B27-associated ankylosing spondylitis is about 30 %. Furthermore, about half of patients with HLA-B27-positive acute anterior uveitis fulfil the criteria of ankylosing spondylitis or reactive arthritis (Linssen et al. 1983).

Characteristics of the patients and controls are summarised in the Table 14.1.

The first three groups of patients with acute anterior uveitis had a complete ophthalmological assessment. The patients in the fourth group had ankylosing spondylitis but had never complained of eye problems and therefore were not examined by an ophthalmologist.

The sex ratio was almost equal in the acute anterior uveitis patients who did not have ankylosing spondylitis.

However, in the patients with ankylosing spondylitis, the male/female ratio was about 2:1.

The sex ratio was not determined in the rheumatoid arthritis patients. The sera from ankylosing spondylitis, acute anterior uveitis and rheumatoid arthritis patients as well as controls were numbered in Amsterdam in such a way that the laboratory in London was not aware of their origin.

The code was broken in Amsterdam after the serological results arrived back from London.

14.4 Serum C-Reactive Protein Levels

Serum C-reactive protein levels were measured by the single radial immunodiffusion method of Mancini.

Table 14.1 Characteristics of the six groups of Dutch patients and the two groups of healthy controls

	AAU only			AS		RA	Controls	
Number of subjects	17	17	17	17	17	25	17	17
Male/female	7/10	8/9	11/6	15/2	12/5	ND	8/7	5/7
Mean age (years)	46	44	37	38	44	ND	37	32
Mean ESR (mm/hour)	ND	ND	ND	ND	ND	ND	56	ND
Mean CRP (mg/litre)	4.9	7.3	11.0	12.0	25.3	25.8	5.9	4.2
HLA-B27	+	–	+	+	+	ND	+	–
Acute anterior uveitis (AAU)	+	–	+	–	ND	ND	–	–

Due to identity protection, sex and age were not known for some controls
Abbreviations: *ESR* erythrocyte sedimentation rate, *CRP* C-reactive protein, *AS* ankylosing spondylitis, *ND* not done

Serum C-reactive protein levels in the two control groups were relatively low (Table 14.1).

Serum C-reactive protein levels were found to be highest in HLA-B27-positive patients with active ankylosing spondylitis and patients with active rheumatoid arthritis when compared to all other disease groups or controls.

Of the remainder, only two groups showed any significant elevation in C-reactive protein levels. The HLA-B27-positive, acute anterior uveitis-positive, ankylosing spondylitis-positive patients had higher levels of C-reactive protein when to compared to HLA-B27-positive controls ($t = 1.60$, $p < 0.05$). The other group consisted of HLA-B27-positive, acute anterior uveitis-negative, ankylosing spondylitis-positive patients who also had an elevated level of C-reactive protein ($t = 2.14$, $p < 0.025$). Furthermore, HLA-B27-positive, acute anterior uveitis-positive, ankylosing spondylitis patients had a higher level of C-reactive protein when compared to HLA-B27-negative controls ($t = 2.02$, $p < 2.60$). A similar significant elevation in C-reactive protein level was observed in the HLA-B27-positive, acute anterior uveitis-negative, ankylosing spondylitis-positive patients when compared to the HLA-B27-negative controls ($t = 2.60$, $p < 0.005$).

14.5 Indirect Immunofluorescence Studies with *Klebsiella* in Ankylosing Spondylitis and Acute Anterior Uveitis Patients and *Proteus* in Rheumatoid Patients from the Netherlands

Indirect immunofluorescence assay was carried out as previously described.

14.5.1 IgA Antibodies to Klebsiella pneumoniae

HLA-B27-positive patients with active ankylosing spondylitis showed the highest levels of IgA antibodies to *Klebsiella pneumoniae*, and this was significantly higher than in HLA-B27-positive healthy controls ($t=6.27, p<0.001$) or HLA-B27-negative healthy controls ($t=11.37$, $p<0.001$) or in patients with rheumatoid arthritis ($t=11.36, p<0.001$) (Fig. 14.1).

Although no other ankylosing spondylitis or acute anterior uveitis showed anti-*Klebsiella* antibody titres above that of the patients with active ankylosing spondylitis, there were elevations above those seen in controls and patients with rheumatoid arthritis.

Patients who were HLA-B27 positive, acute anterior uveitis positive and ankylosing spondylitis positive and those who were HLA-B27 positive, acute anterior uveitis negative and ankylosing spondylitis positive had higher anti-*Klebsiella* antibody titres than patients who were HLA-B27 positive, anterior uveitis positive, ankylosing spondylitis negative, but these differences were not statistically significant when corrected for number of groups examined. The titre of anti-*Klebsiella* antibodies could not be related to exacerbations or remissions in patients with acute anterior uveitis (Blankenberg-Sprenkels et al. 1998).

Furthermore, HLA-B27-negative, acute anterior uveitis-positive and ankylosing spondylitis-negative patients had higher titres of anti-*Klebsiella* antibodies than either HLA-B27-positive controls ($t=2.16, p<0.05$) or HLA-B27-negative controls ($t=6.37, p<0.001$).

14.5.2 IgG Antibodies to Proteus mirabilis

Patients with active rheumatoid arthritis showed significant elevations in IgG antibody titre when compared to either HLA-B27-positive controls ($t=12.3, p<001$) or when compared to HLA-B27-negative controls ($t=10.6, p<0.001$) (Fig. 14.2).

This antibody elevation in anti-*Proteus* titre was also significant when compared to all the other groups: HLA-B27-positive, acute anterior uveitis-positive, ankylosing spondylitis-positive patients ($t=10.8, p<0.001$), HLA-B27-positive, acute anterior uveitis-positive, ankylosing spondylitis-negative patients ($t=9.79$, $p<0.001$), HLA-B27-positive, acute anterior uveitis-negative, ankylosing spondylitis-positive patients ($t=8.6$, $p<0.001$) and HLA-B27-positive patients with active ankylosing spondylitis ($t=8.8, p<0.001$).

14.6 German Studies on *Klebsiella* in Ankylosing Spondylitis

Two centres in northern Germany, in Lübeck and Kiel, have carried out investigations on the involvement of *Klebsiella* bacteria in ankylosing spondylitis.

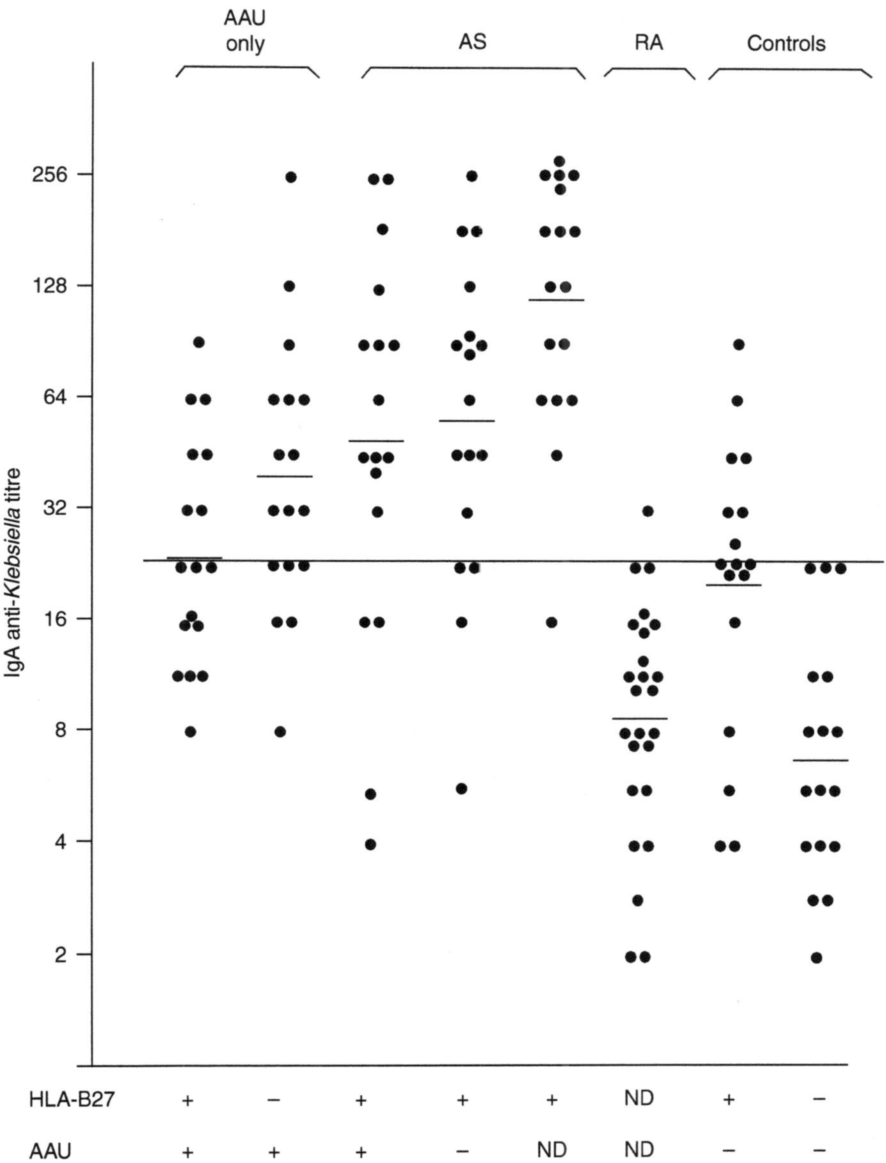

Fig. 14.1 IgA anti-*Klebsiella pneumoniae* antibody titres in sera of patients from groups 1 to 8 (Table 14.1). Each dot represents either a control subject or a patient

14.6.1 Lübeck

Lübeck is the largest German port on the Baltic Sea and has a population of over 200,000.

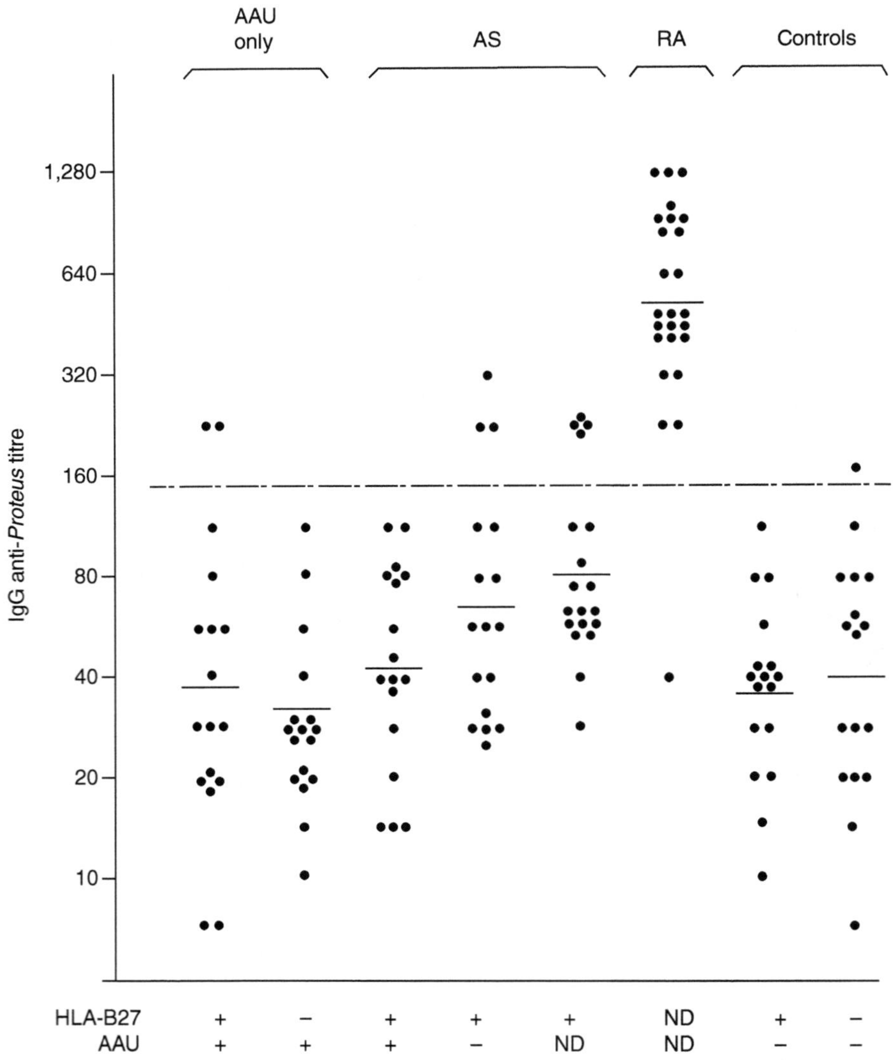

Fig. 14.2 IgG anti-*Proteus mirabilis* antibody titres in sera of patients from groups 1 to 8 (Table 14.1). Each dot represents either a control subject or a patient

It was founded in 1143 by Count Adolf II, and around 1200, it became the point of departure of the Livonian order. In 1226, Emperor Frederick II elevated the town to an Imperial Free City.

In the fourteenth century, it was the main town of the Hanseatic League.

The composer Buxtehude was an organist at the Marienkirche in Lübeck.

During the Second World War, it was heavily bombed, and a firestorm caused severe damage to the centre of the town.

It has a university where Dr. W. L. Gross worked and who emphasized that some strains of *Klebsiella* are involved in ankylosing spondylitis.

14.6.2 Kiel

Kiel is the capital of the state of Schleswig-Holstein and was a member of the Hanseatic League.

The University of Kiel was founded in 1665, and the physicist Max Planck studied there.

Kiel was the centre of the 'sailors' mutiny' which sparked the German Revolution of 1918, and this eventually led to the foundation of the Weimar Republic.

The Kiel Canal joins the North Sea with the Baltic, and the naval installations were damaged during the Second World War.

Dr. H. Sahly from the University of Kiel and Dr. W.L. Gross from the University of Lübeck were the first to report that German ankylosing spondylitis patients had antibodies to *Klebsiella.*

14.7 ELISA Studies on German Patients

Capsular antigens have been shown to be essential for the virulence of *Klebsiella* in animal models (Ehrenworth and Baer 1956).

Serologically, *Klebsiella* series are classified into 77 different capsular types (Orskov and Fife-Asbury 1979).

The study was undertaken to determine which specific capsular *Klebsiella* polysaccharide antigens evoke antibodies in ankylosing spondylitis patients.

Serum samples from 41 ankylosing spondylitis patients who were all HLA-B27 positive were obtained from the Max Planck Institute of Immunology and Rheumatology, University of Erlangen, Nuremberg.

Control samples were obtained from 45 healthy blood donors, who were all HLA-B27 positive, and also from a further group of 40 healthy blood donors, who were all HLA-B27 negative.

Klebsiella isolates of capsular types K1–K82 were prepared by methods similar to those previously described.

Each serum sample was examined to each of the 77 capsular antigens.

Antibodies to *Klebsiella* serotypes K26, K36 and K50 were found frequently in ankylosing spondylitis patients (Sahly et al. 1994).

Some 31 % of the sera from ankylosing spondylitis patients reacted with *Klebsiella* capsular type K26 compared to 4.4 % of the HLA-B27-positive controls and 10 % of the HLA-B27-negative controls.

Some 51 % of the ankylosing spondylitis patients reacted with *Klebsiella* capsular type K36, whereas only 11 % of the HLA-B27-positive and 7.5 % of the HLA-B27-negative controls gave such a response.

A similar result was obtained with *Klebsiella* capsular type K50, where 54 % of the ankylosing spondylitis patients reacted compared to 22 % of the HLA-B27-positive and 2.7 % of the HLA-B27-negative controls.

It would appear that certain types of *Klebsiella* bacteria, possessing capsular types K26, K36 and K50, are predominantly involved in patients with ankylosing spondylitis.

It is possible that such capsular serotypes are present in higher concentrations in the human bowel flora.

Klebsiella microbes can also act as activators of peripheral lymphocytes (Gross et al. 1986), but their role in the pathogenesis of ankylosing spondylitis remains unclear.

14.8 Clinical Implications and Conclusions

Ankylosing spondylitis patients from two different countries, the Netherlands and Germany, have been shown to have elevated levels of antibodies to *Klebsiella* bacteria.

Ankylosing spondylitis and acute anterior uveitis patients had antibodies to *Klebsiella*, and rheumatoid arthritis patients had antibodies to *Proteus*. Each disease group was a specificity control for the other condition. It is clear that ankylosing spondylitis patients had antibodies against *Klebsiella* but not against *Proteus*, whilst the opposite was observed with the rheumatoid arthritis sera which had antibodies against *Proteus* but not against *Klebsiella*.

Professor Bert Feltkamp said he was utterly surprised when his registrar told him that the London studies had picked both groups. The three original centres then refused to retest the ankylosing spondylitis sera.

Here, we are against the problem of simple, commercial test kits not being available to measure anti-*Proteus* or anti-*Klebsiella* antibodies which hampers clinical studies in patients with these diseases. The indirect immunofluorescence assay had been developed in house, in the Immunology Unit of King's College in the University of London by a very capable microbiologist, Dr. Mark Fielder, who carried out the assays on the Dutch sera.

An interesting observation was made in the tissue-typed controls. In those subjects who were HLA-B27 positive and deemed clinically healthy showed higher IgA anti-*Klebsiella* antibody titres than those healthy subjects typed as HLA-B27 negative. Similar observations have been made in England. In Finland, it was found that healthy HLA-B27-positive persons had elevated anti-*Klebsiella* titres of all immunoglobulin classes although only the IgM titres were statistically significantly increased (Toivanen et al. 1993). This may indicate that some subjects in the HLA-B27-positive 'healthy' control group are more likely to develop anti-*Klebsiella* antibodies. The higher anti-*Klebsiella* antibody titre in the HLA-B27 positive control group may also suggest a slow onset of ankylosing spondylitis, but only longitudinal studies with close clinical follow-up and regular measurement of antibody levels to *Klebsiella pneumoniae* would resolve the problem.

14.9 Conclusions

The data presented here show that there are specific and significant antibody elevations against *Klebsiella* in both Dutch and German ankylosing spondylitis patients. Furthermore, Dutch patients with acute anterior uveitis also have elevated levels of antibodies against the *Klebsiella* microbe. There are no antibody elevations against *Proteus mirabilis* in Dutch patients with acute anterior uveitis or ankylosing spondylitis. However, Dutch patients with rheumatoid arthritis have elevated levels of antibodies to the urinary microbe *Proteus mirabilis*.

References

Blankenberg-Sprenkels SHD, Fielder M, Feltkamp TEW, Tiwana H, Wilson C, Ebringer A. Antibodies to *Klebsiella pneumonia* in Dutch patients with ankylosing spondylitis and acute anterior uveitis and to *Proteus mirabilis* in rheumatoid arthritis. J Rheumatol. 1998;25:743–7.

Ehrenworth L, Baer H. The pathogenicity of *Klebsiella pneumoniae* for mice: the relationship to the quantity and rate of production of type-specific polysaccharide. J Bacteriol. 1956;72:713–7.

Gross WL, Lüdemann G, Schmidt K, Ullman U. Lymphocyte response to *Klebsiella* in ankylosing spondylitis. Eur J Clin Invest. 1986;16:338–46.

Linssen A, Dekker-Saeys AJ, Dandrieu MR, Christiaans BJ, Baarsma GS, Tjoa ST, de Jong PTVM, Kijlstra A, Feltkamp TEW. Possible ankylosing spondylitis in acute anterior uveitis. Brit J Rheumatol Suppl. 1983;22 Suppl 2:137–43.

Orskov I, Fife-Asbury MA. New *Klebsiella* capsular antigen K82 and deletion of five of those previously assigned. Int J Syst Bacteriol. 1979;27:386–7.

Sahly H, Podschun R, Sass R, Bröker B, Kekow J, Gross WL, Ullmann U. Serum antibodies to *Klebsiella* capsular polysaccharides in ankylosing spondylitis. Arthritis Rheum. 1994;37: 754–9.

Toivanen P, Koskimies S, Granfors K, Eerola E. Bacterial antibodies in HLA-B27 positive individuals. Arthritis Rheum. 1993;36:1633–5.

Chapter 15
Spanish, Finnish and Swedish Patients with Ankylosing Spondylitis Have Antibodies to *Klebsiella*

15.1 The Spanish Connection: An Introduction

In the early 1990s, an industrious and enthusiastic student from Spain, Mr. A. Marti, came to King's College to study biological sciences under a European Common Market Studentship. When he heard that our research interest involved investigating patients with ankylosing spondylitis, he said that physicians in his native town, Barcelona in Catalonia, a rich and industrial part of Spain, would be very agreeable to carry out a joint study. He introduced us to Dr. Antonio Collado from the Department of Rheumatology in the Hospital Clinic I Provincial de Barcelona who agreed to participate in a study of ankylosing spondylitis in Catalan patients.

15.2 Barcelona: Location and History

Barcelona is located in the north-eastern region of the Iberian peninsula and is the second largest town in Spain after Madrid.

In 218 BC, at the start of the second Punic War, it was occupied by Carthaginian troops under Hamilcar Barca. This military occupation is often cited as the foundation of the modern city of Barcelona.

It was during the second Punic War that Hannibal crossed the Alps with Numidian troops and two dozen elephants. He beat the Romans at the battles of Trasimene and Cannae although he could not take Rome.

Subsequently, Barcelona was occupied by the Romans, Visigoths then Moslems, and finally it was captured by the son of Charlemagne, Louis the Pious.

During the Middle Ages it was part of the Kingdom of Aragon.

Barcelona suffered greatly during the Spanish Civil War, and this is well described by George Orwell in his book *Homage to Catalonia*. Because of its resistance to the Franco regime, the use of the Catalan language was forbidden for many years.

A. Ebringer, *Ankylosing Spondylitis and Klebsiella*,
DOI 10.1007/978-1-4471-4300-0_15, © Springer-Verlag London 2013

Barcelona has a population of about one and half million and has many architectural buildings, such as the unfinished 'Familia Sagrada' designed by Antoni Gaudi.

Dr. Antonio Collado from the Hospital Clinic I Provincial de Barcelona provided serum samples obtained from Spanish ankylosing spondylitis patients as well as controls.

15.3 Catalan Patients and Controls

The aim of this study was to provide new evidence for the association between *Klebsiella* and ankylosing spondylitis, by measuring anti-*Klebsiella* antibodies in a Catalan population with ankylosing spondylitis.

Some 84 patients, 74 males and 10 females, examined between 1987 and 1991 for ankylosing spondylitis, as defined by the New York criteria of 1966, were included in this study. Patients with psoriasis, inflammatory bowel disease or Reiter's syndrome were excluded from the study.

The age of patients ranged from 18 to 66 years, with a mean age of 41 years, and a mean disease duration was 16 years. All patients were HLA-B27 positive.

The clinical and radiological picture was assessed in each patient, and the criteria of disease activity were evaluated in a similar fashion as previously described (Collado et al. 1991).

Two control groups were included in this study: The first group consisted of 41 outpatients (28 males, 13 females) with a mean age of 42 years who were suffering from noninflammatory arthritis. The second group consisted of 22 patients with rheumatoid arthritis (7 males, 15 females) with a mean age of 57 years, as defined by the American Rheumatism Association criteria of 1987.

The erythrocyte sedimentation rate, serum C-reactive protein and total serum IgA were measured as previously described.

Blood from patients and controls was collected at the time of clinical assessment, and serum stored at −30 °C until testing. Serum samples were sent to the Immunology Unit at King's College, in London, for measurement of specific IgA antibodies against *Klebsiella* by the immunofluorescence technique, as previously described.

To measure the titres of IgA anti-*Klebsiella* antibodies, sera were diluted serially from 1/2, 1/4, 1/8, 1/16, 1/32, 1/64, 1/128 to 1/256. Each of these dilutions was arbitrarily taken to represent one unit of binding (U), starting from one unit at 1/2 dilution to 8 at 1/256. No fluorescence at 1/2 was taken as zero unit of binding.

All assays were conducted blind on numbered samples under code.

15.4 Statistical Analysis

Data were analysed with the SPSS-X statistical program. The distribution of variables were checked for normality with the Kolmogorov-Smirnov test. Chi-square

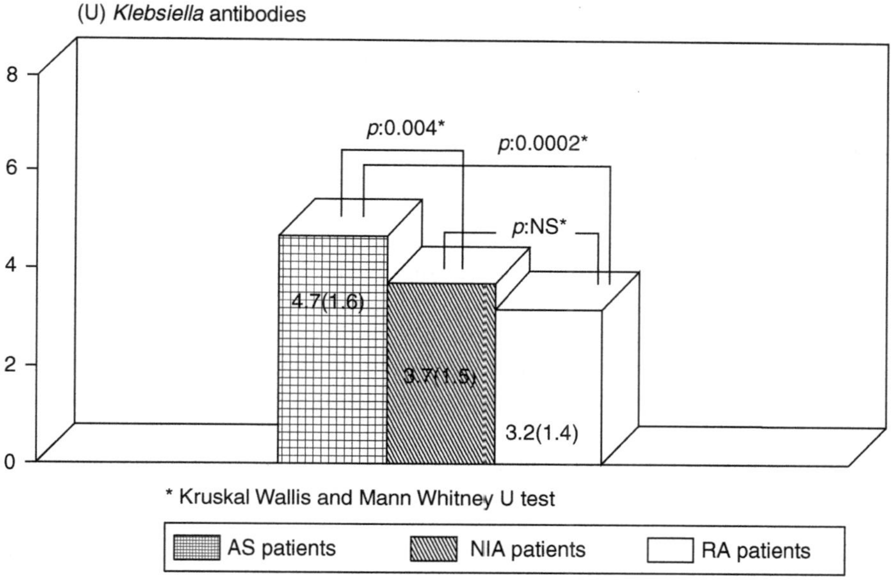

Fig. 15.1 Means (standard deviation) of *Klebsiella pneumoniae* IgA antibody titres (U = units) in sera of ankylosing spondylitis (*AS*) patients, non-inflammatory arthritis (*NIA*) patients and rheumatoid arthritis (*RA*) patients (* indicates statistical calculation)

was used for comparisons of frequencies. The quantitative variables were compared by Student's *t*-test and the Pearson correlation coefficient (*r*). Distributions deemed non-normal were analysed with equivalent non-parametric tests: Kruskal-Wallis for analysis of variance and Mann–Whitney test for comparison between means. Spearman's correlation test was used to analyse correlation between variables.

15.5 Results on Catalan Patients

Patients with ankylosing spondylitis showed higher serum levels of anti-*Klebsiella* IgA antibodies than controls (Fig. 15.1).

The mean serum anti-*Klebsiella* IgA antibodies in ankylosing spondylitis patients were 4.7 units (U), and this was significantly higher than in the non-inflammatory group which was 3.7 U (*p*: 0.004) and in rheumatoid arthritis patients 3.1 U (*p*: 0.002), respectively.

There was no difference in serum levels of anti-*Klebsiella* IgA antibodies between the control groups (Collado et al. 1994).

Anti-*Klebsiella* IgA antibodies at dilutions equal or higher than 1/32 were observed in 36.5 % of ankylosing spondylitis patients in contrast to 17 % of non-inflammatory arthritis patients or 4.5 % in the rheumatoid arthritis group, respectively (*p*: 0.002).

Ankylosing spondylitis patients with active disease had significantly higher levels of erythrocyte sedimentation rates, C-reactive protein, total serum IgA and secretory IgA levels than patients with inactive disease. In this study, no clear relationship between levels of anti-*Klebsiella* antibodies and clinical parameters of disease activity was found.

However, a significant correlation between the levels of IgA against *Klebsiella* and both C-reactive protein and secretory IgA serum levels was found.

Acute uveitis was observed in only one patient at the time of clinical assessment. However, in 14 patients, a history of previous uveitis was recorded. These patients had a higher anti-*Klebsiella* IgA level of 5.6 U compared to a level of 4.4 U (p: 0.01) in those without previous eye inflammation.

In only six ankylosing spondylitis with active peripheral arthritis at the time of clinical evaluation, the mean level of anti-*Klebsiella* IgA antibodies was particularly high at 5.6 U.

No relationship was found between the level of anti-*Klebsiella* IgA antibodies and anti-inflammatory drug intake or duration of disease.

15.6 Turku: The Finland Connection

Turku is a city on the south-west coast of Finland with a population of over 200,000 with surrounding districts.

It is believed to have been settled around the end of the thirteenth century making it the oldest city in Finland. The Dominican monastery was founded in 1249, and the cathedral of Turku was consecrated in 1300.

The first university in Finland was the Royal Academy of Turku which was founded in 1640. Until the time of Napoleon, Finland was part of the Kingdom of Sweden when it was annexed by Russia. For a brief period, Turku was the capital of Finland, but it soon lost this status to Helsinki.

The University of Turku has a renowned Department of Bacteriology where Dr. Kaisa Granfors investigated the link between *Klebsiella* bacteria and ankylosing spondylitis.

15.7 Results of Finnish Patients

Some 99 patients treated for ankylosing spondylitis at the Rheumatism Foundation Hospital in Heinola were investigated for antibodies to *Klebsiella* and other bacteria. The criteria for ankylosing spondylitis were the Rome criteria (Kellgren et al. 1963).

The patients were divided into two groups according to disease activity: Active patients had a sum greater than 30, when erythrocyte sedimentation rate was added to C-reactive protein level when measured in mg/l (Kaarela 1985). Inactive patients had a sum of erythrocyte sedimentation rate plus C-reactive protein of 30 or less. There were 62 patients with active disease and 37 patients with inactive disease.

The mean age of the ankylosing spondylitis patients was 39 years (range: 18–67 years), and the male to female ratio was 74/25.

Antibodies were measured by ELISA, as previously described (Maki-Ikola et al. 1991), to *Salmonella enteritidis*, *Salmonella typhimurium*, *Yersinia enterocolitica* 0.3, *Yersinia enterocolitica* 0.9, *Yersinia pseudotuberculosis* I, *Yersinia pseudotuberculosis* III, *Klebsiella pneumoniae*, *Escherichia coli*, *Proteus mirabilis*, *Borrelia burgdorferi*, *Campylobacter jejuni* and *Chlamydia trachomatis*.

Increased antibody levels in ankylosing spondylitis patients were most often observed against *Klebsiella pneumoniae* (in 33 out of 99 patients) and *Yersinia* (31 patients), followed in frequency by antibodies against *Proteus mirabilis* (21 patients), *Escherichia coli* (18 patients), *Chlamydia trachomatis* (17 patients), *Borrelia burgdorferi* (10 patients), *Campylobacter jejuni* (8 patients) and *Salmonellae* (8 patients).

These figures apply for antibody concentrations exceeding the mean value of blood donors by two standard deviations.

In the present study, prevalence of IgA and IgG class *Klebsiella* antibodies was elevated in ankylosing spondylitis patients from Finland.

In addition, IgA class antibodies against *Escherichia coli* were also observed to be slightly elevated in ankylosing spondylitis, and this could perhaps be explained by the presence of antigens cross-reactive with *Klebsiella.*

Furthermore, the antibody response to *Campylobacter*, *Chlamydia*, *Borrelia*, *Salmonellae*, *Yersinia* and *Proteus* did not differ between ankylosing spondylitis patients and healthy controls.

In *Yersinia*-triggered reactive arthritis, *Yersinia* specific IgA class antibodies persist for long periods, even for several years (Toivanen et al. 1987), but whether a similar situation occurs in ankylosing spondylitis patients is not clear.

15.8 Uppsala and the Swedish Connection

Uppsala is one of the oldest towns in Sweden, situated some 50 miles north of Stockholm.

Since 1164, Uppsala has been the ecclesiastical centre of Sweden, and the large and impressive Gothic cathedral was erected in 1435.

Uppsala University was founded in 1477 and is the oldest centre of higher education in Scandinavia. The renowned botanist Linnaeus lived in the city for many years.

The Department of Rheumatology in the University Hospital was led by Professor Roger Hällgren who investigated the role of *Klebsiella* and other Gram-negative bacteria in patients with ankylosing spondylitis.

15.9 Swedish Studies

A double perfusion device has been developed which allows controlled measuring of gut immunity directly in jejunal fluid (Knutson et al. 1989). Using this direct method, it was found that concentrations of total IgM, IgA, secretory IgA and secretory component were significantly increased in the jejunal perfusion fluids of 19 ankylosing spondylitis patients when compared to controls (Feltelius et al. 1994).

In the current study, the concentrations of IgM, IgG and IgA class antibodies against *Klebsiella pneumoniae*, *Escherichia coli* and *Proteus mirabilis* in the jejunal perfusion fluids of those 19 patients with ankylosing spondylitis as well as in 14 patients with rheumatoid arthritis and 22 healthy controls were measured by ELISA.

The 19 male patients with ankylosing spondylitis that were diagnosed according to the New York criteria had a mean age of 36 years (range 21–66 years) and a mean duration of disease of 11 years (range: 1–25 years).

The 14 rheumatoid arthritis patients suffered from active disease as defined by the presence of at least 3 criteria: duration of morning stiffness longer than 60 min, tenderness or swelling or both in at least 6 joints and an erythrocyte sedimentation rate equal or greater than 30 mm/h.

A segment of intestine was perfused, as previously described, by a small-diameter tube that was 175 cm long and contained 6 channels.

The insertion of the tube, gastric drainage, inflation of the balloons and rinsing of the closed intestinal segment were performed as previously described. ^{11}C-labelled polyethylene glycol was used as a volume marker and phenol-sulphon-phthalein (phenol red) as a marker of the patency of the proximal balloon. The recovery of the volume marker was similar in ankylosing spondylitis patients, rheumatoid arthritis patients and controls.

Proximal leakage into the jejunal segment, as tested by the appearance of phenol red in the perfusion fluid, was less than 2 % of the amount infused in the stomach. The perfusion fluids were collected on ice, centrifuged in cold conditions at 2,500 g and frozen samples submitted for ELISA.

The ankylosing spondylitis patients had statistically significantly higher concentrations of jejunal IgM, IgG and IgA class antibodies against *Klebsiella pneumoniae* 27736 when compared with healthy controls.

When compared with the rheumatoid arthritis patients, the ankylosing spondylitis patients had higher concentrations of IgA and IgG class antibodies against *Klebsiella pneumoniae* 21, as well as higher IgG class concentration with the *Klebsiella pneumoniae* 43 and higher IgA class concentration with the *Klebsiella pneumoniae* 27736 (Mäki-Ikola et al. 1997).

The ankylosing spondylitis had significantly higher jejunal IgM and IgA class antibody concentrations against both *Escherichia coli* and *Proteus mirabilis* when compared with the healthy controls, but no statistically significant differences between patients with ankylosing spondylitis and patients with rheumatoid arthritis.

The rheumatoid arthritis patients had higher IgM class jejunal antibody concentrations against *Proteus mirabilis* when compared with the healthy controls.

These jejunal perfusion studies have demonstrated for the first time direct evidence for an abnormal mucosal humoral immune response against *Klebsiella pneumoniae* in patients with ankylosing spondylitis.

15.10 General Discussion and Conclusions

It would appear that ankylosing spondylitis patients from three different European countries, Spain, Finland and Sweden, have elevated levels of antibodies against the bowel microbe *Klebsiella*, and this is similar to the situation observed in English, Dutch and German patients.

The majority of these ankylosing spondylitis patients in these different countries belong to the HLA-B27 group. Molecular mimicry studies have provided a link between HLA-B27 and *Klebsiella*, but the biochemical mechanism explaining this association requires further examination.

References

Collado A, Sanmartí R, Serra C, Gallart T, Cañete JD, Gratacós J, Vives J, Muñoz-Gomez J. Serum IgA levels of secretory IgA in ankylosing spondylitis. Scand J Rheumatol. 1991;20:153–8.

Collado A, Gratacós J, Ebringer A, Rashid T, Martí A, Sanmartí R, Muñoz-Gomez J. Serum IgA antibodies in ankylosing spondylitis patients from Catalonia. Scand J Rheumatol. 1994; 23:119–23.

Feltelius N, Hvatum M, Brandtzaeg P, Knutson L, Hällgren R. Increased jejunal secretory IgA and IgM in ankylosing spondylitis: normalization after treatment with sulphasalazine. J Rheumatol. 1994;21:2076–81.

Kaarela K. The prognostic factors and diagnostic criteria in early rheumatoid arthritis. Scand J Rheumatol Suppl. 1985;57:1.

Kellgren JH, Jeffrey MR, Ball J. Clinical criteria for ankylosing spondylitis. In: Kellgren JH, Jeffrey MR, Ball J, editors. The epidemiology of chronic rheumatism, vol. 1. Oxford: Blackwell Scientific Publications; 1963. p. 326.

Knutson L, Hällgren R, Odlind B. A new technique for segmental jejunal perfusion in man. Am J Gastroenterol. 1989;84:1278–84.

Mäki-Ikola O, Hällgren R, Kancrud L, Feltelius N, Knutsson L, Granfors K. Enhanced jejunal production of antibodies to *Klebsiella* and other *Enterobacteria* in patients with ankylosing spondylitis and rheumatoid arthritis. Ann Rheum Dis. 1997;56:421–5.

Maki-Ikola O, Lehtinen K, Granfors K, Vainionpaa R, Toivanen P. Bacterial antibodies in ankylosing spondylitis. Clin Exp Immunol. 1991;84:472–5.

Toivanen A, Lahesmaa-Rantala R, Vuento R, Granfors K. Association of persisting IgA response with *Yersinia* triggered reactive arthritis: a study on 104 patients. Ann Rheum Dis. 1987;46: 898–901.

Chapter 16
Molecular Mimicry Between *Klebsiella* Pullulanase Enzyme, HLA-B27 and Collagens I and IV

16.1 Introduction: The Association of HLA-B27 with Ankylosing Spondylitis Is the Central Research Issue in This Disease

The association between ankylosing spondylitis and HLA-B27 has been well established. Over 95 % of ankylosing spondylitis patients possess the histocompatibility antigen HLA-B27, whilst its frequency in the general UK or US population is about 8 %.

There are seven subtypes of HLA-B27 ranging from B*2701 to B*2707.

It has been suggested that the B*2705 is the most common HLA-B27 subtype in Caucasian populations.

Subtypes of HLA-B27, other than B*2705 containing different amino acid sequences, are also involved in ankylosing spondylitis.

It would appear that ankylosing spondylitis patients from many different countries have elevated levels of antibodies against the bowel microbe *Klebsiella pneumoniae.* Any aetiological agent implicated in ankylosing spondylitis must provide an explanation for the link with HLA-B27.

An amino acid homology QTDRED, found in residues 72–77 of B*2705 (Fig. 16.1), has been identified which has molecular identity with residues 188–193 of *Klebsiella pneumoniae* nitrogenase enzyme (Fig. 16.2) (Schwimmbeck et al. 1987). However, for the nitrogenase enzyme to be produced, an extremely low level of fixed nitrogen is required (Brill 1980), and this condition is not achieved in the human gut.

Additionally, extremely anaerobic conditions are necessary for nitrogenase production, and this again may not be achieved in the human gut.

If the inducible enzyme nitrogenase is not produced in *Klebsiella* bacteria in humans, it raises the question whether there are other proteins which may show molecular mimicry with HLA-B27.

A. Ebringer, *Ankylosing Spondylitis and Klebsiella*,
DOI 10.1007/978-1-4471-4300-0_16, © Springer-Verlag London 2013

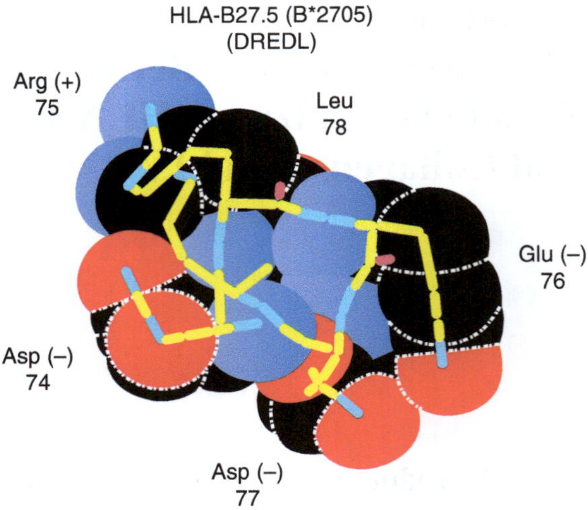

Fig. 16.1 Molecular structure of HLA-B27.5 (B*2705) sequence DREDL

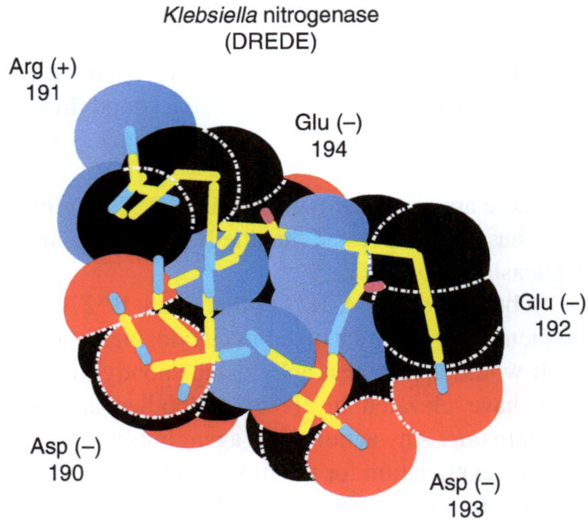

Fig. 16.2 Molecular structure of the sequence DREDE found in *Klebsiella pneumoniae* nitrogenase molecule

16.2 Computer Search for Other *Klebsiella* Proteins Cross-Reacting with HLA-B27

The BLAST database searching program was used to search the PIR protein database (V.33.0) containing 42,215 sequences. The sequence QTDRED from HLA-B27 and *Klebsiella pneumoniae* were compared with all the sequences in the database allowing for mismatches.

The computer search revealed a number of sequence homologies between B*2705 and various microorganisms including the nitrogenase protein of *Klebsiella pneumoniae*.

Table 16.1 Comparison of amino acid sequence homologies between HLA-B27 and proteins from *Klebsiella pneumoniae*

Protein	Residues	Amino acid sequence
HLA-B27	67–82	CKAKAQTDREDLRTLL
Klebsiella pneumoniae nitrogenase	184–199	CNSRQTDREDELIGGC
Klebsiella pneumoniae pulD secretion protein	590–605	RPTVIRDRDEYRQASS

D aspartic acid, *R* arginine, *E* glutamic acid

The mismatch function revealed the presence of another sequence of *Klebsiella pneumoniae* that showed homology with the QTDRED region in B*2705 (Table 16.1).

This sequence was a tetramer DRDE, present in the pullulanase secretion protein pulD (residues 596–599) of a starch-debranching enzyme present in *Klebsiella pneumoniae* (Fig. 16.3).

The pulD sequence was the second amino acid homology to be identified between the hypervariable domain of B*2705 and the Gram-negative microbe *Klebsiella pneumoniae.*

16.3 Peptide ELISA Studies in Ankylosing Spondylitis Patients

Sera were collected from 97 active ankylosing spondylitis patients (New York criteria), attending the 'Ankylosing Spondylitis Research Clinic of the Middlesex Hospital', all having an erythrocyte sedimentation rate greater than 15 mm/h and all being HLA-B27 positive.

Two sets of controls were used. The first group consisted of 25 active rheumatoid arthritis patients (American Rheumatism Association criteria) attending the Department of Rheumatology at the Lister Hospital in Stevenage. The second control group consisted of 25 healthy control sera provided by the London Blood Transfusion Service. All sera were stored at −20 °C until required.

The synthetic peptides were prepared by solid-phase synthesis; purity assays were performed by high-performance liquid chromatography. All peptides had a purity of at least 90 %.

Three 16-mer peptides were constructed:

1. The B*2705 sequence (residues 67–83) CKAKAQTDREDLRTLL
2. The pulD secretion protein (residues 590–605) RPTVIRDRDEYRQASS
3. A control peptide sequence made from a scrambled sequence of the pulD peptide RPTVRSDIDYRQAESR

Sera were tested against the three peptides by non-competitive enzyme-linked immunosorbent assay (ELISA).

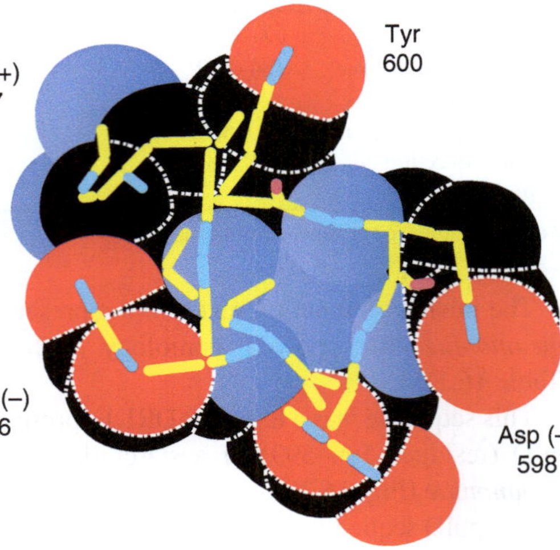

Fig. 16.3 Molecular structure of the sequence DRDEY found in *Klebsiella pneumoniae* pulD secretion protein.

The assays were carried out as follows: Polystyrene microtitre plates (Dynatech) were coated with the synthetic peptide (5 μg/ml) overnight at 4 °C. After absorption and washing with PBS-Tween, the plates were saturated with 2 % casein-PBS-Tween, incubated for 1 h at 37 °C, followed by washing with PBS-Tween.

Serum samples (200 μl at 1/50 dilution in PBS-Tween) were added to the plates, incubated for 90 min at room temperature, followed by washing with PBS-Tween, and peroxidase-conjugated rabbit anti-human class specific IgG, IgA or IgM (Dako Ltd.) diluted 1/500 in PBS-Tween was added, and plates were incubated for 90 min at room temperature.

After washing and enzyme reaction with substrate 2,2′-azinobis(9-ethyl-benzthiazoline-6-sulphonic acid) (ABTS) (Sigma Chemical Co Ltd.) at room temperature for 20 min, the reaction was stopped with sodium fluoride and the optical density (O.D.) measured at wavelength 630 nm.

*16.3.1 B*2705 Results*

ELISA assays performed on the B*2705 synthetic peptide showed significant ($p<0.001$) antibody elevations in ankylosing spondylitis patients in IgG antibody class when compared to control subjects but no significant elevations in IgA or IgM antibodies (Fig. 16.4).

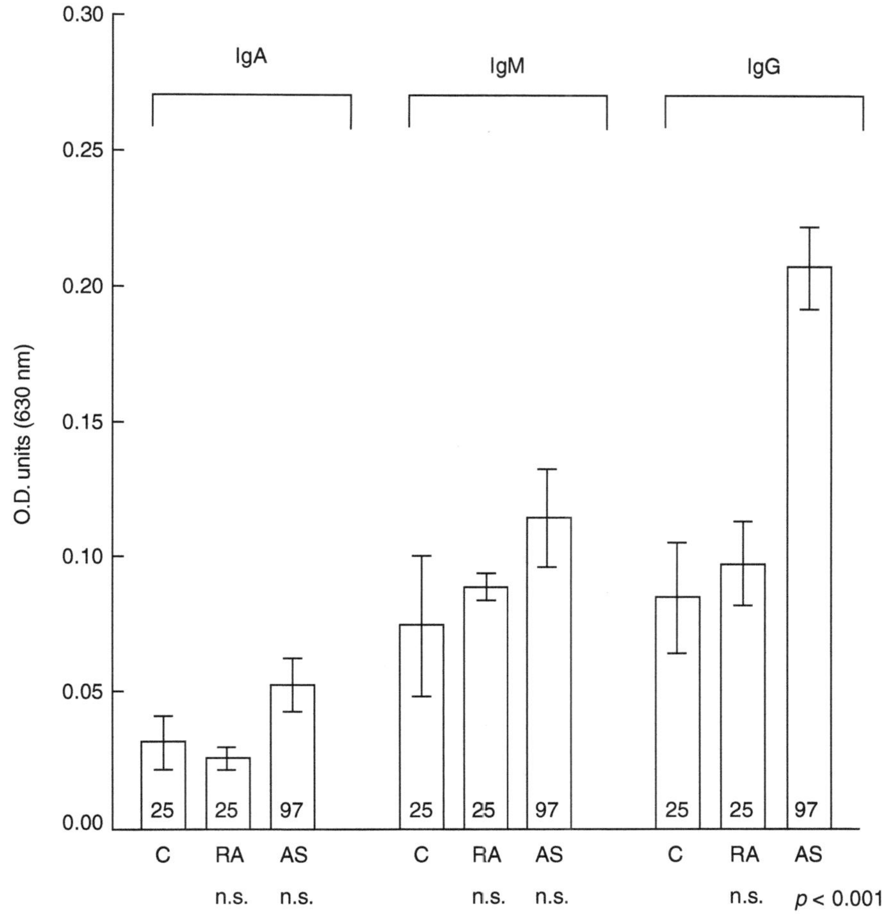

Fig. 16.4 Antibody titres (mean ± standard error of the mean) for IgA, IgM and IgG in 25 controls (*C*), 25 rheumatoid arthritis (*RA*) patients and 97 ankylosing spondylitis (*AS*) when tested by ELISA against 16-mer peptide of HLA-B27 (*O.D.* optical density, *n.s.* not significant)

However, in the rheumatoid arthritis patients, there were no significant elevations in the IgA, IgM or IgG classes when compared to controls (Fielder et al. 1995).

16.3.2 pulD Peptide Results

ELISA assays performed on the pulD peptide demonstrated significant antibody elevations in all three antibody classes, IgA ($p<0.005$), IgM ($p<0.05$) and IgG ($p<0.001$), when compared to controls (Fig. 16.5).

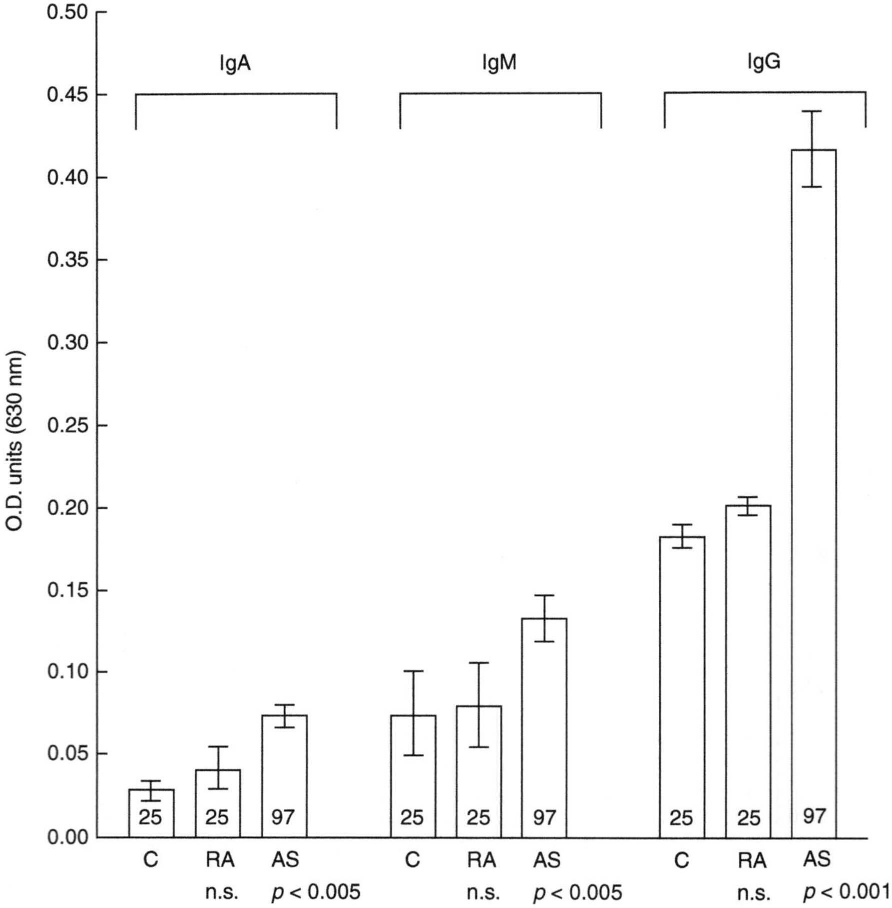

Fig. 16.5 Antibody titres (mean ± standard error of the mean) for IgA, IgM and IgG in 25 controls (*C*), 25 rheumatoid arthritis (*RA*) patients and 97 ankylosing spondylitis (*AS*) when tested by ELISA against 16-mer peptide of pulD (*O.D.* optical density, *n.s.* not significant)

The rheumatoid arthritis patients, again, showed no significant antibody elevations in IgA, IgM or IgG antibody classes.

16.3.3 Scrambled Control Peptide Results

ELISA studies on the scrambled control peptide demonstrated no significant elevations in IgA, IgM or IgG antibody classes in rheumatoid arthritis or ankylosing spondylitis patients when compared to control subjects (Fig. 16.6).

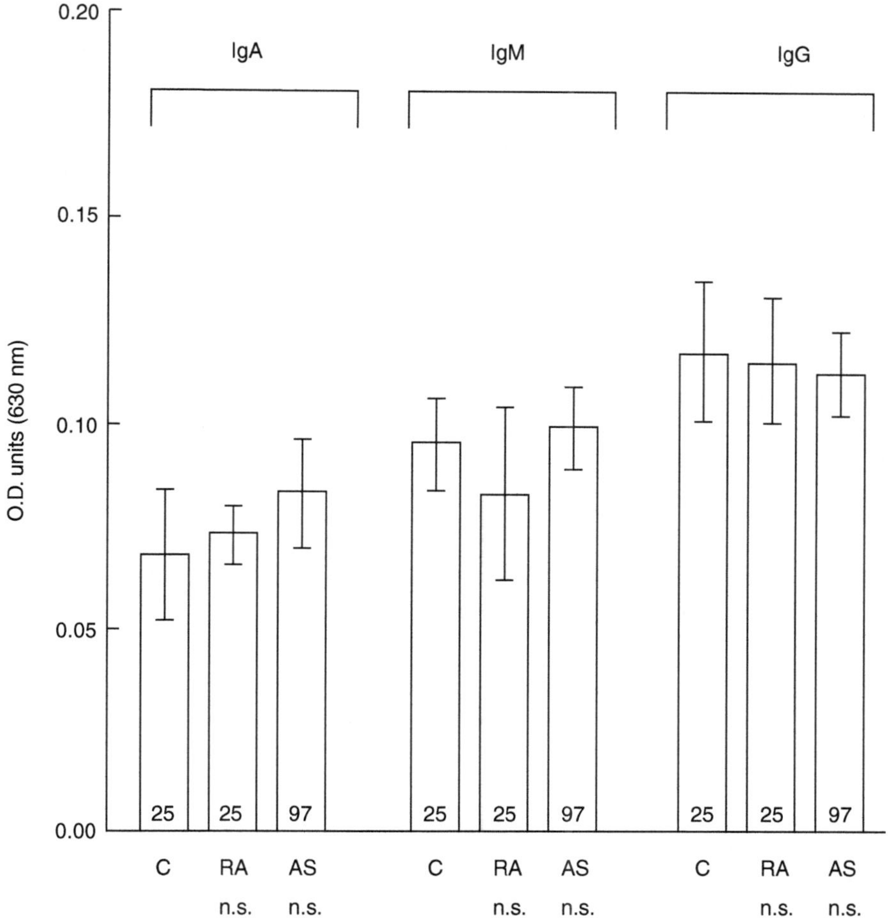

Fig. 16.6 Antibody titres (mean ± standard error of the mean) for IgA, IgM and IgG in 25 controls (*C*), 25 rheumatoid arthritis (*RA*) patients and 97 ankylosing spondylitis (*AS*) when tested by ELISA against 16-mer control peptide (scrambled pulD) (*O.D.* optical density, *n.s.* not significant)

16.4 Pullulan and Pullulanase

Pullulan is an edible, tasteless polysaccharide consisting of maltotriose units. Three glucose units in maltotriose are connected by an α-(1,4) glycosidic link, whereas consecutive maltotriose units are connected to each other by an α-(1,6) glycosidic link.

Pullulan is produced from starch by the ubiquitous fungus *Aureobasidium pullulans*. It is used in various freshener or oral hygiene products and also as a food additive with the E-number E1204. It has also been used in the manufacture of edible films.

Pullulanase is an enzyme that degrades pullulan. It is produced as an extracellular, cell surface-anchored lipoprotein by *Klebsiella* bacteria. Type I pullulanases specifically attack α-(1,6) glycosidic linkages, while type II pullulanases are also able to hydrolyse α-(1,4) linkages.

Carbohydrate polymers consisting of α-(1,4) linkages give rise to long linear chains such as amylose, which are readily degraded by digestive enzymes.

Carbohydrate polymers which contain α-(1,6) as well as α-(1,4) linkages give rise to branched, tree-like molecular structures such as amylopectin. Amylopectin forms 60 to 80 % of dietary starch depending on whether it comes from potatoes or wheat. The α-(1,6) linkages, giving rise to the branched carbohydrate structures, are not readily hydrolysed by digestive enzymes. However, bacteria which contain enzymes that can hydrolyse the α-(1,6) glycosidic links grow very well on such substrates. These enzymes that break the α-(1,6) links are also known as 'debranching enzymes'. The pullulanase enzymes present in *Klebsiella* enable these bacteria to grow on starch substrates.

16.5 ELISA Studies on Effect of Antibody in Bacteria Grown in Presence or Absence of Pullulan

The *Klebsiella pneumoniae* microbe was a clinical isolate kindly provided by the Medical Microbiology Department, Princess Royal Hospital, Haywards Heath, and *Proteus mirabilis* was obtained from the department of microbiology at King's College. The cultures were grown as previously described in minimal media supplemented with 0.005 % yeast extract (Difco).

If induction of the pullulanase enzyme system was required, the starch substrate pullulan with a concentration of 0.3 % w/v (Sigma) was added to the minimal medium.

The cells were harvested by centrifugation (MSE 18; 6 × 250 ml Rotor) and washed in 0.15-M phosphate-buffered saline (PBS). The suspension was centrifuged as before and repeated three times.

After washing, the cells were resuspended in 20 ml of PBS and a stock solution prepared to give an O.D. reading 0.25 on the spectrophotometer (Corning Model 258).

Aliquots of 200 μl of the diluted suspension of bacteria grown on minimal media plus 0.005 % yeast extract were adsorbed onto 96-well ELISA plates (Dynatech) overnight at 4 °C.

The ELISA procedure was carried out as previously described with the exception of the application horseradish peroxidase-conjugated second antibody. In this assay, when *Klebsiella pneumoniae* was used as the antigen, the horseradish peroxidase-conjugated second antibody was of the IgA class, whilst when *Proteus mirabilis* was the antigen, the horseradish peroxidase-conjugated antibody was of the IgG class.

This experiment was repeated with a suspension of bacteria grown on minimal media plus 0.005 % yeast extract (Difco) supplemented with 0.3 % w/v pullulan (Sigma).

16.5.1 Results of ELISA Studies in Ankylosing Spondylitis Patients

Determination of antibody levels in ankylosing spondylitis patients to *Klebsiella pneumoniae* grown in minimal media with yeast extract showed elevation in IgA antibody titres ($p < 0.001$) when compared to controls (Fig. 16.7).

When the experiment was repeated with the addition of the starch component pullulan (Sigma) to the medium (0.3 % w/v), the level of IgA binding in ankylosing spondylitis was again elevated, if not more than in the preceding experiment, when compared to control subjects (Fig. 16.7).

This increase in the level of antibody binding is likely to be due to the development of more capsular polysaccharide on the cell surface of the bacteria when grown with pullulan.

16.5.2 Results of ELISA Studies in Rheumatoid Arthritis Patients

The assay was repeated using another Gram-negative enteric microbe *Proteus mirabilis* as the target, grown exactly under the same conditions as *Klebsiella pneumoniae* in minimal media in absence and presence of pullulan.

Significant and specific IgG antibody elevations were observed in rheumatoid arthritis patients regardless of the absence ($p < 0.001$) or presence ($p < 0.001$) of pullulan when compared to controls (Fig. 16.8).

Furthermore, the levels of antibody titres in the ankylosing spondylitis, rheumatoid arthritis patients or control group, did not appear to be affected by the presence or absence of pullulan in the growth media of *Proteus mirabilis*.

16.6 Serum Antibodies to the Pullulanase (pulA) Enzyme

Aliquots (200 μl) of a solution of pullulanase (Sigma) (3 μg/ml) were adsorbed onto 96-well ELISA plates (Dynatech) overnight at 4 °C.

The ELISA procedure was carried out as previously described; however, only IgA and IgG classes of the horseradish peroxidase-conjugated second antibody were used.

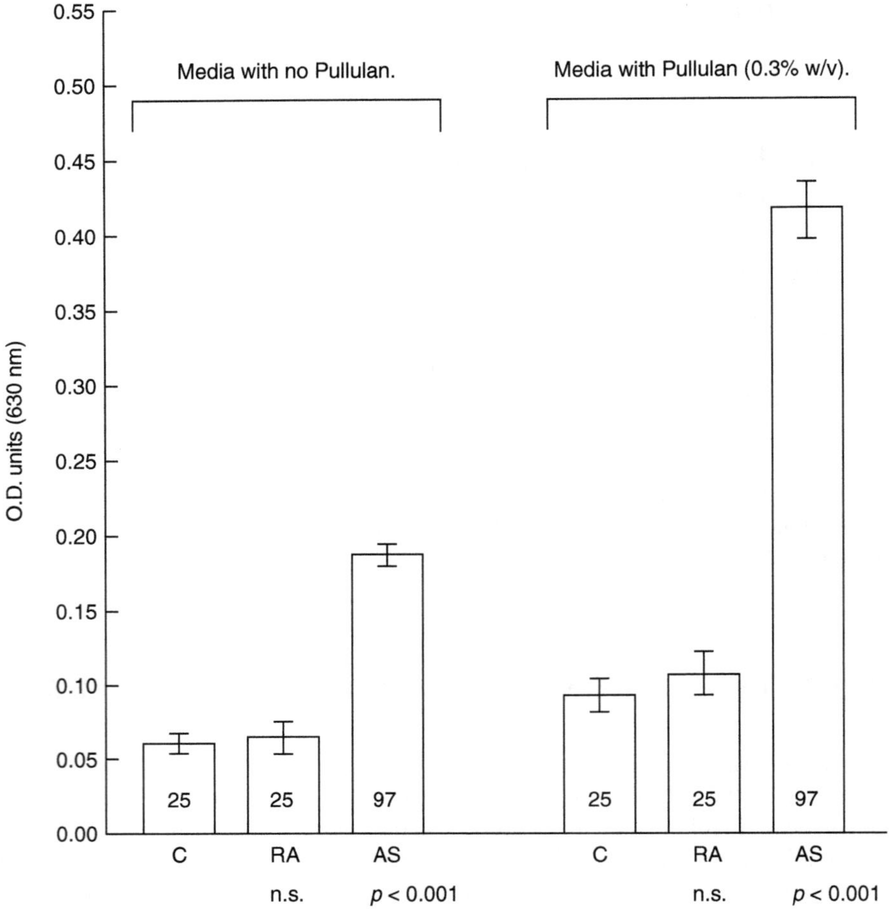

Fig. 16.7 Antibody titres (mean ± standard error of the mean) for IgA, in 25 controls (*C*), 25 rheumatoid arthritis (*RA*) patients and 97 ankylosing spondylitis (*AS*) when tested by ELISA against a clinical isolate of *Klebsiella pneumoniae* grown in the absence and presence of pullulan (*O.D.* optical density, *n.s.* not significant)

Titres of both IgA and IgG antibody classes were determined by ELISA to a pullulanase target.

Ankylosing spondylitis patients showed elevated levels of IgA ($p < 0.001$) and IgG ($p < 0.001$) antibodies to pullulanase when compared to controls (Fig. 16.9).

However, the rheumatoid arthritis patients showed no significant elevations in IgA or IgG antibodies to pullulanase when compared to controls (Fig. 16.9).

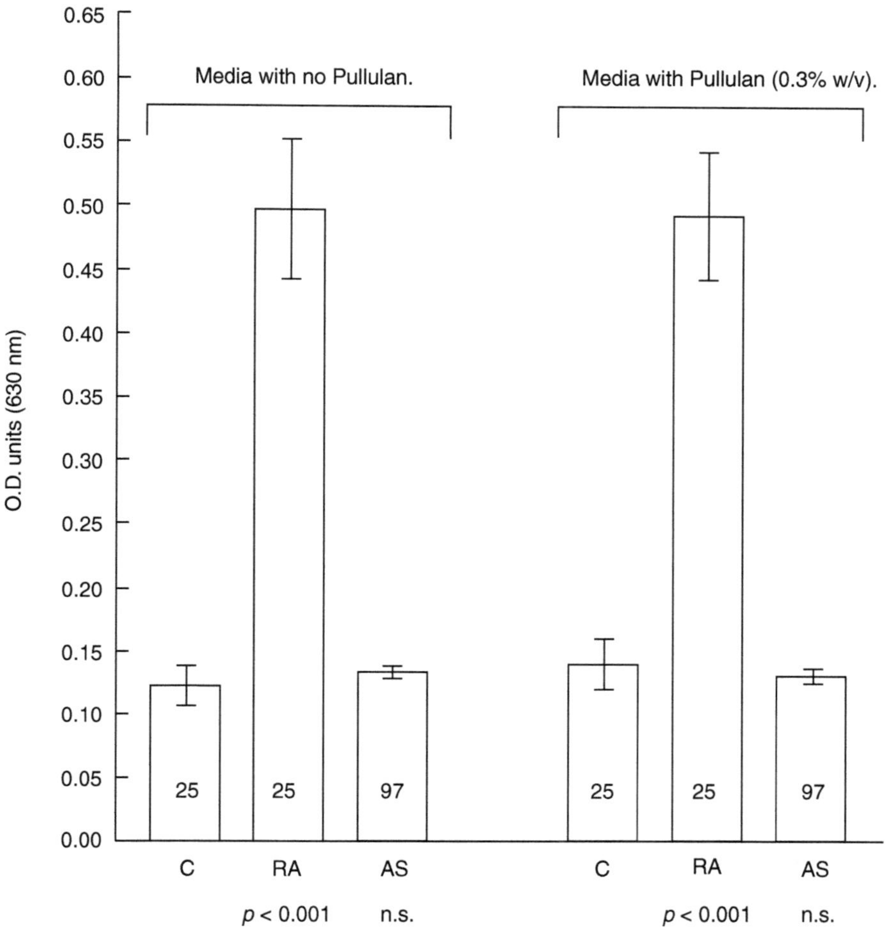

Fig. 16.8 Antibody titres (mean ± standard error of the mean) for IgA, in 25 controls (*C*), 25 rheumatoid arthritis (*RA*) patients and 97 ankylosing spondylitis (*AS*) when tested by ELISA against a clinical isolate of *Proteus mirabilis* grown in the absence and presence of pullulan (*O.D.* optical density, *n.s.* not significant).

16.7 ELISA Studies on Collagen Types I and IV

The levels of cross-reactive antibodies to collagens type I and type IV in the sera of ankylosing spondylitis patients have been measured to assess their relevance in the development of the disease.

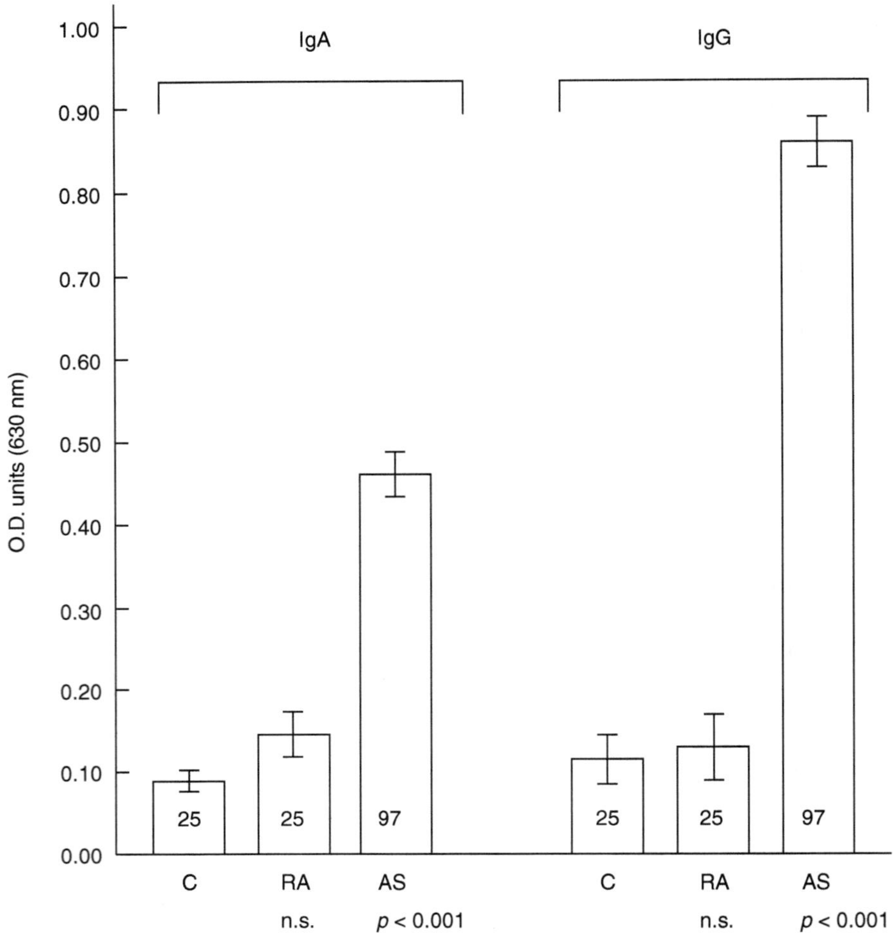

Fig. 16.9 Titres of IgA and IgG antibody titres (mean ± standard error of the in 25 controls (*C*), 25 rheumatoid arthritis (*RA*) patients and 97 ankylosing spondylitis (*AS*) patients when tested by ELISA against pullulanase enzyme (pulA) (*O.D.* optical density, *n.s.* not significant)

Type I collagen is found predominantly in tendons and bone, whilst type IV collagen is present basement membranes, basal lamina, retina, cornea and uvea (Kühn 1987). Episodes of inflammatory uveitis occur in about 30 % of patients with ankylosing spondylitis.

Solutions of collagen type I or type IV (Sigma) (3 μg/ml) were adsorbed onto 96-well ELISA plates (Dynatech) overnight in 200 μl volumes. The ELISA plate was washed and saturated with 2 % casein-PBS-Tween as described previously; however, incubation for 1 h was performed at room temperature.

Additionally, only IgA and IgG classes of the horseradish peroxidase-conjugated secondary antibody were used in this assay.

IgA elevations to both type I collagen ($p<0.001$) and type IV collagen ($p<0.001$) were observed in ankylosing spondylitis patients in comparison to control subjects (Fig. 16.10).

IgG responses to collagen type I ($p<0.001$) and to collagen type IV ($p<0.001$) were also elevated in ankylosing spondylitis patients when compared to control subjects (Fig. 16.11).

However, the rheumatoid arthritis patients showed no significant elevations in IgA or IgG antibodies against either type I collagen or type IV collagen when compared to controls (Figs. 16.10 and 16.11).

16.8 Discussion and Conclusions

A strong association between HLA-B27 and ankylosing spondylitis has been known since 1973. These two observations were later linked when an amino acid homology was demonstrated between HLA-B*2705 and the inducible nitrogenase enzyme found in *Klebsiella pneumoniae* (Schwimmbeck et al. 1987). The link to *Klebsiella pneumoniae* was specific since antibodies to other Gram-negative microorganisms such as *Escherichia coli*, *Proteus mirabilis*, *Salmonella* spp., *Shigella* spp. and *Yersinia enterocolitica* have not been found to be elevated in ankylosing spondylitis patients.

A further sequence homology has been identified between HLA-B*2705 and another protein present in *Klebsiella pneumoniae*, the pulD secretion protein of the starch-debranching pullulanase enzyme system (Table 16.1). Whilst the pulD sequence does not display the 100 % homology shown with *Klebsiella pneumoniae* nitrogenase, a similarity is nonetheless present in the form of a tetramer, DRDE (residues 596–599) and HLA-B*2705 (DRED).

The pulD sequence (residues 596–599) only differs from the DRED sequence in HLA-B*2705 (residues 74–77) by two conservative substitutions, one a ‘D’ (aspartic acid) for an ‘E’ (glutamic acid) at position 598 and the second of an ‘E’ (glutamic acid) for a ‘D’ (aspartic acid) at position 599. It is clear that these substitutions involving negatively charged amino acids provide a powerful antigenic determinant to the pulD molecule of *Klebsiella pneumoniae.*

Once the host is exposed to the enteric peptides of *Klebsiella pneumoniae* having sequences resembling HLA-B27, an immune response will be evoked which may target the HLA molecules.

Although similar sequences may be present in other Gram-negative bacteria, antibody levels in ankylosing spondylitis patients revealed no specific elevations in immunoglobulin levels against other bacteria with respect to controls with the exception of *Klebsiella pneumoniae* (Ebringer 1992).

The pulD is the terminal secretion protein of the pullulanase system and is known to have regions said to form strongly amphipathic β-sheets which confer membrane-spanning properties to outer membrane proteins (Scofield et al. 1993).This suggests

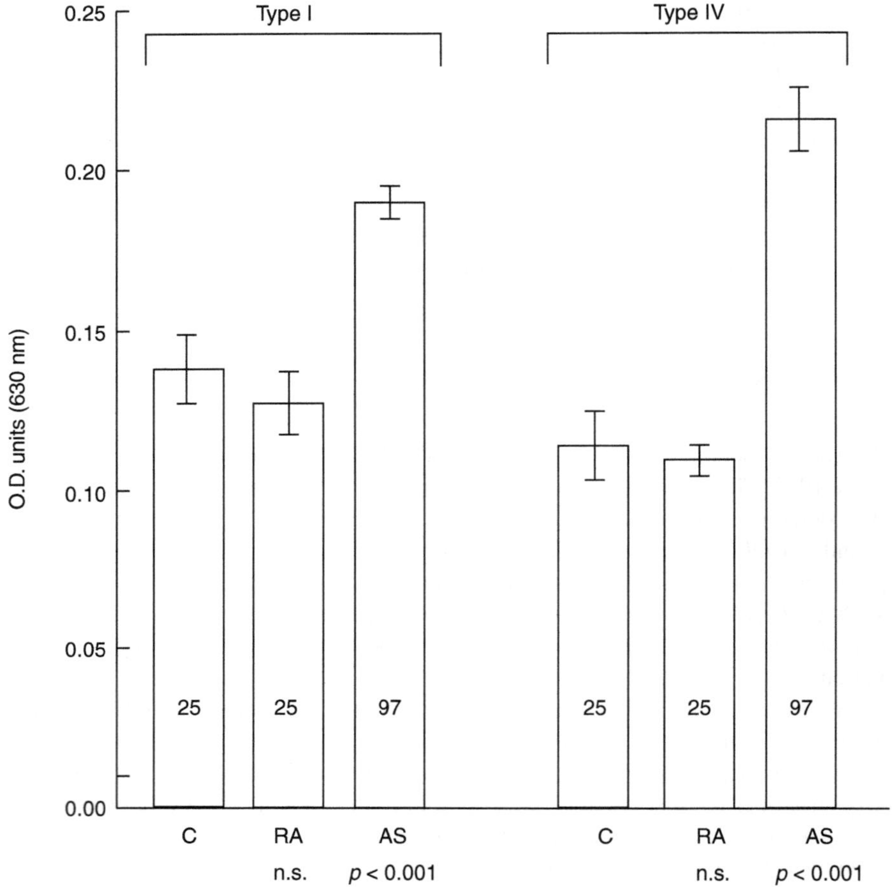

Fig. 16.10 Titres of IgA antibody titres (mean ± standard error of the in 25 controls (*C*), 25 rheumatoid arthritis (*RA*) patients and 97 ankylosing spondylitis (*AS*) patients when tested by ELISA against type I collagen and type IV collagen (*O.D.* optical density, *n.s.* not significant)

that the protein should be on the surface of the microbe and accessible to the cells of the immune system.

The ELISA studies with the synthetic peptides demonstrate that the ankylosing spondylitis patients have antibodies to the 16-mer B*2705 and pulD peptides. The ankylosing spondylitis patients showed significant elevations in both IgA and IgG classes to the B*2705 peptide. This binding to a peptide of a self protein demonstrates the presence of autoantibodies in the sera of ankylosing spondylitis patients. It is therefore possible that these antibodies may bind HLA-B27 positive cells, fix complement when present in high concentration and thereby initiate inflammation.

The microbial source evoking these antibodies could be in the form of pulD protein of *Klebsiella pneumoniae*. The ELISA data with the pulD synthetic peptide yielded similar results to that obtained with B*2705. The pulD antibody elevations were seen in all three antibody classes, whilst with the control peptide

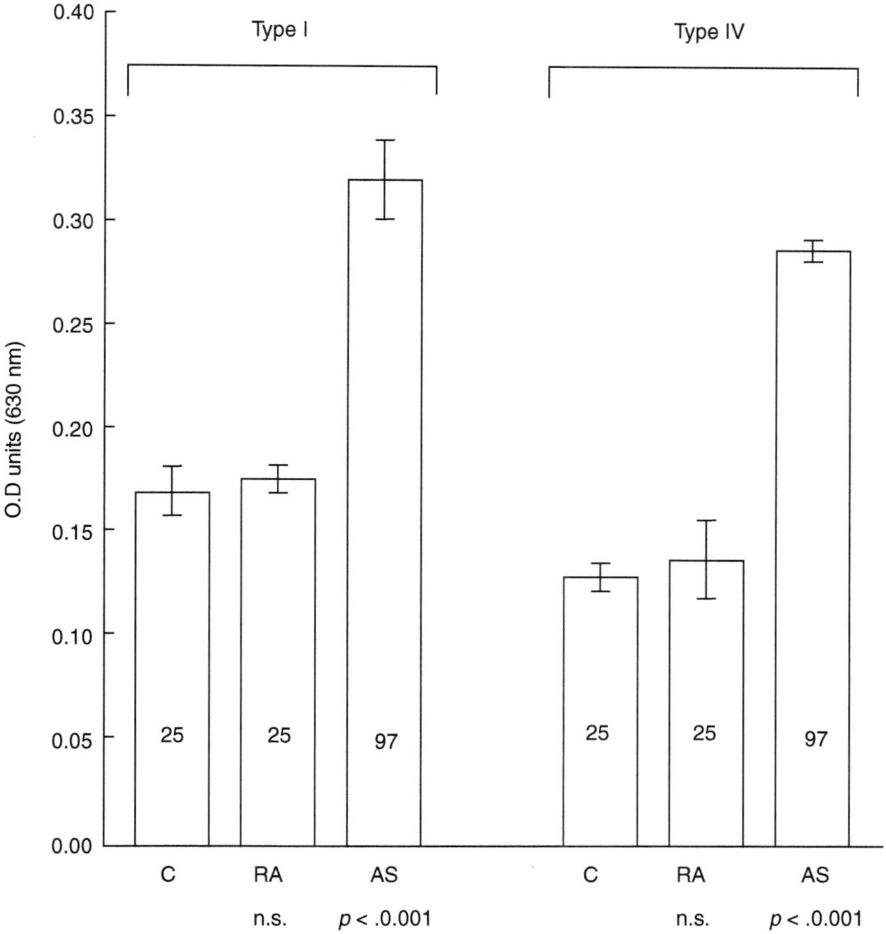

Fig. 16.11 Titres of IgG antibody titres (mean ± standard error of the in 25 controls (*C*), 25 rheumatoid arthritis (*RA*) patients and 97 ankylosing spondylitis (*AS*) patients when tested by ELISA against type I collagen and type IV collagen (*O.D.* optical density, *n.s.* not significant)

(scrambled pulD peptide), no antibody elevations were observed in any patient group to any antibody class.

The data derived from the B*2705 and pulD peptide binding suggests that there is some degree of molecular mimicry or cross-reactivity between the two sequences, one self and the other one microbial in origin.

The presence of the pullulanase system in *Klebsiella pneumoniae* allows the microorganism to cleave α(1–6) bonds in α(1–4) and α(1–6)-branched starches such as glycogen and amylopectin, found in potatoes and wheat-derived products such as bread or pasta and rice. The effect of this property is that the microorganism gains access to another carbon source, which can alter the type of antigens presented on the surface of the bacteria leading to the development of the polysaccharide capsular layer and alter the level of antibody binding by sera obtained from patients.

This can be seen when the *Klebsiella pneumoniae* are grown in minimal medium with 0.005 % yeast extract (Fig. 16.7). When organisms grown in these media were exposed to sera from ankylosing spondylitis patients and healthy and disease rheumatoid arthritis controls, an elevation in antibody titre is observed.

However, if the microorganisms are grown on the same media supplemented with pullulan (0.3 % w/v) as the carbon source, the degree of antibody binding in ankylosing spondylitis patients is greatly increased. This increase also shows that the capsule is highly antigenic and is one of the predominant antigens recognised by ankylosing spondylitis patients. A similar observation has been made by other workers from Germany, investigating antibodies to *Klebsiella* microbes in ankylosing spondylitis patients.

In the control experiment, where *Proteus mirabilis* is grown under the same conditions, with and without pullulan, antibody elevations are only seen in the rheumatoid arthritis patients but not the ankylosing spondylitis patients or healthy controls. Importantly, there is no significant difference in the antibody-binding capacity of *Proteus mirabilis* microorganisms when grown in presence or absence of pullulan, regardless of whether the sera is from patients or healthy controls (Fig. 16.8).

IgA and IgG antibody titres were also found to be elevated against the extracellular enzyme pullulanase (pulA) in ankylosing spondylitis patients when compared to controls. The pulA enzyme would appear to have a very important property in relation to arthritic disease. At the N-terminal end of the pulA protein in some strains of *Klebsiella pneumoniae*, there are repeats of the tripeptide Gly-X-Pro, characteristic of collagens type I, type III and type IV (Charalambous et al. 1988) (Table 16.2). In the case of pullulanase from *Klebsiella pneumoniae*, there is an unusual N-terminal amino acid sequence which includes 6 repeats of the tripeptide Gly-X-Pro. This type of sequence is characteristic of animal collagens and collagen-like proteins which form triple-helical structures.

Pullulanase is exported from these bacteria via a rather unusual route involving transient localisation at the outer cell surface where the enzyme is exposed to the environment and able to hydrolyse the substrate pullulan and other starch-derived compounds.

IgA and IgG antibody elevations to both type I and type IV collagens have been demonstrated compared to controls. It is interesting to note that type I collagen is present predominantly in tendons and bone.

The possibility of antibodies cross-reacting between pulA and type I collagen may be important in the deposition of fibrous tissue in the axial skeleton and the development of inflammation at the entheses or enthesitis.

Histological changes in thigh muscle biopsies of ankylosing spondylitis patients have previously been reported, and type III collagen is present in muscle tissues.

Type IV collagen is present in basement membranes, basal lamina, retina and cornea. Ankylosing spondylitis patients suffer from acute anterior uveitis which could be triggered by these anti-collagen antibodies. The antibody binding to pulA, type I and type IV collagen demonstrated here, as well as the suggested

Table 16.2 Comparison of amino acid sequence homologies between *Klebsiella* pullulanase (pulA) and collagens I, III and IV

Protein	Residues	Amino acid sequence
pulA	11–29	GXP-GXP-GXP-GXP-GXP-GXP
Collagen I		GXP-GXP-GAD-GPA-GXP-GXP
Collagen III		GXP-GXP-GXP-GXP-GXP
Collagen IV		GAE-GXP-GXP-GXP

G glycine, *X* any other amino acid, *P* proline, *A* alanine, *D* aspartic acid, *E* glutamic acid

cross-reactivity between pulA and collagen type III may explain some of the pathological features of ankylosing spondylitis.

Ankylosing spondylitis patients are usually treated with anti-inflammatory drugs, but the demonstration that pullulanase enzymes of *Klebsiella pneumoniae* are involved in using starch dependent substrates for the growth of these microorganisms may explain the observed patterns of exacerbations and remissions. The possibility arises further that this could even open a new approach to therapy involving dietary starch restriction.

References

Brill WJ. Biochemical genetics of nitrogen fixation. Microbiol Rev. 1980;44:449–58.

Charalambous BM, Keen JN, McPherson MJ. Collagen-like sequences stabilize homotrimers of a bacterial hydrolase. EMBO J. 1988;7:2903–9.

Ebringer A. Ankylosing spondylitis is caused by *Klebsiella*. Evidence from immunogenetic, microbiologic and serologic studies. Rheum Dis Clin North Am. 1992;18:105–21.

Fielder M, Pirt SJ, Tarpey I, Wilson C, Cunningham P, Ettelaie C, Binder A, Bansal S, Ebringer A. Molecular mimicry and ankylosing Spondylitis: possible role of a novel sequence in pullulanase of *Klebsiella pneumoniae*. FEBS Lett. 1995;369:243–8.

Kühn K. In: Mayne R, Burgeson RE, editors. Structure and function of collagen types. London: Academic; 1987.

Schwimmbeck PL, Yu DTY, Oldstone MBA. Autoantibodies to HLA-B27 in the sera of HLA-B27 patients with ankylosing spondylitis and Reiter's syndrome: Molecular mimicry with *Klebsiella pneumoniae* as potential mechanism of autoimmune disease. J Exp Med. 1987;166:173–81.

Scofield RH, Warren WL, Koelsch G, Harley JB. A hypothesis for HLA-B27 immune dysregulation in spondyloarthropathy: Contributions from enteric organisms, B27 structure, peptides bound by B27 and convergent evolution. Proc Natl Acad Sci. 1993;90:9330–4.

Chapter 17
Antibodies to *Klebsiella* and HLA-B27 Peptides in Ankylosing Spondylitis Patients from Southern Japan

17.1 The Japanese Connection: An Introduction

In the early 1980s, the Immunology Unit of King's College had shown that there were elevated levels of antibodies to the Gram-negative bowel microbe *Klebsiella* in patients suffering from ankylosing spondylitis. These patients were being investigated in the 'Ankylosing Spondylitis Research Unit' of the Middlesex Hospital which had been set up in 1976 to study why up to 96 % of ankylosing spondylitis with this disease possessed the HLA-B27 major histocompatibility group antigen, whilst the frequency of this antigen in the general population of England or of the United States was only 8 %.

However, immunological studies in Japan showed that HLA-B27 was present in only 0.4 % of the Japanese population, one of the lowest frequencies throughout the world.

Furthermore, ankylosing spondylitis, as a disease, is extremely rare in Japan, so rare that when the disease is observed, it is referred to orthopaedic surgeons, because of their interests in backache and not to rheumatologists (Tujimoto 1978). However, Japanese ankylosing spondylitis patients show also a high prevalence of the HLA-B27 as do similar patients in other parts of the world (Sonozaki et al. 1975).

In 1993, I was approached by Professor Sinsuke Hukuda from Shiga University that a promising research worker and orthopaedic surgeon Dr. Yoshitaka Tani had been awarded a visiting scholarship from the Rheumatism Foundation of Japan to come to London and study antibodies to *Klebsiella* in Japanese ankylosing spondylitis patients.

Since ankylosing spondylitis belonged to the orthopaedic medical community in Japan because of its rarity, it attracted the attention of this talented and hard-working orthopaedic surgeon, Dr. Yoshitaka Tani, as a research project.

He collected all the ankylosing spondylitis patients in the southern parts of Japan and decided to determine whether they had elevated levels of antibodies to *Klebsiella* as had been reported in ankylosing spondylitis patients in England.

A. Ebringer, *Ankylosing Spondylitis and Klebsiella*,
DOI 10.1007/978-1-4471-4300-0_17,

Dr. Yoshitaka Tani came to London with his ankylosing spondylitis sera and blood donor control sera. The ankylosing spondylitis and control sera were stored in a freezer, and he was told he should go back to Japan and bring back as well sera from active rheumatoid arthritis patients to be used as 'disease controls' together with the Japanese blood bank controls from healthy individuals.

Active rheumatoid arthritis patients were defined as those having at least an erythrocyte sedimentation rate in excess of 30 mm/h (ESR > 30 mm/h) at the time when the blood sample was obtained. Then, both ankylosing spondylitis sera and rheumatoid arthritis sera would be tested simultaneously against both *Klebsiella* and *Proteus* bacteria, under blind conditions in London. Each microbe would be acting as a 'disease control' for the other condition.

Dr. Yoshitaka Tani returned to Japan and brought back to London a set of sera obtained from Japanese active rheumatoid arthritis patients from the Otsu area in southern Japan.

All the sera, from rheumatoid arthritis and ankylosing spondylitis patients as well as from the blood donors, were then tested under blind conditions against both *Klebsiella* and *Proteus* microorganisms, as well as against *Escherichia coli.*

17.2 Otsu: Location and History

Otsu is the capital city of the Shiga province in southern Japan. In 2006, Shiga was merged with Otsu, and the size of the merged population was approximately 350,000.

In the years 667–672, Omi Otsu palace was founded in Otsu by Emperor Tenji. During the Edo period (1603–1867), when the Tokugawa shoguns were rulers of Japan, the poet Matsuo Basho frequented Otsu and took on apprentices.

On 11th May 1891, the 'Otsu incident' occurred, during a failed assassination attempt on Tsarevich Nicholas Alexandrovich of Russia.

The Shiga University is in the Shiga Prefecture of Japan. It comprises campuses from the cities of Otsu and Hikone.

The ankylosing spondylitis and rheumatoid arthritis patients came from the Shiga province in Japan.

17.3 Patients and Controls

Serum samples from 152 Japanese subjects were studied.

There were 29 sera from active ankylosing spondylitis patients selected according to the New York criteria. There were 27 men and 2 women, and the male/female ratio was 13.5/1. The mean age of the active ankylosing spondylitis patients was 42 years (range 20–69 years).

The mean (± standard error) erythrocyte sedimentation rate of the active ankylosing spondylitis patients was 49.0±9.7 mm/h. The mean (± standard error) C-reactive protein level of the active ankylosing spondylitis patients was 24.8±9.1 mg/l.

There were also 23 ankylosing spondylitis patients with inactive disease 21 men/2 women), and the male/female ratio was 10.5/1. The mean age of the inactive ankylosing spondylitis patients was 42 years (range 25–68 years). The mean (± standard error) erythrocyte sedimentation rate of the inactive ankylosing spondylitis was 12.2±2.1 mm/h. The mean (± standard error) C-reactive protein level of the inactive ankylosing spondylitis patients was 3.9±1.1 mg/l.

There were 30 patients with active rheumatoid arthritis as defined by the American Rheumatism Association criteria. There were 5 men and 25 women. The female/male ratio was 5/1. The mean age of the active rheumatoid arthritis patients was 51 years (range 23–70 years). The mean (± standard error) erythrocyte sedimentation rate of the active rheumatoid arthritis was 77.7±5.9 mm/h. The mean C-reactive protein level of the active rheumatoid arthritis patients mean (± standard error) was 40.2±5.2 mg/l.

There were also 20 rheumatoid arthritis patients with probably active disease, 5 men and 15 women. The female/male ratio was 3/1. The mean age of the probably active rheumatoid arthritis patients was 55 years (range 30–77 years). The mean (± standard error) erythrocyte sedimentation rate of the probably active rheumatoid arthritis patients was 38.3±9.4 mm/h. The mean (± standard error) C-reactive protein level of the probably active rheumatoid arthritis patients was 5.9±1.3 mg/l.

Furthermore, sera from 50 healthy controls (25 men and 25 women) were supplied by the Red Cross Blood Centre in Otsu, Japan.

All ankylosing spondylitis patients except one were HLA-B27 positive.

Some 93.3 % of the active rheumatoid arthritis patients possessed either HLA-DR1 or HL-DR4. Furthermore, some 40 % of the rheumatoid arthritis patients had both HLA-DR1 and DR4.

Control subjects were not tissue typed.

17.4 Results of ELISA Studies on Bacteria

ELISA studies were carried out as previously described against 3 different microbes: *Proteus mirabilis*, *Escherichia coli* and *Klebsiella pneumoniae.* All assays were carried out under code so that the status of each serum sample under investigation was not known to the tester.

Ankylosing spondylitis patients with active disease had elevated levels of IgA antibodies against *Klebsiella pneumoniae*, and this difference was statistically significant when compared to controls ($t = 5.72$, $p < 0.001$) (Fig. 17.1).

Active and inactive ankylosing spondylitis had no elevations in IgG or IgM antibodies against *Klebsiella pneumoniae.*

Inactive ankylosing spondylitis patients showed no elevations in IgA, IgG or IgM antibodies against *Klebsiella pneumoniae.*

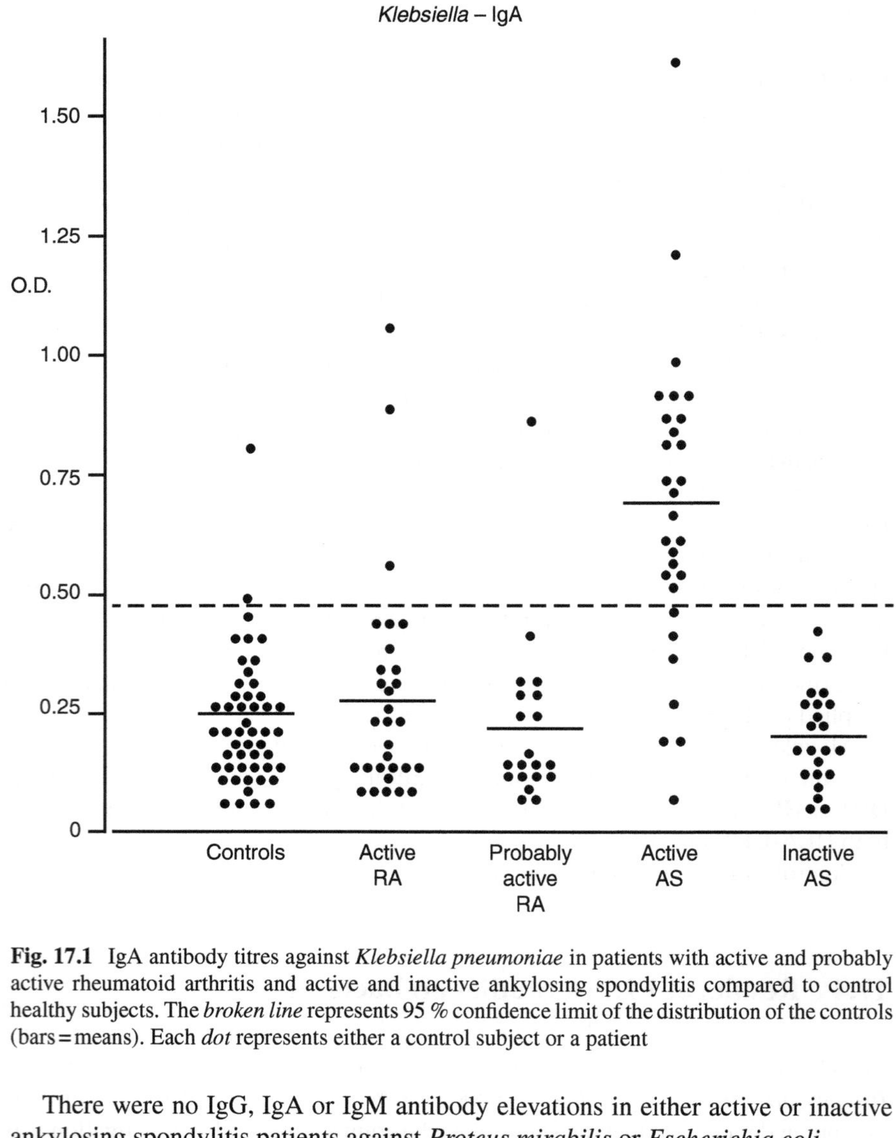

Fig. 17.1 IgA antibody titres against *Klebsiella pneumoniae* in patients with active and probably active rheumatoid arthritis and active and inactive ankylosing spondylitis compared to control healthy subjects. The *broken line* represents 95 % confidence limit of the distribution of the controls (bars = means). Each *dot* represents either a control subject or a patient

There were no IgG, IgA or IgM antibody elevations in either active or inactive ankylosing spondylitis patients against *Proteus mirabilis* or *Escherichia coli.*

Patients with active rheumatoid arthritis showed elevated levels of IgG antibodies against *Proteus mirabilis* when compared to controls, and this difference was statistically significant ($t = 14.10$, $p < 0.001$) (Fig. 17.2).

Similar results were seen in probably active rheumatoid arthritis patients when compared to controls, and this difference was also statistically significant ($t = 8.30$, $p < 0.001$).

Active rheumatoid arthritis patients also had elevated levels of IgM antibodies against *Proteus mirabilis* when compared to controls, and again, this difference was statistically significant ($t = 3.72$, $p < 0.001$).

Probably active rheumatoid arthritis patients did not exhibit IgM antibody elevations against *Proteus mirabilis.*

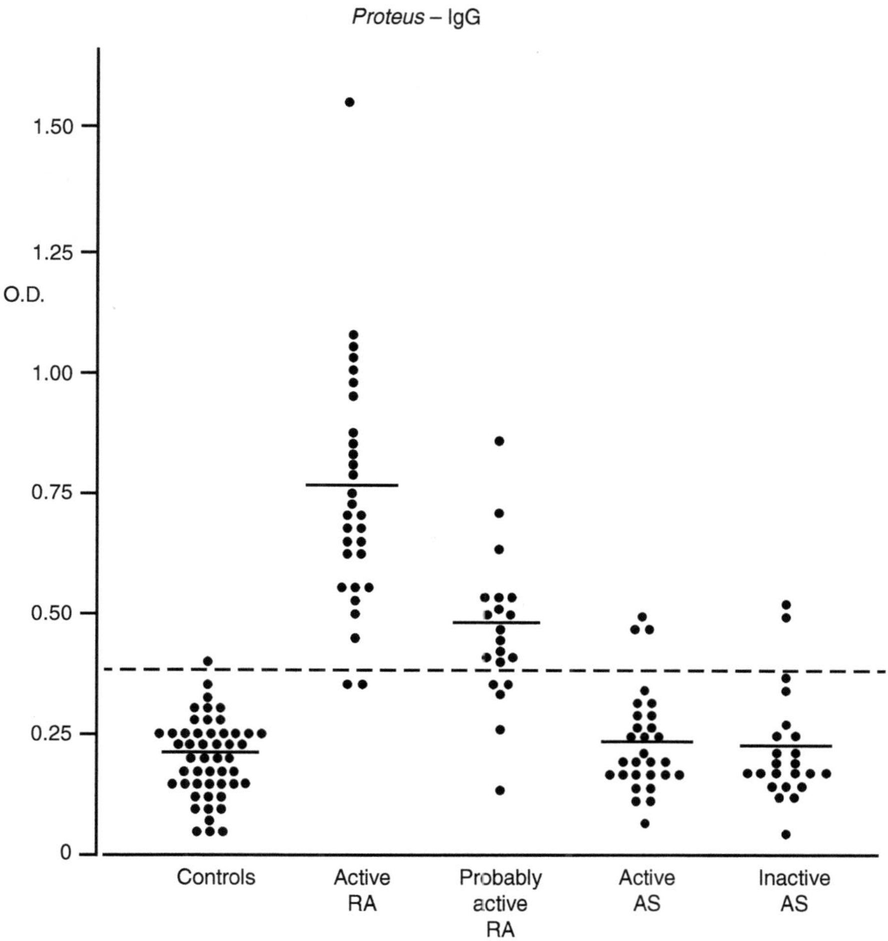

Fig. 17.2 IgG antibody titres against *Proteus mirabilis* in patients with active and probably active rheumatoid arthritis and active and inactive ankylosing spondylitis compared to healthy control subjects. The *broken line* represents 95 % confidence limit of the distribution of the controls (bars = means). Each *dot* represents either a control subject or a patient

There were no IgG, IgA or IgM antibody elevations in active or probably active rheumatoid arthritis patients when tested against *Klebsiella pneumoniae* or *Escherichia coli* bacteria.

17.5 Results of ELISA Studies on HLA-B27 and Pullulanase Peptide Sequences

Three 16-mer peptide sequences were constructed:

1. The HLA-B27 sequence (residues 67–83) CKAKAQ**DRED**LRTLL
2. The pullulanase-D (pulD) secretion protein (residues 590–605) RPTVIR**DRDE**YRQASS

3. Control peptide made from scrambled sequence of pulD RPTVRSDIDYRQAESR

All synthetic peptides were prepared by solid-phase synthesis; purity assays were performed by high-performance liquid chromatography. All had a purity of at least 90 %.

All assays against the three synthetic peptides were carried out by ELISA, as previously described and carried out under code, so that the status of each serum sample under investigation was not known to the tester.

17.5.1 Antibodies to the HLA-B27 Sequence

Active ankylosing spondylitis patients showed significant elevations in all antibody classes against the HLA-B27 peptide when compared to controls.

The mean IgG level optical density units (O.D. units) (mean ± standard error) against the HLA-B27 peptide in active ankylosing spondylitis patients was 0.446 ± 0.027 O.D. units, and this was significantly higher than the level of 0.159 ± 0.010 O.D. units found in control subjects ($t = 11.94$, $p < 0.001$) (Fig. 17.3).

The mean IgA level in active ankylosing spondylitis patients against the HLA-B27 peptide was 0.195 ± 0.012 O.D. units, and this was again significantly higher than the level of 0.076 ± 0.008 O.D. units found in control subjects ($t = 8.298$, $p < 0.001$).

The mean IgM level in active ankylosing spondylitis patients against the HLA-B27 peptide was 0.261 ± 0.018 O.D. units, and this was again statistically higher than the level of 0.136 ± 0.007 O.D. units found in control subjects ($t = 7.503$; $p < 0.001$).

Somewhat similar results were seen in inactive ankylosing spondylitis patients. The mean IgG level was 0.281 ± 0.024 O.D. units, and this was statistically higher than the level of 0.159 ± 0.010 O.D. units found in control subjects ($t = 5.908$, $p < 0.001$).

The mean IgA level in inactive ankylosing spondylitis patients was 0.161 ± 0.015 O.D. units, and this was statistically higher than the level of 0.076 ±0.008 O.D. units found in control subjects ($t = 5.775$, $p < 0.001$).

There was no statistically significant elevation in IgM antibodies in inactive ankylosing spondylitis patients against the HLA-B27 peptide when compared to controls.

There was also a small correlation between the IgG antibody levels to the HLA-B27 peptide and serum C-reactive protein ($r = +0.332$, $p < 0.05$), but there was no correlation with erythrocyte sedimentation rates.

There were no antibody elevations against the HLA-B27 peptide in active and inactive rheumatoid arthritis patients when compared to control subjects.

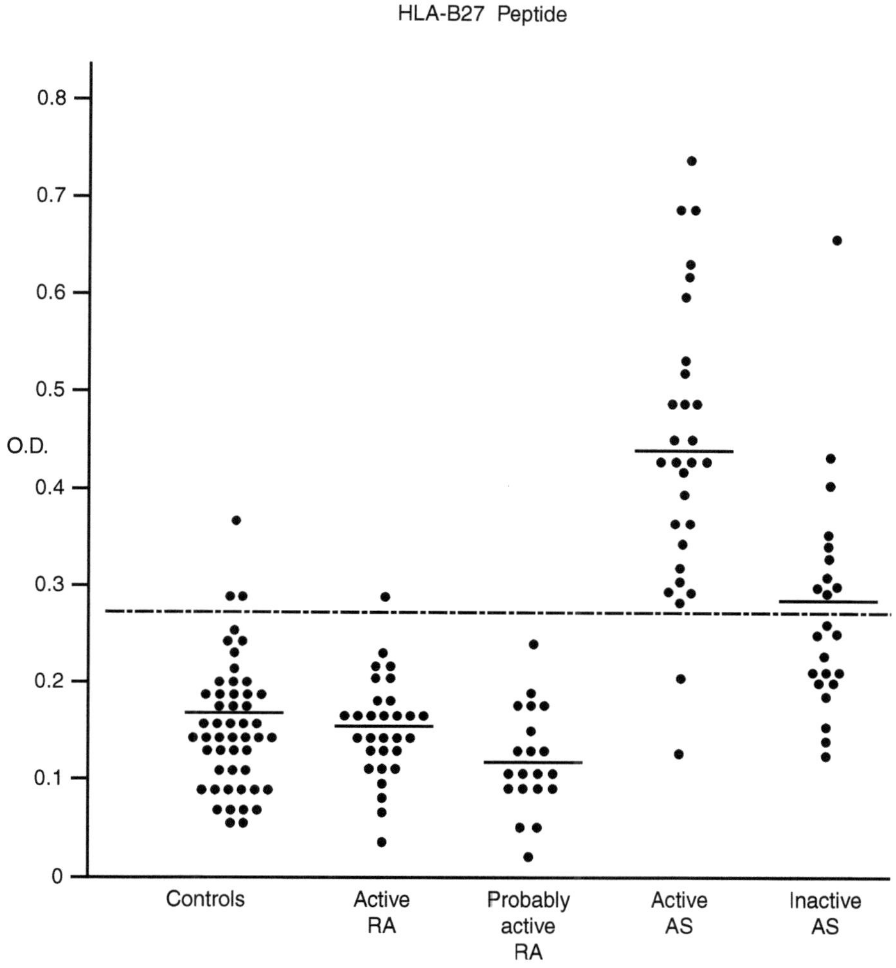

Fig. 17.3 IgG antibody titres against the HLA-B27 peptide in active and probably active rheumatoid arthritis patients and active and inactive ankylosing spondylitis patients compared to healthy control subjects. The *broken line* represents 95 % confidence limit of the distribution of the controls bars = means). Each *dot* represents either a control subject or a patient

17.5.2 Antibodies to the Pullulanase-D Peptide

Active ankylosing spondylitis patients showed significant elevations in IgG and IgA antibody but not IgM classes against the pullulanase-D peptide.

The mean IgG level against the pulD peptide in active ankylosing spondylitis patients was 0.505 ± 0.034 O.D. units, and this was significantly higher than the level of 0.215 ± 0.009 O.D. units found in control subjects ($t = 10.37$, $p < 0.001$) (Fig. 17.4).

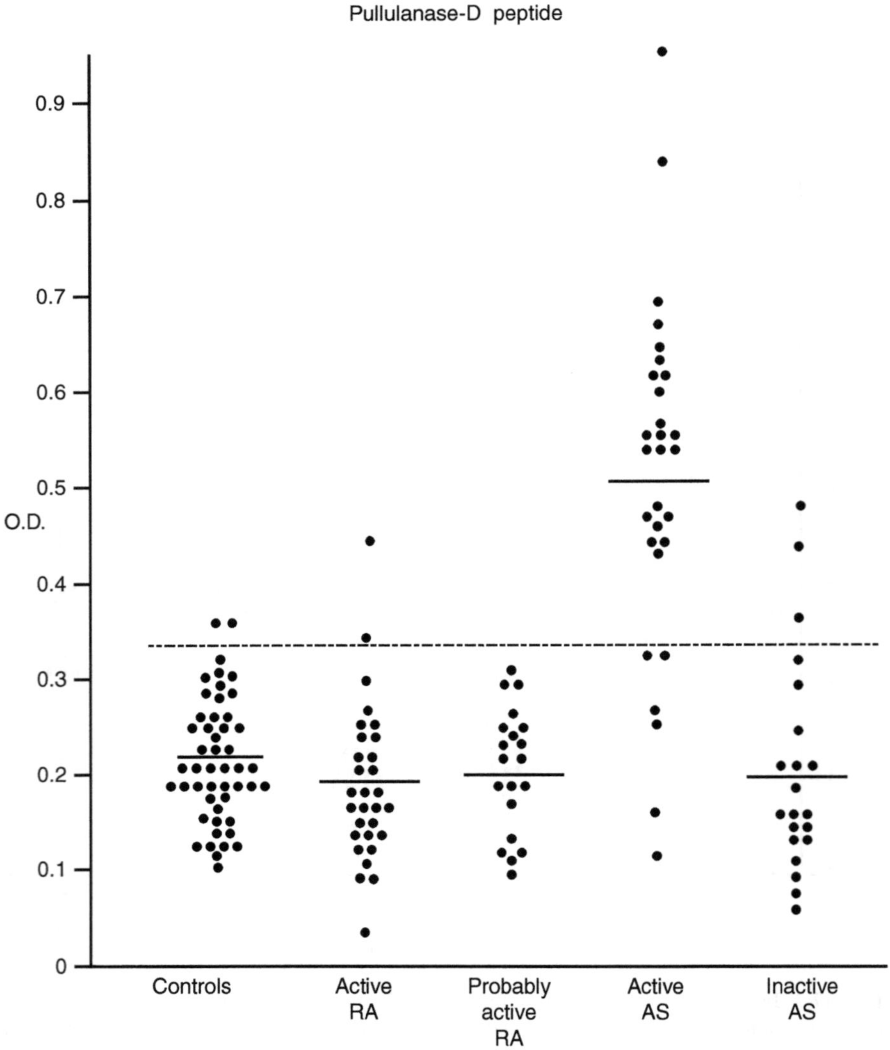

Fig. 17.4 IgG antibody titres against the pulD peptide in active and probably active rheumatoid arthritis patients and active and inactive ankylosing spondylitis patients compared to healthy control subjects. The *broken line* represents 95 % confidence limit of the distribution of the controls (bars = means). Each *dot* represents either a control subject or a patient

The mean IgA level against the pulD peptide in active ankylosing spondylitis patients was 0.224 ±0.035 O.D. units, and this was again significantly higher than the level of 0.064 ± 0.007 O.D. units found in control subjects ($t = 5.646$, $p < 0.001$).

There was also a significant correlation between the IgG antibody levels to pullulanase-D peptide and erythrocyte sedimentation rates ($r = +0.498$, $p < 0.001$) as well as C-reactive protein levels ($r = +0.426$, $p < 0.01$).

Furthermore, there was also a small correlation between IgA antibody levels to pullulanase-D peptide and erythrocyte sedimentation rates ($r = +0.339$, $p < 0.05$).

There were no antibody elevations against the pullulanase-D peptide in active and inactive rheumatoid arthritis patients when compared to control subjects.

17.5.3 Antibodies to Scrambled pulD Control Peptide

No antibody elevation of any class was seen against the control scrambled pulD peptide in ankylosing spondylitis patients or rheumatoid arthritis patients when compared to control subjects (Fig. 17.5).

17.6 Discussion and Conclusions

The data presented here show that there are specific and significant antibody elevations against *Klebsiella pneumoniae* in Japanese ankylosing spondylitis patients from Otsu in southern Japan.

These results would appear to be specific, since Japanese rheumatoid arthritis had antibody elevations against *Proteus mirabilis* but not against *Klebsiella pneumoniae*, whilst the reverse was observed with Japanese ankylosing spondylitis patients who had antibodies against *Klebsiella pneumoniae* but not against *Proteus mirabilis*.

This would appear to be the first time that Japanese ankylosing spondylitis patients have been found to have elevated levels of specific antibodies against the bowel microbe *Klebsiella pneumoniae* (Tani et al. 1997).

Similar Japanese studies have shown that antibodies to 'common enterobacterial antigens' are present in the serum and synovial fluids of patients with rheumatoid arthritis (Aoki et al. 1996).

These relationships between ankylosing spondylitis, rheumatoid arthritis and bacterial infections could be explained by cross-reactivity and molecular similarity in amino acid sequences between leucocyte HLA antigens and bacterial proteins (Ebringer and Wilson 2000).

In rheumatic fever, anti-*streptococcal* antibodies are associated with pathological damage to cardiac tissues (Zabriskie et al. 1970), and a similar mechanism could operate in ankylosing spondylitis in both Japanese and European patients.

Some 51 of the 52 Japanese ankylosing spondylitis patients were HLA-B27 positive, giving a percentage of 98 % HLA-B27 positivity in this disease. This is similar to the 96 % HLA-B27 positivity found in European ankylosing spondylitis patients. Clearly we are dealing with a condition which is characterised by the presence of the HLA-B27 marker.

Although the majority of HLA-B27 positive individuals do not have ankylosing spondylitis, when these individuals are exposed to *Klebsiella* bacteria, an inflammatory

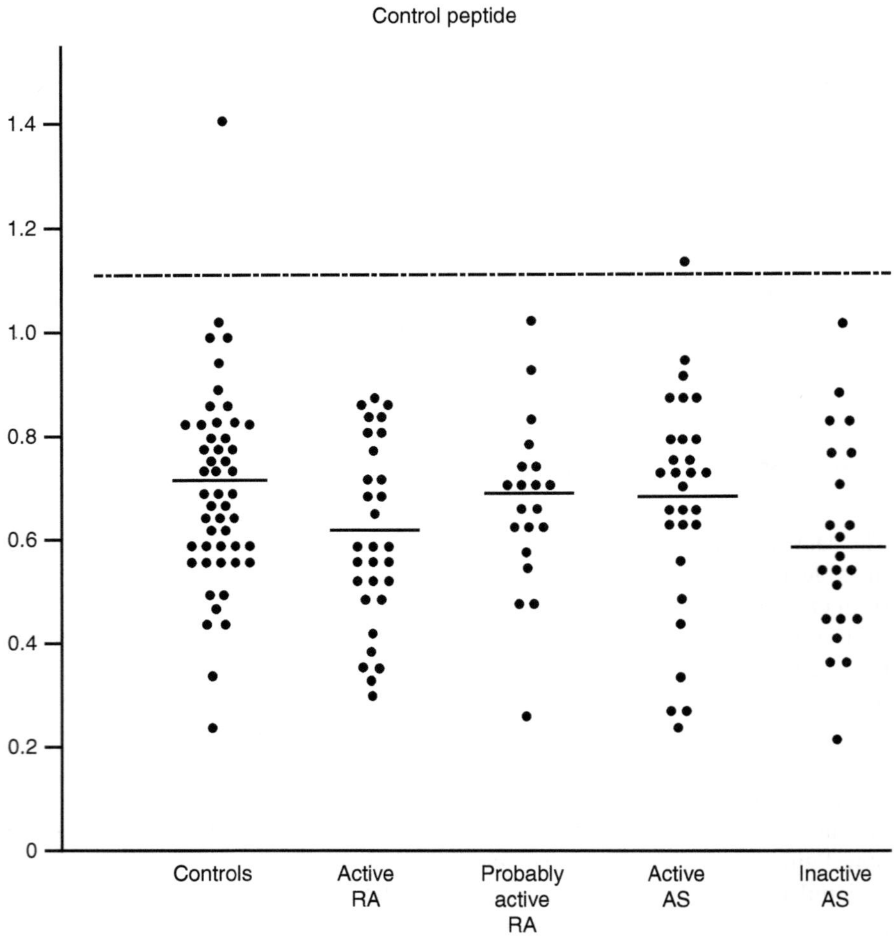

Fig. 17.5 IgG antibody titres against the control, scrambled pulD peptide in active and probably active rheumatoid arthritis patients and active and inactive ankylosing spondylitis patients compared to healthy control subjects. The *broken line* represents 95 % confidence limit of the distribution of the controls (bars = means). Each *dot* represents either a control subject or a patient

rheumatic disease develops, which can be called 'B27 disease' (Ebringer and Rashid 2007). Any patient presenting with vague symptoms of pains in large joints, backache and morning muscle stiffness should be tested for the presence of the HLA-B27 marker because this could influence therapy before irreversible bony changes develop in the lumbar spine and sacroiliac joints.

These results would seem to suggest that the Gram-negative microbe *Klebsiella pneumoniae* is somehow involved in the onset and pathogenesis of ankylosing spondylitis at least in Japanese patients coming from Otsu and surrounding areas.

Furthermore, Japanese ankylosing spondylitis patients have elevated levels of antibodies directed against both a specific HLA-B27 peptide and against the peptide from *Klebsiella* pullulanase which is an important debranching enzyme involved in providing substrates from dietary starch for bacterial growth in the colon.

Since rice is a common component of the Japanese diet, it raises the interesting question whether the low level of HLA-B27 found in Japan could be linked to the high consumption of dietary starch.

The results from these Japanese patients appear to be similar to those obtained from ankylosing spondylitis patients in European (Sahly and Podschun 1997) and American studies.

The general tentative conclusion can be proposed that *Klebsiella pneumoniae* is involved in the causation of ankylosing spondylitis in populations throughout the world.

References

Aoki S, Yoshikawa K, Yokoyama T, Nonogaki T, Wasaki S, Mitsui T, Niwa S. Role of enteric bacteria in the pathogenesis of rheumatoid arthritis: evidence for antibodies to enterobacterial common antigens in rheumatoid sera and synovial fluids. Ann Rheum Dis. 1996;55:363–9.

Ebringer A, Rashid T. "B27 disease" is a new autoimmune disease that affects millions of people. Ann N Y Acad Sci. 2007;1110:112–20.

Ebringer A, Wilson C. HLA molecules, bacteria and autoimmunity. J Med Microbiol. 2000; 49:305–11.

Sahly H, Podschun R. Clinical, bacteriological and serological aspects of *Klebsiella* infections and their spondylarthropathic sequelae. Clin Diagn Lab Immunol. 1997;4:393–9.

Sonozaki H, Seki H, Chang S, Okuyama M, Juji T. HLA-A27 in Japanese patients with ankylosing spondylitis. Tissue Antigens. 1975;5:131–6.

Tani Y, Tiwana H, Hukuda S, Nishioka J, Fielder M, Wilson C, Bansal S, Ebringer A. Antibodies to *Klebsiella, Proteus* and HLA-B27 peptides in Japanese patients with ankylosing spondylitis and rheumatoid arthritis. J Rheumatol. 1997;24:109–14.

Tujimoto M. Epidemiological research on the prevalence of ankylosing spondylitis. Med J Osaka Univ. 1978;28:363–81.

Zabriskie JB, Hsu KC, Seegal BC. Heart reactive antibody associated with rheumatic fever: characterization and diagnostic significance. Clin Exp Immunol. 1970;7:147–59.

Chapter 18
Ankylosing Spondylitis Sera Are Cytotoxic to Cells Bearing HLA-B27 Sequences

18.1 Introduction: The Association of HLA-B27 with the *Klebsiella* Nitrogenase and *Klebsiella* Pullulanase Enzymes

Ankylosing spondylitis is a chronic inflammatory disorder affecting predominantly the lumbar spine where 95 % of patients are HLA-B27 positive. Increased levels of antibodies to the gut microbe *Klebsiella pneumoniae* have been reported, suggesting an aetiological role for this microbe in the pathogenesis of this disease. Sera from patients with this condition have been investigated in cytotoxicity studies, and sera from patients with rheumatoid arthritis have been used as 'disease controls' together with sera obtained from healthy blood donor subjects.

Amino acid sequence homologies have been identified between HLA-B*2705 (QTDRED) and two enzymes present in *Klebsiella pneumoniae* nitrogenase reductase (QTDRED) and pullulanase secretion protein pulD (DRDE) (Fielder et al. 1995).

Patients with active ankylosing spondylitis have been shown to have elevated levels of antibodies to all three peptide sequences compared to control groups.

The cytotoxic activity of sera from ankylosing spondylitis and rheumatoid arthritis patients has been investigated to determine whether tissue-damaging properties were present in patients when compared to sera obtained from healthy individuals.

We have reported that rheumatoid arthritis patients with active disease have elevated levels of antibodies to the urinary microbe *Proteus mirabilis*, and this has been confirmed by several independent groups, one from the UK (Senior et al. 1995) and another one from the USA (Newkirk et al. 2005).

Amino acid homologies and immunological cross-reactivity between the susceptibility motif EQR(K)RAA and *Proteus mirabilis* haemolysin ESRRAL as well as type XI collagen LRREI and *Proteus mirabilis* urease IRRET have been demonstrated in studies from the Immunology Unit at King's College in London. We have used sera from rheumatoid arthritis patients as 'disease controls' in studying the cytotoxic properties of ankylosing spondylitis sera.

A. Ebringer, *Ankylosing Spondylitis and Klebsiella*,
DOI 10.1007/978-1-4471-4300-0_18,

18.2 Antibodies to *Klebsiella* Nitrogenase Reductase in Patients with Ankylosing Spondylitis

The variable region of HLA-B27 peptide contains the sequence QTDRED (residues 72–77) which is also found in *Klebsiella pneumoniae* nitrogenase reductase (residues 188–193) (Schwimmbeck et al. 1987). Although it has been suggested that the inducible *Klebsiella* nitrogenase enzyme is unlikely to be found in microbes at body temperature, we have measured antibodies to it in patients with ankylosing spondylitis.

Antibody elevations were measured against the KP2 component of *Klebsiella pneumoniae* nitrogenase reductase which contains the QTDRED sequence. The KP2 component was kindly provided by Dr. M. Buck of the Nitrogen Fixation Laboratory, Sussex University, and had been prepared as previously described (Eady et al. 1972).

Serum samples were obtained from 100 English ankylosing spondylitis patients attending the 'Ankylosing Spondylitis Research Clinic of the Middlesex Hospital' and compared to 50 rheumatoid arthritis patients attending the Rheumatology Department at the Lister Hospital, Stevenage, and 50 control sera provided by the Blood Transfusion Service in London.

The groups examined were as follows: 100 patients with ankylosing spondylitis (71 male, 29 female; mean age 47 years), 50 rheumatoid arthritis patients (15 male, 35 female; mean age 57 years) and 50 healthy control subjects (30 male, 20 female; mean age 44 years).

Antibody levels against the KP2 component of the *Klebsiella pneumoniae* nitrogenase reductase were measured by 'enzyme-linked immunosorbent assay' (ELISA). All assays were carried out under code, so that the status of each serum sample under investigation was not known to the tester (Ahmadi et al. 1998). C-reactive protein levels were determined as previously described.

The mean (± standard error of the mean) IgG antibody level to the KP2 component in ankylosing spondylitis patients was 0.32 ± 0.01 OD (optical density at 630 nm) units, and this was significantly higher than the level of 0.22 ± 0.01 OD units found in control subjects ($t = 6.12$; $p < 0.001$) or the level of 0.25 ± 0.01 OD units found in rheumatoid arthritis patients ($t = 4.33$; $p < 0.001$).

The mean IgA antibody level to the KP2 component in ankylosing spondylitis patients was 0.42 ± 0.02 OD units, and this was significantly higher than the level of 0.15 ± 0.02 OD units found in control subjects ($t = 8.84$; $p < 0.001$) or the level of 0.17 ± 0.02 OD units found in rheumatoid arthritis patients ($t = 7.97$; $p < 0.001$).

However, there was no significant elevation in IgM antibody concentrations against the *Klebsiella* nitrogenase protein in ankylosing spondylitis patients.

The rheumatoid arthritis patients showed no significant antibody increases against the KP2 component in all immunoglobulin classes IgG, IgA or IgM with respect to control subjects.

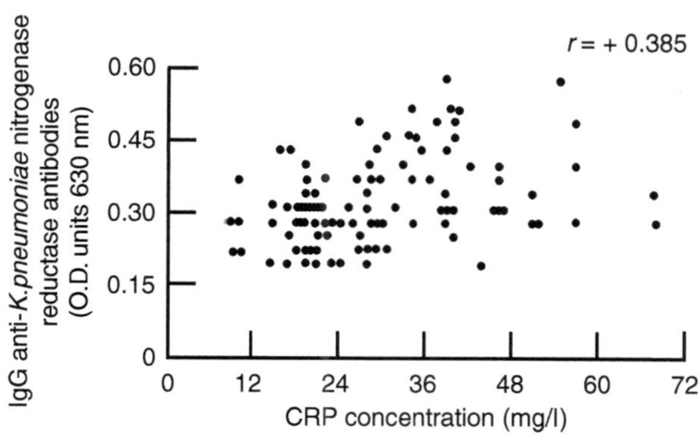

Fig. 18.1 Correlation analysis between class-specific IgG anti-*Klebsiella pneumoniae* (KP2) nitrogenase reductase antibodies and C-reactive protein concentrations in serum of ankylosing spondylitis patients

There was a significant correlation between IgG anti-*Klebsiella pneumoniae* nitrogenase reductase and the level of C-reactive protein in the ankylosing spondylitis patients ($r = +0.385$; $p < 0.001$) (Fig. 18.1) as well as between IgA anti-*Klebsiella pneumoniae* nitrogenase reductase and C-reactive protein ($r = +0.442$; $p < 0.001$) (Fig. 18.2).

However, there was no correlation between any antibody levels and C-reactive protein in the rheumatoid arthritis patients.

These results suggest that ankylosing spondylitis patients may have also been exposed to the *Klebsiella* nitrogenase reductase enzyme as well as to the *Klebsiella* pullulanase enzyme.

Clearly both the *Klebsiella* nitrogenase reductase enzyme and the *Klebsiella* pullulanase enzyme could contribute to the anti-HLA-B27 immunological activity found in ankylosing spondylitis patients.

18.3 Sera from Ankylosing Spondylitis and Rheumatoid Arthritis Patients

The cytotoxicity studies were carried out in the following patients.

There were 34 patients with ankylosing spondylitis, diagnosed by the New York criteria, attending the 'Ankylosing Spondylitis Research Clinic of the Middlesex Hospital', 26 men and 8 women with a mean age of 46 years (range: 23–69 years). Their mean (± standard error) erythrocyte sedimentation rate was 48.2 ± 3.7 mm/h.

Sera were also collected from patients with active rheumatoid arthritis, (erythrocyte sedimentation rate > 15 mm/h) attending the Department of Rheumatology at the Lister Hospital in Stevenage.

The diagnosis of rheumatoid arthritis was made according to the American Rheumatism Criteria.

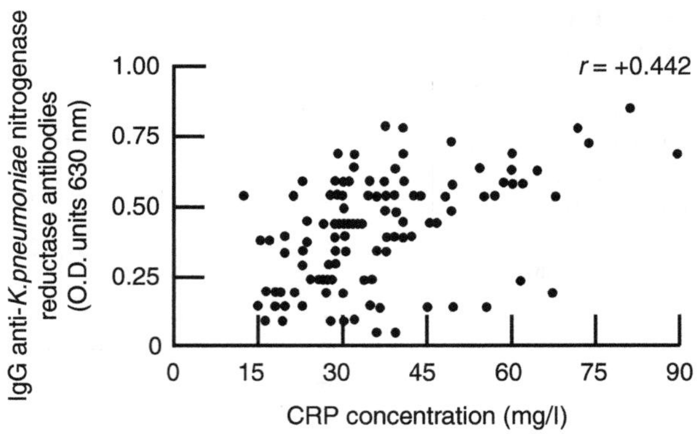

Fig. 18.2 Correlation analysis between class-specific IgA anti-*Klebsiella pneumoniae* (KP2) nitrogenase reductase antibodies and C-reactive protein concentrations in serum of ankylosing spondylitis patients

There were 51 patients with rheumatoid arthritis, 18 men and 33 women with a mean age of 49 years (range: 28–70 years). Their mean (± standard error) erythrocyte sedimentation rate was 45.4 ± 9.6 mm/h.

Sera were also obtained from 38 healthy blood donors, 18 men and 28 women with a mean age of 40 years (range: 24–57 years).

Antibodies against synthetic peptides 15/16 mer peptides containing ESRRAL, EQRRAA, LRREI, IRRET, EDERAA, QTDRED and DRED as well as control sequences were measured in the sera obtained from ankylosing spondylitis and rheumatoid arthritis patients.

18.4 Synthetic Peptides and ELISA

Peptides were prepared by solid-phase synthesis and analysed for purity by high-performance liquid chromatography as previously described. All peptides had at least 90 % purity. The molecular mimicry sequences are shown in bold.

The test peptides were:

1. SQKDLL**EQRRAA**VDTY of HLA-DRB1*0404
2. LGSS**ESRRAL**QDSQR of *Proteus mirabilis* haemolysin
3. QSLDS**LRREI**EQMRR of type XI collagen
4. FAESR**IRRET**IAAED of *Proteus mirabilis* urease
5. Control peptide SQKDIL**EDERAA**VDTY of HLA-DRB1*0402
6. CKAKA**QTDRED**LRTLL of HLA-B*2705
7. RPTVIR**DRDE**YRQASS of *Klebsiella pneumoniae* pullulanase
8. ASLEHEEGKILRAQLE of human myosin
9. KKLTEKEAELQAKLE of *Streptococcus pyogenes*
10. LGSISRSELARQDSQR of scrambled haemolysin
11. RPTVRSDIDYRQAESR of scrambled pullulanase

The ELISA was carried out as previously described.

All assays were carried out in duplicate and under code, so that the status of each serum sample under investigation was not known to the tester.

18.5 Antibodies to Peptide Antigens in Ankylosing Spondylitis Patients

18.5.1 Antibodies to the HLA-B27 Peptide

Levels of IgG antibodies to the HLA-B27 peptide CKAKAQ**QTDRED**LRTLL in ankylosing spondylitis patients were significantly elevated compared to rheumatoid arthritis patients and healthy blood donor controls.

The mean (± standard error) in ankylosing spondylitis patients was 0.491 ± 0.011 OD units, and this was significantly greater than the level of 0.181 ± 0.012 OD units found in rheumatoid arthritis patients ($t = 18.52$, $p < 0.0001$) or the level of 0.223 ± 0.015 OD units ($t = 14.15$, $p < 0.0001$) found in healthy controls.

There was no significant difference in the level of antibodies to the HLA-B27 peptide between rheumatoid arthritis patients and healthy blood donors.

18.5.2 Antibodies to the Klebsiella pneumoniae Nitrogenase Peptide

Levels of IgG antibodies to the *Klebsiella pneumoniae* nitrogenase peptide CNSR**QTDRED**ELIIA were significantly elevated in ankylosing spondylitis patients compared to rheumatoid arthritis patients and healthy blood donors.

The mean (± standard error) in ankylosing spondylitis patients was 0.529 ± 0.011 OD units, and this was significantly greater than the level of 0.197 ± 0.012 OD units found in rheumatoid arthritis patients ($t = 18.89$, $p < 0.0001$) or the level of 0.233 ± 0.014 OD units ($t = 15.96$, $p < 0.0001$) found in healthy controls. There was no significant difference in the level of antibodies to the *Klebsiella pneumoniae* nitrogenase peptide between rheumatoid arthritis patients and healthy blood donors.

18.5.3 Antibodies to the Klebsiella pneumoniae Pullulanase Peptide

Levels of IgG antibodies to the *Klebsiella pneumoniae* pullulanase peptide RPTVIR**DRDE**YRQASS were significantly elevated in ankylosing spondylitis patients compared to rheumatoid arthritis and healthy blood donors.

The mean (± standard error) in ankylosing spondylitis patients was 0.530 ± 0.010 OD units, and this was significantly greater than the level of 0.183 ± 0.0.012 OD units found in rheumatoid arthritis patients ($t = 20.15$, $p < 0.0001$) or the level of 0.218 ± 0.016 OD units ($t = 16.32$, $p < 0.0001$) found in healthy controls.

There was no significant difference in the level of antibodies to the *Klebsiella pneumoniae* pullulanase peptide between rheumatoid arthritis patients and healthy blood donors.

There was no significant reactivity of rheumatoid arthritis and ankylosing spondylitis sera when compared to the sera from healthy blood donors to the following peptides from: human myosin, *Streptococcus pyogenes* and the scrambled peptides from haemolysin or pullulanase.

18.6 Antibodies to Peptide Antigens in Rheumatoid Arthritis Patients

*18.6.1 HLA-DRB1*0404 Peptide*

The levels of IgG antibodies to the HLA-DRB1*0404 peptide SQKDLL**EQRRAA**VDTY of the IgG class were significantly elevated in rheumatoid arthritis patients when compared to ankylosing spondylitis patients or healthy controls. The mean (± standard error) level in rheumatoid arthritis patients was 0.537 ± 0.013 OD units, and this was significantly higher than the level of 0.134 ± 0.006 OD units found in ankylosing spondylitis patients (t=23.65, p<0.0001) or the level of 0.152 ± 0.010 OD units found in healthy controls (t=21.62, p<0.0001).

There was no significant difference between ankylosing spondylitis patients and healthy controls when tested against the DRB1*0404 peptide.

18.6.2 Proteus mirabilis Haemolysin Peptide

The levels of IgG antibodies to the *Proteus mirabilis* haemolysin peptide LGSIS**ESRRAL**QDSQR were significantly elevated in rheumatoid arthritis patients when compared to ankylosing spondylitis patients or healthy controls. The mean (± standard error) level in rheumatoid arthritis patients was 0.590 ± 0.015 OD units, and this was significantly higher than the level of 0.155 ± 0.008 OD units found in ankylosing spondylitis patients (t=22.17, p<0.0001) or the level of 0.170 ± 0.010 found in healthy controls (t=21.38, p<0.0001). There was no significant difference between ankylosing spondylitis patients and healthy controls when tested against the *Proteus mirabilis* haemolysin peptide.

18.6.3 Type XI Collagen Peptide

The levels of IgG antibodies to the type XI collagen peptide GSLD**LRREI**EQMRR were significantly elevated in rheumatoid arthritis patients when compared to the ankylosing spondylitis or healthy controls.

The mean (± standard error) level in rheumatoid arthritis patients was 0.490 ± 0.009 OD units, and this was significantly higher than the level of 0.133 ± 0.007 OD units found in ankylosing spondylitis patients ($t = 30.08$, $p < 0.0001$) or the level of 0.136 ± 0.007 OD units found in healthy controls ($t = 26.17$, $p < 0.0001$).

There was no significant difference between the ankylosing spondylitis patients and healthy controls when tested against the type XI collagen peptide.

18.7 Preparation of Sheep Red Blood Cells for Cytotoxicity Assay

A 20-ml aliquot of sheep blood (Unipath Ltd, Hampshire, UK) was washed twice with 0.85 % sodium chloride (saline) solution in a centrifuge (Heraeus, minifuge) at 750 × g (3,000 rpm) for 15 min.

Supernatant was discarded, and 600 μl of the packed cells were removed and placed into each of 2 universal containers. The cells in each container were resuspended in 10-ml saline, and 10 ml of a 1/20,000 tannic acid (Aldrich Chemical Co, Dover, UK) in saline was added to each container, followed by mixing and incubation for 15 min at 37 °C in a water bath. After centrifugation for 5 min, the supernatant was discarded, and cells were resuspended in 20 ml saline and washed. One container was later used as a negative control.

The cells in the other container were resuspended in 10-ml saline, and 10-ml antigen (2 mg/ml) was added, followed by mixing and incubation for 30 min at 37 °C in a water bath. After washing by centrifugation for 5 min, the supernatant was discarded; the cells were washed three times with saline and both coated and uncoated (control) cells resuspended in 50 ml of saline.

Serum samples were inactivated in a water bath at 56 °C for 30 min.

The cytotoxicity assay was carried out as follows: 100 ml of serum diluted 1/8 in saline was added to 96-well microtitre plates (Dynatech) together with 100 μl of peptide-coated sheep red blood cells, and the plates were incubated at 37 °C for 30 min. A 100-μl aliquot of guinea pig complement (Calbiochem Ltd., Nottingham, UK) diluted 1/10 in saline was added followed by mixing, then incubation at 37 °C for 30 min and later at 4 °C overnight to allow the unlysed cells to settle.

A 100-μl aliquot of test supernatant was removed and placed into wells of a microtitre plate and absorbance measured 570 nm.

Minimum lysis was calculated from peptide coated cells treated with saline plus complement, and absorbance value obtained from the minimum lysis was subtracted from each test value. One hundred percent lysis was calculated from 100 μl of uncoated cells treated with 200 μl of distilled water, and this was labelled as 'maximum lysis'.

Percentage lysis was determined using the following formula:

$$\% \text{ Lysis} = \frac{(\text{Test lysis} - \text{Minimum lysis})}{(\text{Maximum lysis} - \text{Minimum lysis})} \times 100$$

All assays were carried in duplicate and under code, in that the tester did not know which sera came from patients or control subjects.

18.8 Cytotoxicity Studies in Ankylosing Spondylitis Patients

Sera from ankylosing spondylitis and rheumatoid arthritis patients, as well as sera from healthy controls, were tested for complement-mediated cytotoxicity against sheep red cells coated with HLA-B27*2705 synthetic peptide.

The sera from ankylosing spondylitis patients showed significantly higher percentage lysis for sheep red blood cells coated with CKAKA**QTDRED**LRTLL of HLA-B*2705 peptide when compared to rheumatoid arthritis patients or healthy controls (Fig. 18.3).

The mean (± standard error) percentage lysis in ankylosing spondylitis patients was 69.2±3.1 %, and this was significantly higher than the level found in rheumatoid arthritis patients which was 14.8±1.1 % (t=19.28, p<0.0001) or the level of 16.3±1.4 % (t=16.13, p<0.0001) found in healthy blood donors (Wilson et al. 2003).

There was no significant difference in the cytotoxic activity of rheumatoid arthritis sera or the ones obtained from healthy donors when tested against sheep red blood cells coated with the HLA-B*2705 peptide.

No significant differences were found between ankylosing spondylitis and rheumatoid arthritis patients or healthy controls when testing sheep red blood cells coated with either human myosin, haemolysin-scrambled or pullulanase-scrambled peptides.

There was a significant correlation between anti-nitrogenase antibodies and percentage lysis of sheep red blood cells coated with HLA-B*2705 (QTDRED) peptides for the ankylosing spondylitis and rheumatoid arthritis as well as the healthy control subjects (r=+0.826, p<0.0001) (Fig. 18.4).

There was also a significant correlation between anti-pullulanase (DRDE) antibodies and percentage lysis of sheep red blood cells coated with HLA-B*2705 (QTDRED) peptide for the ankylosing spondylitis and rheumatoid arthritis patients as well as the healthy control subjects (r=+0.823, p<0.0001) (Fig. 18.5).

There was also a significant correlation between anti-HLA-B*2705 antibodies and percentage lysis of sheep red blood cells coated with HLA-B*2705 (QTDRED) peptide for the ankylosing spondylitis and rheumatoid arthritis patients as well as the healthy control subjects (r=+0.817, p<0.0001).

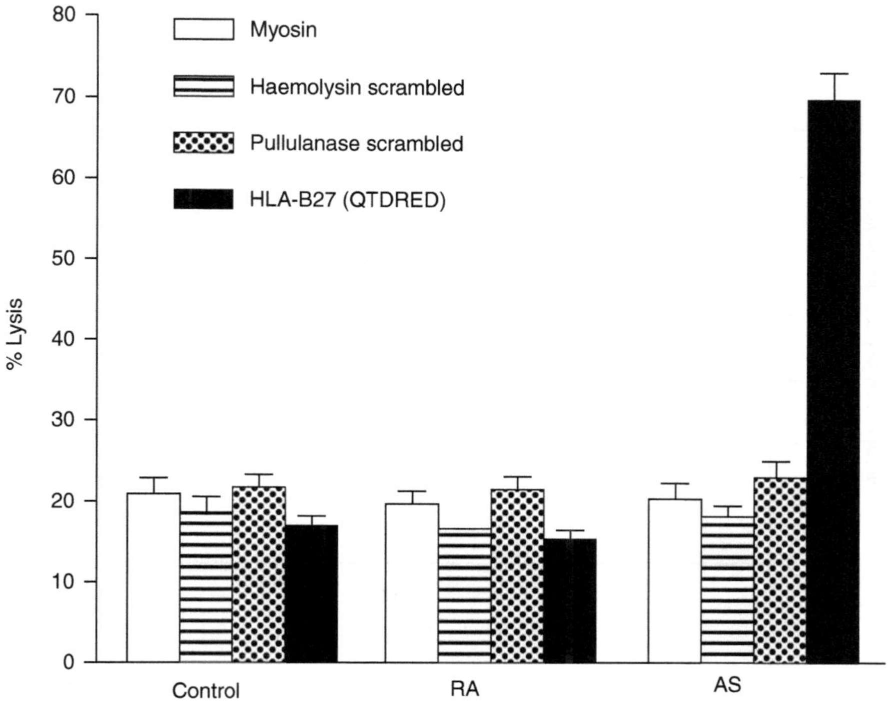

Fig. 18.3 Percentage lysis of sheep red blood cells coated with HLA-B27 peptide (QTDRED) and other peptides via complement-mediated cytotoxicity by control sera and sera from patients with rheumatoid arthritis (*RA*) and ankylosing spondylitis (*AS*)

18.9 Cytotoxicity Studies in Rheumatoid Arthritis Patients

Sera from rheumatoid arthritis and ankylosing spondylitis patients as well as sera from healthy blood donors were tested for reactivity in a complement-mediated cytotoxicity assay with sheep red blood cells coated with HLA-DRB1*0402 (EDERAA) peptide, type XI collagen (LRREI) peptide and HLA-DRB1*0404 (EQRRAA) peptide (Fig. 18.6).

18.9.1 EQRRAA Peptide

The sera from rheumatoid arthritis patients showed significantly higher levels of cytotoxic activity against sheep red blood cells coated with SQKDLL**EQRRAA**VDTY from HLA-DRB1*0404 when compared to ankylosing

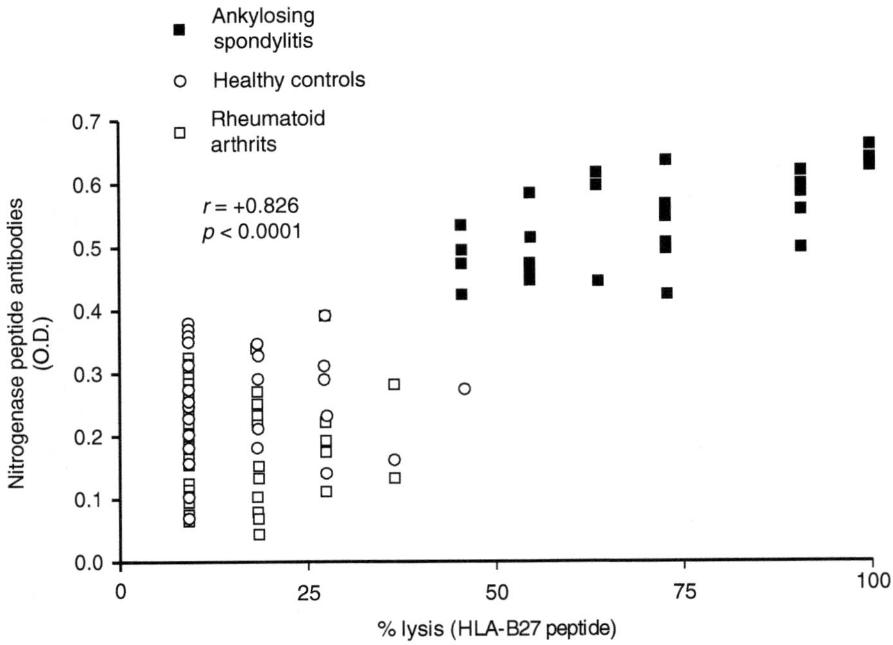

Fig. 18.4 Correlation of anti-*Klebsiella* nitrogenase peptide IgG antibody levels for ankylosing spondylitis and rheumatoid arthritis patients and controls with percentage lysis of sheep red blood cells coated with HLA-B27 peptide

spondylitis patients or healthy controls. The mean (± standard error) percentage lysis in rheumatoid arthritis patients was 83.3±2.2 %, and this was significantly higher than the level 13.7±0.8 % found in ankylosing spondylitis patients (t=25.63, p<0.0001) or the level of 15.5±1.2 % (t=25.06, p<0.0001) found in healthy controls.

There was no significant difference in the cytotoxic activity of the ankylosing spondylitis sera or the ones obtained from healthy controls, when tested against sheep red blood cells coated with the HLA-DRB1*0404 (EQRRAA) peptide.

18.9.2 LRREI Peptide

The sera from rheumatoid arthritis patients showed significantly higher levels of cytotoxic activity against sheep red blood cells coated with GSLDS**LRREI**EQMRR from type XI collagen when compared to ankylosing spondylitis patients or healthy controls.

The mean (± standard error) percentage lysis in rheumatoid arthritis patients was 65.7±2.2 %, and this was significantly higher than the level of 11.5±0.9 % found in ankylosing spondylitis patients (t=19.16, p<0.0001) or the level of 13.7±1.3 % found in healthy controls (t=18.43, p<0.0001).

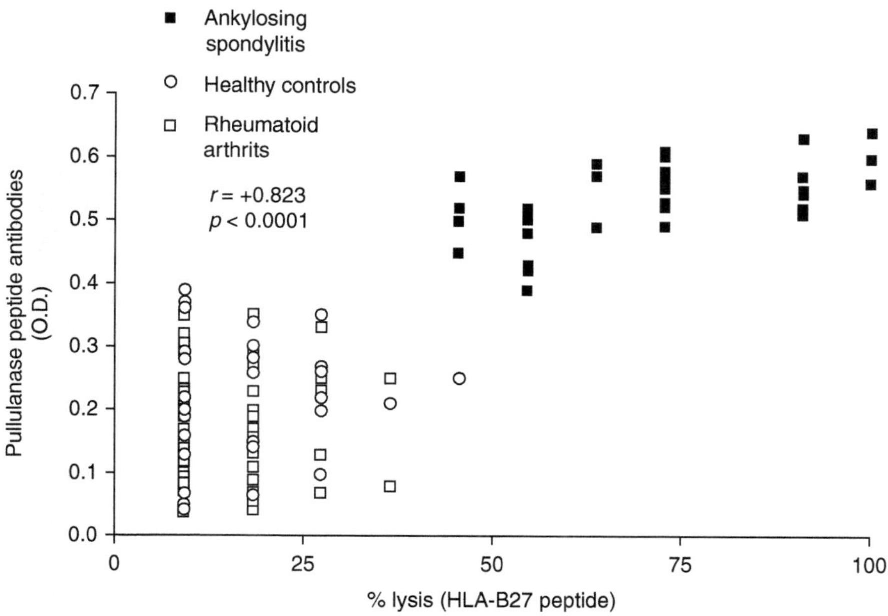

Fig. 18.5 Correlation of anti-*Klebsiella* pullulanase peptide IgG antibody levels for ankylosing spondylitis and rheumatoid arthritis patients and controls with percentage lysis of sheep red blood cells coated with HLA-B27 peptide

There was no significant difference in the cytotoxic activity of the ankylosing spondylitis sera or the ones obtained from healthy controls when tested against sheep red blood cells coated with the type XI collagen peptide.

18.9.3 EDERAA Peptide

There was no significant cytotoxic reactivity against sheep red blood cells coated with SQKDIL**EDERAA**VDTY of HLA-DRB1*0402 in the rheumatoid arthritis or ankylosing spondylitis sera when compared to sera from healthy blood donors.

18.10 Discussion and Conclusions

Ankylosing spondylitis patients have been shown to have increased levels of antibodies against synthetic peptides derived from *Klebsiella pneumoniae* and HLA-B*2705, and there was significant correlation between anti-HLA-B*2705 antibodies and percentage lysis of sheep red cells coated with HLA-B*2705 peptide.

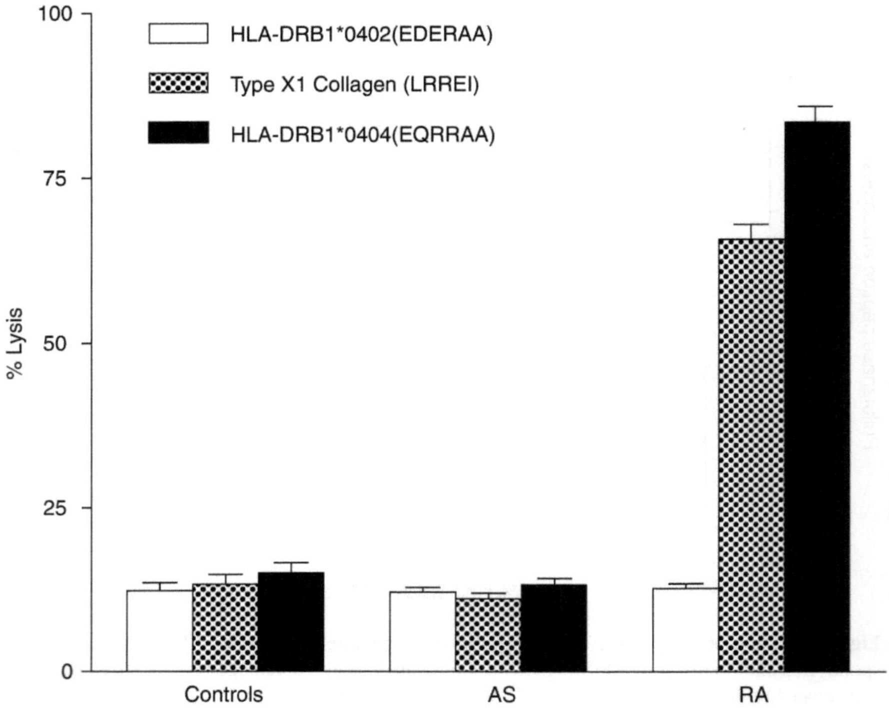

Fig. 18.6 Percentage lysis of sheep red blood cells coated with HLA-DRB1*0404 (EQRRAA), 0402 (EDERAA) and type XI collagen (LRREI) peptides via complement-mediated cytotoxicity by control sera and sera from patients with ankylosing spondylitis (*AS*) and rheumatoid arthritis (*RA*)

Furthermore, there was a significant correlation between cytotoxic activity against sheep red cells coated with HLA-B*2705 peptide and antibodies to both *Klebsiella* nitrogenase reductase and *Klebsiella* pullulanase enzymes. Studies with overlapping peptides from *Klebsiella pneumoniae* nitrogenase reductase involving the epitope KAKAQTDR proximal to the NH2 terminus of QTDRED had previously been shown to have increased antibody activity in HLA-B27-positive ankylosing spondylitis patients (Ewing et al. 1990).

A similar situation is known to occur in rheumatic fever, where anti-*streptococcal* antibodies have been found to be cytotoxic for heart and fibroblast cell lines, because of molecular similarity between the *streptococcal* M protein and human cardiac myosin (Cunningham et al. 1992).

The sera from ankylosing spondylitis and rheumatoid arthritis patients used in our studies were deemed to be active in that their erythrocyte sedimentation rates were elevated. The high levels of *Proteus mirabilis* haemolysin, urease, HLA-DRB1*0404 and type XI collagen peptide antibodies were not due to non-specific effects of inflammation because although ankylosing spondylitis patients were active, their levels of antibodies were similar to those found in healthy control subjects.

Similarly, rheumatoid arthritis patients have been shown to have increased levels of antibodies against synthetic peptides derived from *Proteus mirabilis* haemolysin (ESRRAL), HLA-DRB*0404 (EQRRAA), type XI collagen (LRREI) and *Proteus mirabilis* urease (IRRET).

However, we were unable to find any significant increase in levels of antibodies to HLA-DRB1*0402 (EDERAA) peptide, a histocompatibility group not linked to rheumatoid arthritis.

The pathological sequence in ankylosing spondylitis patients could be summarised as follows: Anti-*Klebsiella* antibodies bind to HLA-B27 chondrocytes and, in presence of high concentration of antibodies, activate the complement cascade and eventually cause tissue damage.

HLA-B27 epitope ► *Klebsiella* infection in the gut ► Anti-*Klebsiella* antibodies ► Joint damage involving collagens I and IV

Antibodies against type I collagen would target the large joints and spine giving rise to enthesitis whilst antibodies to collagen IV would target the uvea and produce acute anterior uveitis.

Sera from rabbits immunised with whole *Klebsiella* microorganisms were found to bind labelled vitreous humour antigens (Avakian et al. 1981). Radioimmunoassay of calf and cow vitreous humour could be inhibited by *Klebsiella* ultrasonicates thereby suggesting that microbial antigens may resemble some eyeball components (Welsh et al., 1981). Increased isolation of faecal *Klebsiella* was demonstrated in the first 2 weeks after the onset of uveitis symptoms (White et al., 1984). It was suggested that acute anterior uveitis of ankylosing spondylitis could be produced by some Gram-negative bacteria such as *Klebsiella*.

The bacterial antigens carrying the shared sequences to HLA-B27 will be immunogenic especially around the edges of the shared sequences because it is at these sites that the immune system will not recognise that it is dealing with a self antigen.

If for instance the bacterial shared sequence QTDRED is spanning residues of the nitrogenase molecule, then the edge antigenic pentamer, 187-188-189-190-191, will not be recognised as a self antigen, because of the haptenic effect of the nonself amino acid at position 187.

The antibodies produced against such an edge determinant, however, may well bind to HLA-B27. There is no breakdown of tolerance, and the evocation of bacterial antibodies having antiself or autoimmune activity is part of the immune normal when encountering partially cross-reacting antigens (Ebringer 1992).

When present in small quantities, such antibodies would not activate the complement cascade because two adjacent Fc portions of immunoglobulins are necessary for initiation of complement activity.

Therefore, there will be no cytotoxic event and thus no inflammation. However, when such antibodies are present in high concentrations, they could activate the complement cascade with consequent development of inflammation that will result in localised tissue damage and fibrosis, especially in the entheses around the lumbar spine and sacroiliac joints (Fig. 18.7).

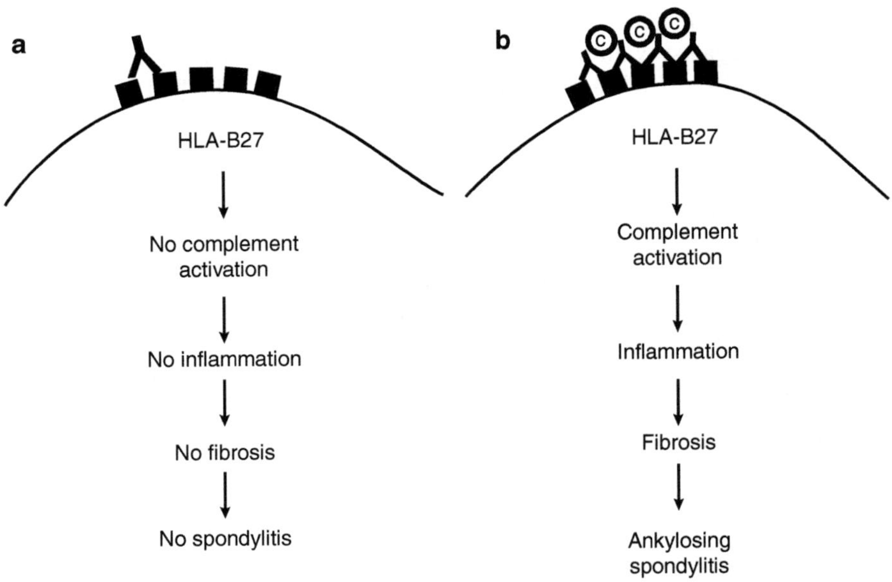

Fig. 18.7 (**a**) Anti-*Klebsiella* antibody, present at low concentration, binds to HLA-B27 lymphocytes, but complement cascade is not activated and therefore no inflammation occurs (**b**) Anti-*Klebsiella* antibodies, present at high concentration, bind to HLA-B27 lymphocytes. Proximity of 2 Fc parts of immunoglobulins leads to complement activation with cell death and therefore inflammation occurs. The result of inflammation is deposition of fibrous tissue, thereby limiting joint mobility and producing spinal ankylosis

The clear demonstration that anti-*Klebsiella* sera in patients with ankylosing spondylitis have specific cytopathic properties could be relevant in the pathogenesis of this disease and also of acute anterior uveitis.

References

Ahmadi K, Wilson C, Tiwana H, Shanmuganathan S, Binder A, Ebringer A. Antibodies to Klebsiella pneumoniae nitrogenase reductase in patients with ankylosing spondylitis. Ann Rheum Dis. 1998;57:441.

Avakian H, Abuknesha R, Welsh J, Ebringer A. Uveitis, vitreous humour and *Klebsiella*. I. Binding studies with rabbit antisera. Br J Ophthalmol. 1981;65:315–22.

Cunningham MW, Antone SM, Gulizia JM, McManus BM, Fischetti VA, Gaunt CJ. Cytotoxic and viral neutralising antibodies cross-react with streptococcal M protein, enteroviruses and human cardiac myosin. Proc Natl Acad Sci USA. 1992;89:1320–4.

Eady R, Smith B, Cook K, Postgate J. Nitrogenase of *Klebsiella pneumoniae*. Biochem J. 1972; 128:655–75.

Ebringer A. Ankylosing spondylitis is caused by *Klebsiella*. Rheumatic Dis Clin North Am. 1992; 18:105–21.

Ewing C, Ebringer R, Tribbick G, Geysen HM. Antibody activity in ankylosing spondylitis sera to two sites on HLA-B27.1 at the MHC groove (within sequence 65–85) and to a *Klebsiella pneumoniae* nitrogenase reductase peptide (within sequence 181–199). J Exp Med. 1990;171:1635–47.

Fielder M, Pirt SJ, Tarpey I, Wilson C, Cunningham P, Ettelaie C, Binder A, Bansal S, Ebringer A. Molecular mimicry and ankylosing spondylitis: possible role of a novel sequence in pullulanase of *Klebsiella pneumoniae*. FEBS Lett. 1995;369:243–8.

Newkirk MM, Goldbach-Mansky R, Senior BW, Klippel J, Schumacher HR, El-Gabalawy HS. Elevated levels of IgA and IgM antibodies to *Proteus mirabilis* and IgM antibodies to *Escherichia coli* are associated with early rheumatoid factor (RF) positive rheumatoid arthritis. Rheumatology (Oxford). 2005;44:1433–41.

Schwimmbeck P, Yu DT, Oldstone M. Autoantibodies to HLA-B27 in the sera of HLA-B27 positive patients with ankylosing spondylitis and Reiter's syndrome. J Exp Med. 1987;166:173–81.

Senior BW, McBride RDP, Morley KD, Kerr MA. The detection of raised levels of IgM to *Proteus mirabilis* in sera from patients with rheumatoid arthritis. J Med Microbiol. 1995;43:176–84.

Welsh J, Avakian H, Ebringer A. Uveitis, vitreous humour and *Klebsiella*: II. Cross-reactivity studies with radioimmunoassay. Br J Ophthalmol. 1981;65:323–8.

White L, McCoy R, Tait B, Ebringer R. A search for gram-negative enteric micro-organisms in acute anterior uveitis: association of *Klebsiella* with recent onset of disease, HLA-B27 and B7 CREG. Br J Ophthalmol. 1984;68:750–5.

Wilson C, Rashid T, Tiwana H, Beyan H, Hughes L, Bansal S, Ebringer A, Binder A. Cytotoxicity responses to peptide antigens in rheumatoid arthritis and ankylosing spondylitis. J Rheumatol. 2003;30:972–8.

Chapter 19
Pathogenesis of Ankylosing Spondylitis and *Klebsiella* Substrates

19.1 Introduction: The Association of Serum IgA in Ankylosing Spondylitis Points to a Bowel Microbe

Elevation of serum IgA has been recognised for some time as a feature in patients with active ankylosing spondylitis. Plasma cells in the gut-associated lymphoid tissues are the major sources of serum IgA.

The frequency of *Klebsiella* isolation in ankylosing spondylitis patients was found to correlate with the objective parameters of inflammation, namely, erythrocyte sedimentation rate and C-reactive protein levels.

In a study involving 159 ankylosing spondylitis patients, there was a clear correlation between the level of serum IgA and erythrocyte sedimentation rate (Fig. 19.1). These results clearly indicate that presence of inflammation, as assessed by elevation in an acute phase reactant, is associated with elevation in serum IgA, an immunoglobulin class that is usually triggered by an antigen acting across a mucous membrane.

Absorption studies have been carried out with *Klebsiella* and other microorganisms such as *Proteus* and *Streptococcus* on sera obtained from 91 ankylosing spondylitis patients and 20 healthy controls. Total serum IgA was measured before and after overnight absorption on a continuous roller and amount of IgA bound by the microorganisms determined. There was an increased absorption of IgA antibodies by *Klebsiella*, whereas absorption by equal numbers of other microorganisms did not exceed 40 mg/dl (Fig. 19.2). This was not due to non-specific protein binding, since total serum proteins, as estimated by the Folin method, were comparable in both groups.

As a result of these studies and the specific antibodies previously described from many countries, it is our hypothesis that the Gram-negative microbe *Klebsiella* is the main initiating external agent in the pathogenesis of ankylosing spondylitis.

In the pathogenetic mechanism, antibodies to *Klebsiella* microbes are directly involved, in the same way as anti-*Streptococcal* antibodies are the causative agents in rheumatic fever and Sydenham's chorea.

A. Ebringer, *Ankylosing Spondylitis and Klebsiella*,
DOI 10.1007/978-1-4471-4300-0_19, © Springer-Verlag London 2013

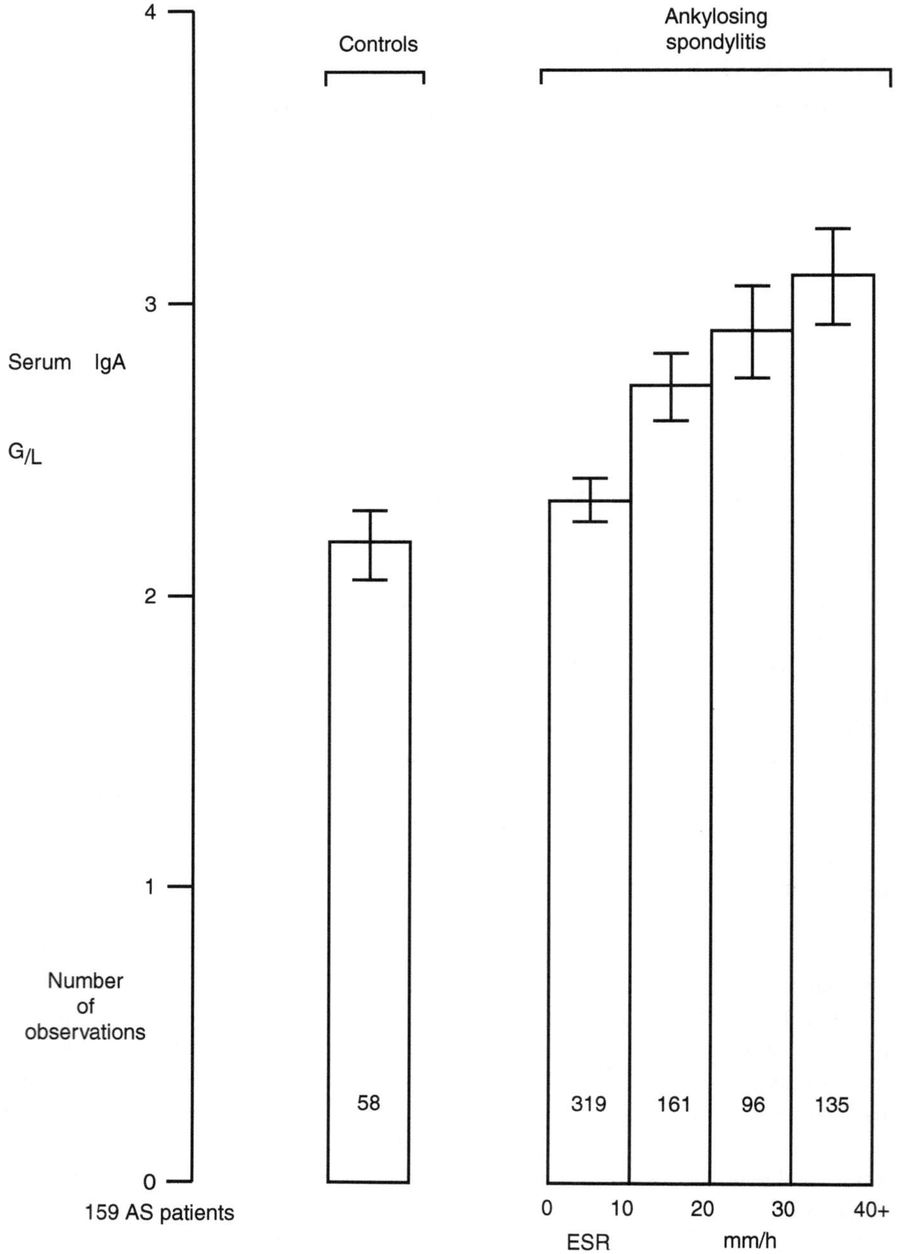

Fig. 19.1 Total serum IgA (mean ± standard error) in patients with ankylosing spondylitis and controls. Erythrocyte sedimentation rate (ESR) measured only in ankylosing spondylitis patients

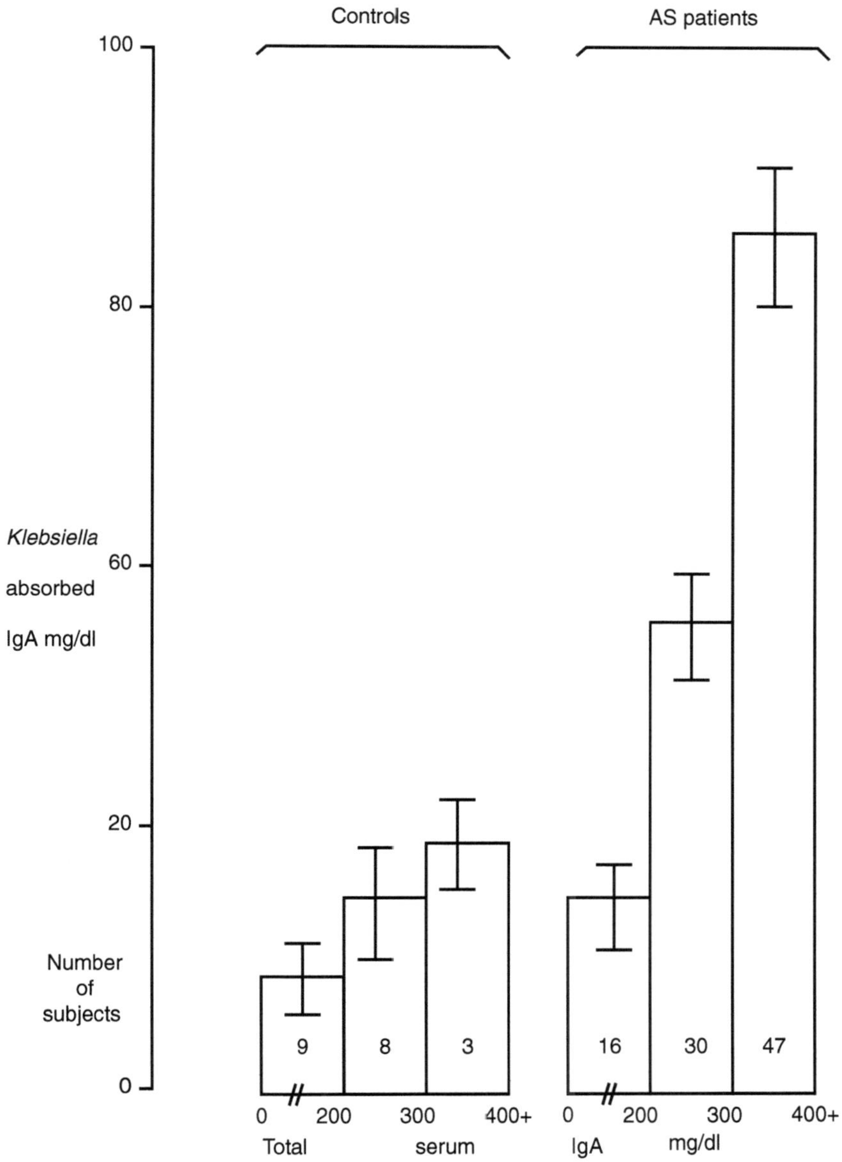

Fig. 19.2 Serum IgA absorption (mean ± standard error) with whole *Klebsiella pneumoniae* microorganisms in ankylosing spondylitis patients and healthy controls

The involvement of antibodies in ankylosing spondylitis was suggested by the classical lymphangiographic studies carried out by Professeur Alain Fournier from Marseille.

19.2 Marseille: Location and History

Marseille is the second largest city in France with a population of over one million and bordering the Mediterranean. It was known in antiquity as Massilia and was founded by Greeks from Phocea in 600 BC.

In 49 BC, Julius Caesar conquered the city which came under direct Roman rule. During the early Middle Ages, it was conquered by the Visigoths and later Charlemagne granted the city civic powers.

In 1348, the city was struck by the bubonic plague.

Marseille was united with Provence in 1481 and then was incorporated into the kingdom of France.

The local population joined the French Revolution in 1792 and sent 500 volunteers to Paris. Their rallying cry on their march from Marseille to Paris became known as 'La Marseillaise' which then became the national anthem of France.

Professeur Alain Fournier directed and supervised the lymphangiographic studies in ankylosing spondylitis.

19.3 Lymphangiographic Studies

It is interesting to consider that the lymphatic drainage of the colon and rectum occurs through the pre-sacral and para-aortic lymph nodes, which are closely related to the sacroiliac joints and lumbar spine.

Over 40 years ago, Fournier's group from Marseille described lymphangiographic studies conducted over a period of 8 years in 25 ankylosing spondylitis patients.

They noted that some patients had gross lymph node abnormalities, starting with lymphadenopathy in the early stages then followed by sclerofibrosis which produced obstructions to the free flow of lymph, and these changes were appearing even before there were any definite bony changes (Fournier et al. 1969):

> Un certain nombre des patients peuvent présenter de grosses altérations ganglionnaires au moment où l'on constate les premiers signes osseux et cette constatation témoigne de l'existence d'un stade pré-clinique et en quelque sorte pré-radiologique.

Fournier and co-workers went on to conclude:

> Le processus pathogène atteint d'abord l'appareil lymphatique et celui-ci le transmit ensuite aux sacro-iliaques et a la colonne vertébrale.

Fournier makes the suggestion, in 1969, that the pathological process first affects the lymph nodes and only then does the disease spreads to the sacroiliac joints and the lumbar spine.

Dr. Alain Delagrange, who was supervised by Professeur Fournier, describes the sclerotic changes in the lymph nodes and their close association with the lumbar spine in his medical thesis:

> Cette adeno-sclérose est parfois si totale que le ganglion, non seulement se ratatine et devient irrégulier, mais encore disparaît complètement ou du moins ne donne plus d'images

radiologiques. Ce sont les éléments de la chaîne lombo-aortique qui sont les plus atteints et cela coincide presque toujours avec de gros dégâts vertébraux: syndesmophytose, aspect en tige de bambou, ostéoarthrophie, calcifications discales, destruction des interlignes postérieurs, épaississement du ligament sur-épineux et une ligamentite peri-vertébrale. (Delagrange 1968).

It is clear that lymph nodes are affected before the sacroiliac joints and the lumbar spine.

19.4 The Proposed Model for the Pathogenesis of Ankylosing Spondylitis

The pathogenesis of ankylosing spondylitis, according to the molecular mimicry hypothesis, can be divided into five stages (Fig. 19.3). It is relevant to note that in this pathogenetic model, there are no bacterial fragments or antigens at sites of inflammation, around the entheses, in the spine or the uvea.

The 5 stages are as follows:

Stage 1: Infection by *Klebsiella* microbes

Antibodies to *Klebsiella* microorganisms in patients with ankylosing spondylitis have been reported from 17 different countries (Table 19.1). The world wide distribution of increased *Klebsiella* antibodies in ankylosing spondylitis patients would strongly support the hypothesis that exposure to this microbe occurs in this disease. In this primary stage, antibodies are produced against *Klebsiella* antigens.

Epitopes expressed on the surface of bacterial molecules are more likely to be involved in humoral immune responses than epitopes that are internalised and consist of hydrophobic sequences. One of the main targeted antigens to *Klebsiella* antibodies is to capsular lipopolysaccharides which constitute the main part of the outer membrane wall of these microbes.

Stage 2: Production of anti-QTDRED, anti-DRDE antibodies and anti-collagen antibodies:

The various antigenic molecules present on the surface of *Klebsiella* microorganisms including capsular polysaccharides or enzymes produced by these microbes, such as pullulanase or nitrogenase reductase, may all be triggering the disease development in ankylosing spondylitis.

The anti-QTDRED antibodies evoked by nitrogen reductase, the anti-DRDE antibodies evoked by pulD and the anti-collagen I, III and IV antibodies evoked by pulA are the main pathogenic agents which are produced in the local lymph nodes draining the colon.

When these autoantibodies leave the lymph nodes and localise in the nearby related tissues through Batson's plexus, as suggested by the work of Professeur Fournier, an anatomical connection has been made to the lumbar spine and associated joints.

Stage 3: Binding of anti-QTDRED and anti-DRDE to HLA-B27 and anti-pulA antibodies binding to collagens I, III and IV

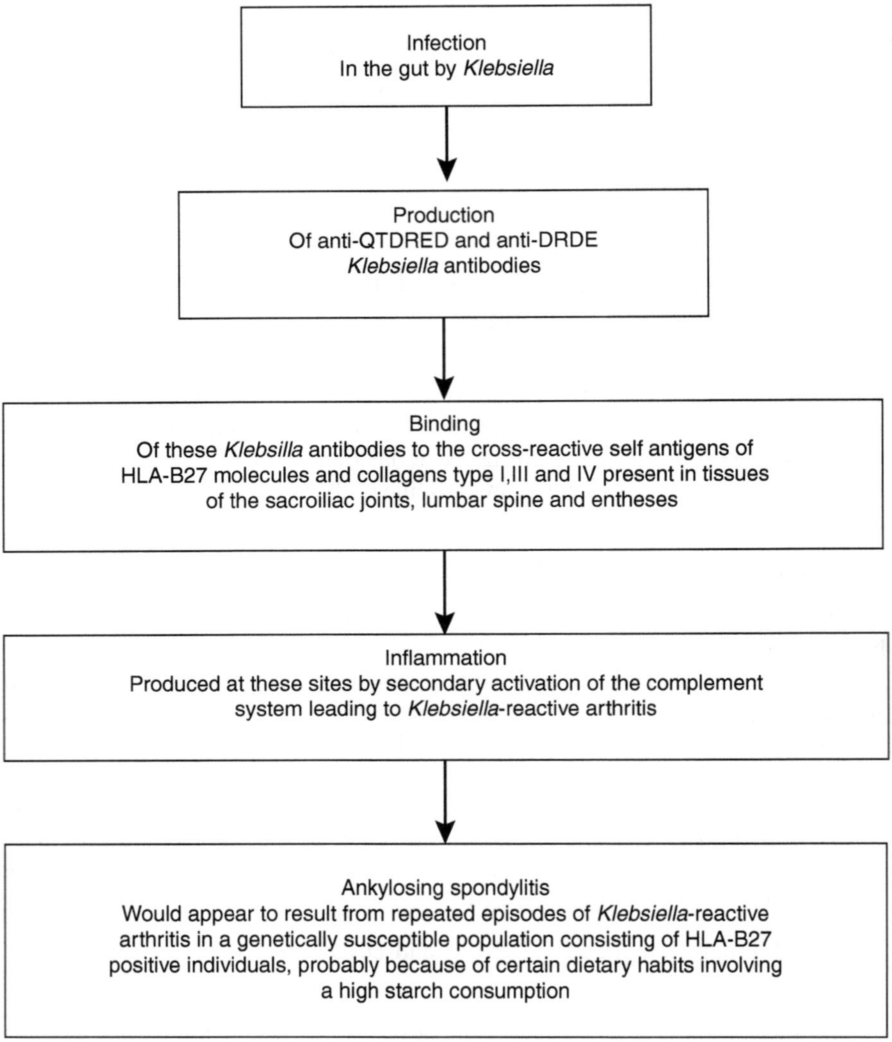

Fig. 19.3 Proposed sequential pathogenetic events in the development of ankylosing spondylitis

If the anti-pulD and anti-pulA antibodies are present in sufficiently high concentrations, then two adjacent IgG molecules will activate the complement cascade, which will lead to a cytopathic event and the triggering of inflammation, with interleukin and cytokine production.

Thus the antibacterial antibodies are acting as autoantibodies, and this makes ankylosing spondylitis an autoimmune disease.

The use of biologicals at this stage, that is, 'stage 3', will limit the damage caused by the bacterially evoked autoantibodies.

Table 19.1 Geographical distribution of anti-*Klebsiella* antibodies in ankylosing spondylitis patients when compared to controls and year of publication

	Country	Year	Number of patients	Statistical p-value
1.	England	1984	107	$p<0.01$
2.	USA	1987	24	$p<0.001$
3.	Scotland	1988	59	$p<0.001$
4.	Slovakia	1989	20	$p<0.05$
5.	Australia	1990	50	$p<0.001$
6.	Canada	1993	31	$p<0.001$
7.	China	1993	60	$p<0.001$
8.	Germany	1994	41	$p<0.01$
9.	Sweden	1994	19	$p<0.001$
10.	Spain	1994	84	$p<0.005$
11.	Turkey	1996	40	$p<0.001$
12.	Netherlands	1998	34	$p<0.001$
13.	Finland	1998	184	$p<0.001$
14.	Mexico	1998	44	$p<0.001$
15.	Taiwan	1998	52	$p<0.001$
16.	Russia	1989	25	$p<0.005$
17.	India	2002	20	$p<0.005$

However, it is relevant to note that the disease can also be interfered with, by blocking or targeting the 'stage 1' of the pathogenic pathway.

This could be done by reducing the quantities of *Klebsiella* bacteria in the colon by using antibiotics, such as sulphasalazine or reducing the quantity of substrates on which these bacteria grow and proliferate.

Stage 4: Inflammation by autoantibodies produces enthesitis and uveitis

The presence of anti-pulD antibodies will bind to the HLA-B27 chondrocytes and in presence of high concentration of antibodies and complement will cause tissue damage which in turn will set off localised inflammation.

The presence of anti-pulA antibodies will bind to collagens I and III found in the lumbar spine and also to collagen IV found in the basal membranes and the uvea and give rise to enthesitis, Crohn's like lesions in the small bowel and uveitis.

Stage 5: Repeated episodes of colonic *Klebsiella* infection will lead to recurrent inflammation, fibrosis and eventually classical ankylosing spondylitis

Repeated episodes of bacterial infection by *Klebsiella* bacteria in the colon will lead to waves of high titres of anti-*Klebsiella* antibodies which will produce intermittent but recurrent inflammation characterised by backache, morning muscle stiffness and occasionally uveitis.

Progressive lying down of fibrous tissue will lead to stiffness, rigidity of the spine and ribs, formations of syndesmophytes, the development of the characteristic radiological manifestations of sacroiliitis till eventually the spine becomes completely fused and the patient exhibits the classical features of advanced, irreversible ankylosing spondylitis.

19.5 Importance for Early Diagnosis of Ankylosing Spondylitis

Several years are required for the classical, clinical features of ankylosing spondylitis, particularly radiological evidence of sacroiliitis to appear before the diagnosis can be established. Often, by the time the disease is diagnosed, the destructive pathological events have occurred, and at this late stage, it appears to be difficult to reverse the damaging effects of the disease.

It should be emphasised that association of inflammatory back pain together with certain other features such as enthesitis, arthritis and acute anterior uveitis, as well as the presence of HLA-B27, greatly increase the probability of 'undifferentiated spondyloarthritis' to be considered as 'ankylosing spondylitis' (Rudwaleit et al. 2004).

In a 10-year follow-up study of a group of probable ankylosing spondylitis patients, it was observed that the progression from 'undifferentiated spondyloarthritis' to definite ankylosing spondylitis would occur after some 9 years (Mau et al. 1988).

It is the theme of this book that the great majority of ankylosing spondylitis patients who carry HLA-B27 and who live in a relatively salubrious environment have been infected by the commensal microbe *Klebsiella*, a microbe that does not cause overt gastroenteritic symptoms and not by *Salmonella*, *Shigella* or *Yersinia* microorganisms, microbes known to be associated with 'Gram-negative reactive arthritis'.

It is therefore relevant to review the concept of 'Gram-negative reactive arthritis'.

19.6 The Concept of 'Gram-Negative Reactive Arthritis' and HLA-B27

The three main Gram-negative microorganisms associated with 'reactive arthritis' are *Salmonella*, *Shigella* and *Yersinia*, and the majority of affected patients are carriers of HLA-B27 (Aho et al. 1973).

Several epidemiological studies have been carried out that clearly establish a temporal relationship between a colonic infection and the subsequent 'reactive arthritis' in a genetically susceptible host.

19.6.1 Paronen's Study

In 1944, during the Russo-Finnish war, a *Shigella* dysentery epidemic occurred on the Karelian front, affecting over 150,000 soldiers, and Paronen reported 344 cases of Reiter's disease which developed after the gastroenteritis (Paronen 1948). Over 20 years later, 100 of the original 344 were traced, and 32 were found to have ankylosing spondylitis or sacroiliitis (Sairanen et al. 1969).

Six years later, after Paronen had died, and when the relevance of tissue typing had become recognized, 16 out of the 32 patients with ankylosing spondylitis or sacroiliitis were further traced, and 15 (or 94 %) were found to possess HLA-B27 (Sairanen and Tiilikainen 1975).

19.6.2 The 'USS Little Rock' Epidemic

In the notorious post-dysenteric cases of Reiter's disease which occurred among the members of the crew of the 'USS Little Rock', the 'reactive arthritis' developed predominantly in individuals carrying the appropriate HLA antigens. An epidemic of *Shigella* gastroenteritis which affected about half the sailors out of a crew of 1,200 was followed by 9 cases of Reiter's disease, and all of these had suffered from gastroenteritis (Noer 1966).

Subsequently eight out of the original nine individuals with Reiter's disease were traced; seven were HLA-B27 positive and one carried HLA-B7, an allele which belongs to the B7-CREG group and crossreacts with HLA-B27 (Calin and Fries 1976).

19.6.3 Salmonella Reactive Arthritis in Finland

In a study of 63 Finnish patients, diagnosed with '*Salmonella* reactive arthritis', between 1970 to 1986, 95 % had abdominal pains, and stool cultures were positive for *Salmonella* strains in 93 % of patients.

Subsequently low back pain occurred in 44 % of patients, but HLA-B27 was present in 88 % of the patients.

In a follow-up of 50 of those patients, 8 had developed chronic spondyloarthropathy. In a radiological examination 6 out of 44 patients had developed sacroiliitis (Leirisalo-Repo et al. 1997).

19.6.4 Yersinia Reactive Arthritis

In *Yersinia* reactive arthritis, the majority of patients carry HLA-B27, and this implies the involvement of genetic factors in the development of the disease (Aho et al. 1974).

It would appear that individuals who are HLA-B27 positive are susceptible to develop a 'Gram-negative reactive arthritis' following a gastroenteritis infection by Gram-negative bacteria such as *Shigella*, *Salmonella* or *Yersinia*.

Since the majority of ankylosing spondylitis patients throughout the world have specific antibodies to the Gram-negative microbe *Klebsiella*, and not against

Shigella, *Salmonrella* or *Yersinia*, it would not be inappropriate to say that such patients suffer from '*Klebsiella* reactive arthritis'.

Furthermore, the question of how *Klebsiella* bacteria proliferate in the human gut raises the problem of substrates required for microbial growth.

19.7 Starch as the Source of the Main Bacterial Substrate in the Gut

Early studies in patients with ankylosing spondylitis using low doses of antibiotics such as co-trimoxazole and phthalyl-sulphathiazole did not lead to any significant improvements, although some patients admitted that the use of antibiotics decreased the dose of "non-steroidal anti-inflammatory drugs (NSAID's) required to control their symptoms. Clearly another approach was required to control the *Klebsiella* bowel flora.

19.7.1 A Patient Provides an Important Clue

In 1982, an ankylosing spondylitis patient was placed on a low residue diet (only steak and tomatoes) for weight reasons and 4 months later when he was reviewed in the Outpatient Ankylosing Spondylitis Research Clinic, he pointed out, that not only had he lost weight but his 'backache had gone'.

As soon as he said it, I had a E ρικοα moment, as Archimedes said it some 2000 years ago, 'I found it'. I had starved the bugs of nutrients. The bugs were growing on what the patients had eaten in the preceding few hours. Something I had been trying to do for some 5 years, to reduce the quantity of the bowel flora, since we had identified *Klebsiella* microbes as the trigger agents in ankylosing spondylitis but did not know how to do it. It was the diet. It was that simple, why had I not thought of it earlier.

19.7.2 Fecal Flora in Vegetarian Seventh Day Adventists

A review of the literature showed that subjects on high carbohydrate diets have high levels of *Klebsiella* microorganisms in their stools. Seventh Day Adventists are predominantly vegetarians. Fecal studies were carried on 47 on subjects who were on a high carbohydrate/low protein diet and compared to 45 subjects on a low carbohydrate/high protein diet. The mean number of *Klebsiella* microorganisms in the 'high carbohydrate group' was 30,000/g of faeces compared to a value of 700 *Klebsiella* microbes per gram of faeces in the 'low carbohydrate group' (Finegold et al. 1977).

Here was proof that a high starch diet affected the quantity of *Klebsiella* microbes recovered in stool specimens.

19.7.3 Carbohydrates as Bacterial Substrates

The substrates available in the gut for fermentation are the major factors in determining the microbial population in the various regions of the gastrointestinal tract. These substrates include simple sugars, polysaccharides such as starch or cellulose, proteins, peptides, fats and other lipids.

Klebsiella microbes do not grow on cellulose derived from plants (Deschamps et al. 1983) but can grow readily on simple sugars.

Equal amounts (5 g/L) of simple sugars and amino acids were compared for their ability to act as nutrients for the growth of *Klebsiella pneumoniae* in 24-h cultures and the number of bacteria obtained compared for the different simple substrates.

The mean number of *Klebsiella* microbes for 3 different sugars (glucose, sucrose and lactose) per gram of substrate was 8.7 ± 1.0 (mean ± standard error) ($\times 10^9$) ($p < 0.001$) compared to a value of 0.8 ± 0.2 ($\times 10^9$) obtained following incubation with 11 different amino acids (Fig. 19.4) (Ebringer et al. 1985).

Thus, *Klebsiella* microorganisms grow better on carbohydrate than on protein substrates.

19.7.4 Ileostomy Studies

One way of finding which substrates are available for bacterial proliferation in the ileo-caecal region is to analyse ileostomy fluids obtained from patients whose colon had been removed surgically.

In a study of 26 ulcerative colitis patients, who had undergone proctocolectomy with ileostomy, it was found that the 'ileostomy fluid' contained significant amounts (5–10 G/day) of mono and disaccharides (McNeil et al. 1982). The source of these carbohydrates could be dietary starch.

19.7.5 Oral Hydrogen Excretion Studies

Nearly all normal subjects fail to absorb appreciable amounts (5–20 %) of starch in wheat flour, commonly present in bread and pasta, as assessed by oral hydrogen excretion studies, following a test meal. This is due to the formation of insoluble complexes between some carbohydrate and protein components of wheat.

Breath hydrogen concentration were measured for 5 h after an overnight fast, followed by a test meal containing equal amounts of either sucrose, bread or pasta. Oral hydrogen is a measure of bacterial proliferation in the colon. The sucrose meal produced no increase in oral hydrogen since it would have been absorbed in the stomach and upper small bowel. However, significant amounts of oral hydrogen were detected at 4 and 5 h after a test meal with bread and pasta (Fig. 19.5) (Anderson et al. 1981).

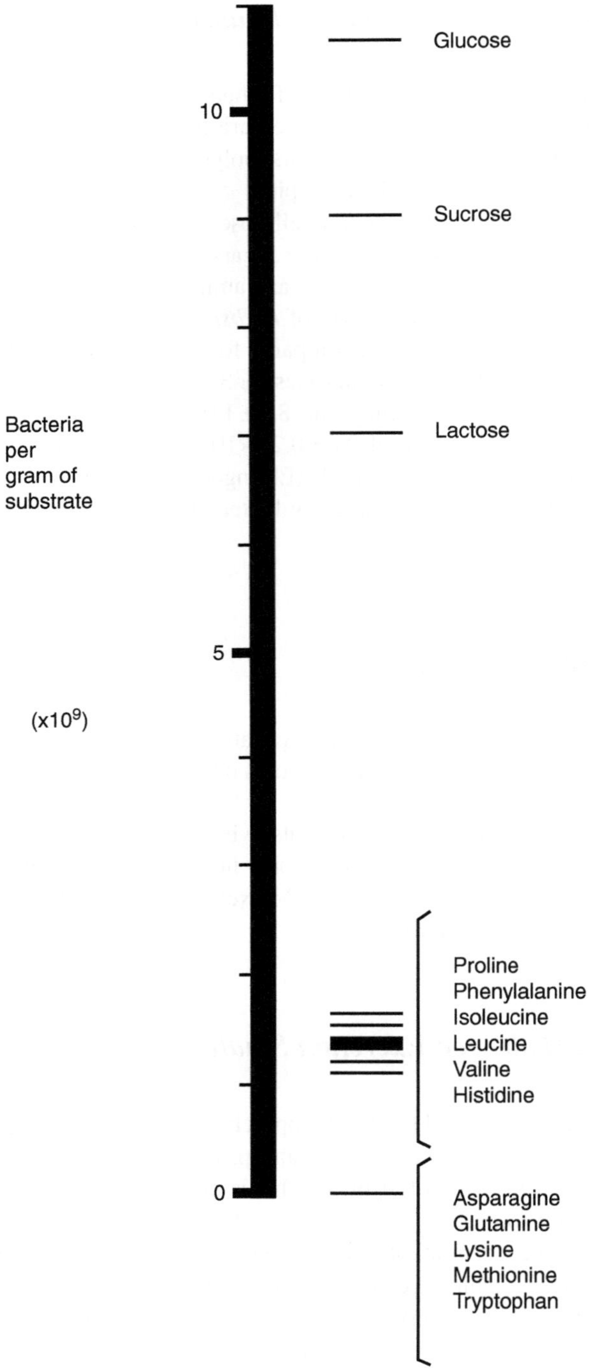

Fig. 19.4 Mean number of *Klebsiella pneumoniae* microorganisms following 24-h culture using different carbohydrates and amino acids as substrates

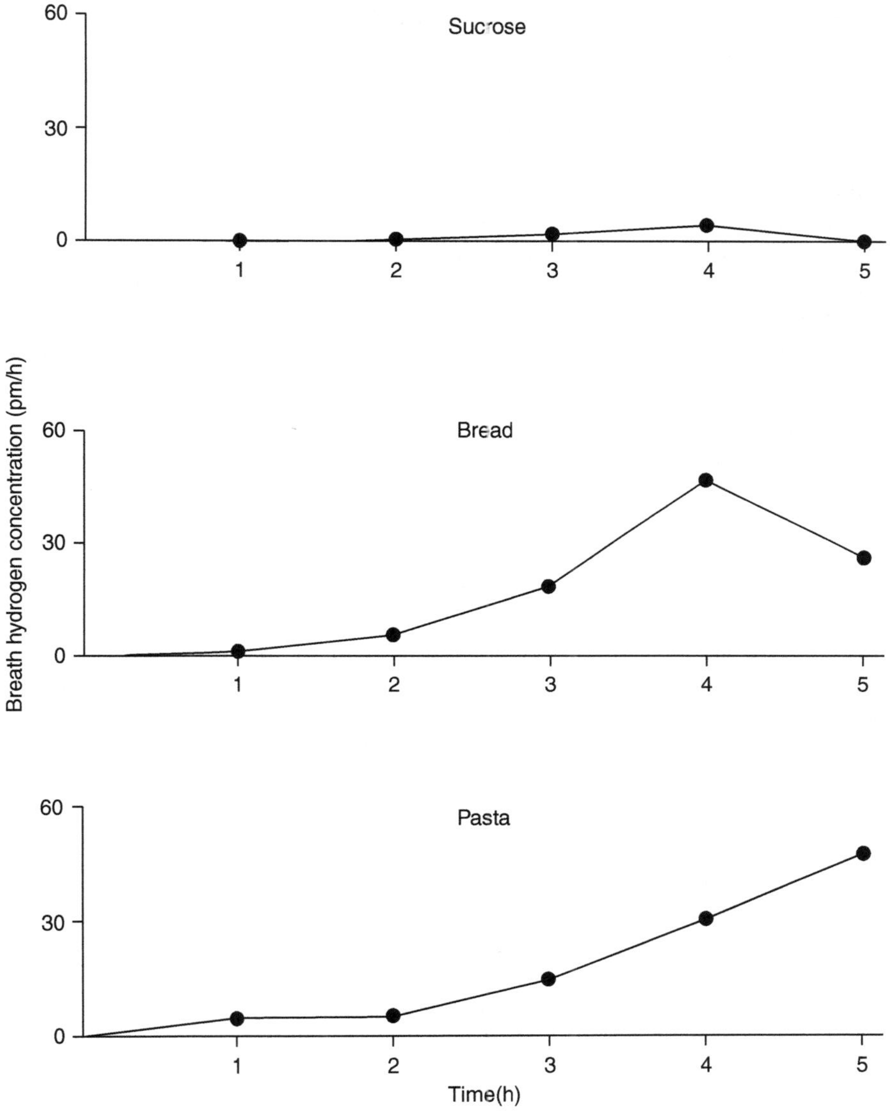

Fig. 19.5 Breath hydrogen concentrations after an overnight fast followed by a test meal containing equal amounts of either sucrose or bread and pasta (Adapted from Anderson, with permission)

It would appear that dietary mono- and disaccharides, such as sugar, can be readily absorbed in the stomach and upper part of the small bowel and therefore are not available as substrates for bacterial fermentation in the colon. The carbohydrates detected in the 'ileostomy fluids' would appear to be derived from complex carbohydrates.

These observations could form the basis of a 'low starch diet' for ankylosing spondylitis patients.

19.8 Composition of the 'Low Starch Diet'

The carbohydrates detected in the 'ileostomy fluids' would appear to be derived from starch present in flour and potatoes. Therefore, an exclusion diet removing complex carbohydrates but not simple carbohydrates such as dietary glucose and sucrose might inhibit the growth of *Klebsiella* and therefore could affect disease activity in patients with ankylosing spondylitis.

A simple 'low carbohydrate diet' was devised, the main emphasis being in advising ankylosing spondylitis patients to significantly reduce their intake of 'bread, potatoes, cakes, pasta and rice' (Fig. 19.6).

To compensate for the calorie loss incurred by reducing starch intake, subjects were advised to increase their intake of meat, fish, fruits and vegetables but excluding potatoes.

The diet was tried in two groups of healthy subjects before studies were carried in ankylosing spondylitis patients.

19.9 Discussion and Conclusions

The observation that only antibodies to *Klebsiella* microbes can be detected in ankylosing spondylitis patients throughout the world leads to the hypothesis that these are the causative agents of this disease.

A pathogenetic mechanism is proposed, involving five stages which lead to the development of spondyloarthropathy and eventually in advanced cases to a fixed spine.

The discovery that HLA-B27 is present in most of these patients has led through the concept of molecular mimicry to identify the Gram-negative microbe *Klebsiella* as the main trigger of this disease and that ankylosing spondylitis could be considered a form of '*Klebsiella* reactive arthritis'.

It was found that dietary starch was the substrate for the growth of colonic bacteria including *Klebsiella* and a simple 'low starch diet' was devised for treating ankylosing spondylitis patients.

Ankylosing Spondylitis Research Clinic (Professor Alan Ebringer)
Department of Rheumatology,The Middlesex Hospital, UCH School of Medicine
and Infection and Immunity Group,Division of Life Sciences,King's College,London,UK

THE LONDON "AS" DIET.

Low starch/High protein diet for ankylosing spondylitis patients.

It is thought that in a some cases a diet low in starches found in flour products and potatoes, and high in proteins and vegetables is of benefit to AS patients.

Ankylosing spondylitis (AS) is considered to be a form of "reactive arthritis" following an infection in the terminal ileum and ascending colon by the bowel microbe klebsiella. Specific anti-Klebsiella antibodies, in AS patients have now been reported from 17 different countries: England, Scotland, Netherland, Spain, Finland, India, Japan, Taiwan, Germany, Belgium, Slovakia, Russia, Turkey, Australia, USA, Canada and Argentina.

Over 95% of AS patients possess the HLA-B27 blood group whilst it is present only in 8% of the general population. The Klebsiella microbe has molecules which resemble HLA-B27 and this is the reason why AS patients belong to the HLA-B27 group.

When one eats large amounts of starch foods (bread,potatoes,cakes, pasta and rice) the Klebsiella bacteria feed on it, multiply and then the immune system makes antibodies against the microbe and some of these antibodies will also have activity against HLA-B27 and against collagens found in the spine and uvea, thereby acting as tissue damaging autoantibodies - hence the need to abstain from these foods.

Since the mesentery of the bowel is attached to the front of the lumbar spine, it is inevitable that BACKACHE in the lumbar area will be a feature of AS.

One simple way of reducing this inflammation is to reduce the daily intake of STARCH FOODS. However consult your doctor before going on the diet.

However if the AS in inactive the diet can be less rigidly followed.

Essentially it means REDUCE: BREAD,POTATOES, CAKES AND PASTA, and also manufactured foods which often contain starch and INCREASE: the intake of MEAT, FISH, FRUITS AND VEGETABLES.

References:
1. Ebringer A and Wilson C. The use of a low starch diet in the treatment of patients suffering from ankylosing spondylitis. Clinical Rheumatology 1996,15:Sup. 1:61-65.

Fig. 19.6 The 'low starch diet' sheet given to ankylosing spondylitis patients attending the 'Ankylosing Spondylitis Research Clinic of the Middlesex Hospital' in London

References

Aho K, Ahvonen P, Lassus A, Sievers K, Tiilikainen A. HLA-27 in reactive arthritis. Lancet. 1973;ii:157.

Aho K, Ahvonen P, Lassus A, Sievers K, Tiilikainen A. HLA-B27 in reactive arthritis. A study of *Yersinia* arthritis and Reiter's disease. Arthr Rheum. 1974;17:521-6.

Anderson LH, Levine AS, Levine MD. Incomplete absorption of carbohydrate in all purpose wheat flour. New Engl J Med. 1981;304:891–2.

Calin A, Fries JF. Epidemic Reiter's syndrome: genetics and environment. Arthritis Rheum. 1976;18:390.

Delagrange A. La lymphographie dans la spondylarthrite ankylosante. Thèse de Doctorat en Médecine, Faculté de Médecine et de Pharmacie, Marseille; 1968.

Deschamps AM, Richard C, Lebeault JM. Bacteriology and nutrition of environmental strains of *Klebsiella pneumoniae* involved in wood and bark decay. Ann Microbiol (Inst Past). 1983;134A:189–96.

Ebringer A, Baines M, Childerstone M, Ghuloom M, Ptaszynska T. Etiopathogenesis of ankylosing spondylitis and the cross-tolerance hypothesis. Adv Inflamm Res. 1985;3:101–28.

Finegold SM, Sutter VL, Sugihara PT, Elder HA, Lehmann SM, Phillips RL. Fecal microbial flora in Seventh Day Adventists populations and control subjects. Am J Clin Nutr. 1977;30:1781–92.

Fournier AM, Denizet D, Delagrange A. La lymphographie dans la spondylarthritie ankylosante. J Radiol Electrol Med Nucl. 1969;50:773–84.

Leirisalo-Repo M, Helenius P, Hannu T, Lehtinen A, Kreula J, Taavitsainen M, Koskimies S. Long term prognosis of reactive *Salmonella* arthritis. Ann Rheum Dis. 1997;56:516–20.

Mau W, Zeidler H, Mau R, Majewski A, Freyschmidt J, Stangel W, Deicher H. Clinical features and prognosis with possible ankylosing spondylitis. Results of a 10-year follow-up. J Rheumatol. 1988;15:541–6.

McNeil NI, Bingham S, Cole TJ, Grant AM, Cummings JH. Diet and health of people with an ileostomy. 2. Ileostomy function and nutritional state. Br J Nutr. 1982;47:407–15.

Noer HR. An "experimental epidemic" of Reiter's syndrome. J Amer Med Ass. 1966;198:693–8.

Paronen I. Reiter's disease: a study of 344 cases observed in Finland. Acta Med Scand. 1948;131(Suppl):1–114.

Rudwaleit M, van der Heijde D, Khan MA, Braun J, Sieper J. How to diagnose axial spondyloarthritis early. Ann Rheum Dis. 2004;63:535–43.

Sairanen E, Paronen I, Mähönen H. Reiter's syndrome: a follow-up study. Acta Med Scand. 1969;185:57–63.

Sairanen E, Tiilikainen A. HLA-27 in Reiter's disease following *Shigellosis*. Scand J Rheumatol. 1975;(Suppl.8) Eur Rheum Cong. Abst. 30/11.

Chapter 20
Ankylosing Spondylitis and the 'Low-Starch Diet'

20.1 Introduction: The Therapeutic Imperative

It is the theme of this book that the discovery of HLA-B27 in ankylosing spondylitis in 1973, by the London and Los Angeles groups, has provided rheumatology with the possible cause of this disease, namely, commensal *Klebsiella* proliferation in the ileo-caecal region and ascending colon following a high intake of dietary starch.

Therefore, therapeutic efforts should be directed towards the removal of the primary cause of this disease, in an endeavour to prevent the irreversible consequences of bony ankylosis.

It is thus pertinent to review the main features of therapy in ankylosing spondylitis.

The treatment of patients with ankylosing spondylitis is based on the use of a variety of drug regimens involving sulphasalazine, 'non-steroidal anti-inflammatory drugs' (NSAID's) such as phenylbutazone, 'disease-modifying arthritic drugs' (DMARD's) such as methotrexate and more recently a number of biologicals which inhibit inflammatory cytokines and interleukins (Braun et al. 2003).

However some of these drugs are associated with many deleterious side effects such as an increased risk of serious infections (Kroessen et al. 2003).

20.2 Current Therapeutic Interventions

Several forms of therapy are currently used in the treatment of ankylosing spondylitis patients.

20.2.1 Physiotherapy and Exercise

All ankylosing spondylitis patients in most centres are advised on various physical methods involving physiotherapy, spa exercises, postural education to improve

A. Ebringer, *Ankylosing Spondylitis and Klebsiella*,
DOI 10.1007/978-1-4471-4300-0_20, © Springer-Verlag London 2013

mobility and prevent stiffness as well as deformities which are the main disabling sequelae occurring in this disease (Van Tubergen et al. 2001).

20.2.2 Sulphasalazine

Sulphasalazine is one of the oldest drug used in the treatment of ankylosing spondylitis patients.

It is considered to be an effective and well-tolerated drug with not many side effects when administered in low doses.

A 26-week placebo-controlled trial showed that enteric coated sulphasalazine seemed to be an effective and well-tolerated drug in ankylosing spondylitis patients (Nissila et al. 1988).

A 6-month, multi-centre, double-blind placebo-controlled trial of the drug in ankylosing spondylitis patients resistant to 'non-steroidal anti-inflammatory drugs' (NSAIDS) showed that sulphasalazine had greater efficacy than placebo (Dougados et al. 1995).

Swedish ankylosing spondylitis patients treated with sulphasalazine showed a significant decrease in total serum IgA and secretory IgA in the jejunal perfusion fluids when compared to healthy controls (Feltelius et al. 1994).

In a 3-year placebo-controlled trial of sulphasalazine, a reduced frequency of peripheral arthritis was observed in the treated but not in the control group of ankylosing spondylitis patients (Kirwan et al. 1993).

It would appear that the antimicrobial component in sulphasalazine is sulphapyridine (Taggart et al. 1996) and could be acting against the bowel microbial flora.

20.2.3 Sulphasalazine and Klebsiella

A significant decrease in the concentration of *Klebsiella pneumoniae* IgA antibodies during 26 weeks treatment with sulphasalazine has been reported in Finnish ankylosing spondylitis patients when compared to controls (Nissila et al. 1994).

20.2.4 Moxifloxacin in Ankylosing Spondylitis

In an open study from Turkey, 76 ankylosing spondylitis patients, 88 % of whom were HLA-B27 positive, were treated with the broad spectrum fluoroquinolone antibiotic moxifloxacine, 400 mg daily for 12 weeks.

Most patients showed clear clinical improvements, and the objective parameters of inflammation decreased significantly: erythrocyte sedimentation rate ($p<0.001$) and C-reactive protein ($p<0.001$) when compared to values at the start of the trial (Ogrendik 2007).

These studies demonstrate that drugs having antibiotic properties are effective in the treatment of ankylosing spondylitis patients.

20.3 'Low-Starch Diet' in Controls

Another approach could be by reducing the quantities of *Klebsiella* bacteria in the colon. This could be done by reducing the quantity of substrates on which these bacteria grow and proliferate.

The 'low-starch diet' was tried in two groups of healthy subjects before studies were carried out in ankylosing spondylitis patients.

20.3.1 Open Study with 21 Healthy Controls

A group of 21 healthy subjects, namely, University students and hospital staff, attempted the 'low-starch diet' for a period of 8 weeks.

The 'low-starch diet' was defined as 'No bread, no potatoes, no cakes, no pasta and no rice'.

To compensate for the calorie loss incurred in reducing starch intake, the healthy control subjects were advised to increase their intake of meat, fish, fruits and vegetables but excluding potatoes.

There were no restriction on their drinking habits, an important point with some of the University students.

Blood samples were taken at the beginning and end of the study. Total serum IgA was measured by the immunodiffusion method of Mancini, as previously described.

Total serum IgA was considered to be an estimate of the quantity of bowel flora present in the colon, evoking an immune response.

Total serum IgA significantly dropped from 255 mg/dl at the start of the study to 212 mg/dl ($p<0.001$) by the end of 8 weeks (Fig. 20.1).

The C-reactive protein levels were also measured before and after the end of the diet. All control subjects had zero C-reactive protein levels before and after the completion of the diet.

20.3.2 Nutritionally Controlled Study with 11 Healthy Subjects

In a second study, 39 healthy volunteers were recruited from Town Hall staff, local police and University students.

All underwent a 1-week measured food intake assessment by a qualified nutritionist under the supervision of the Department of Nutrition at King's College.

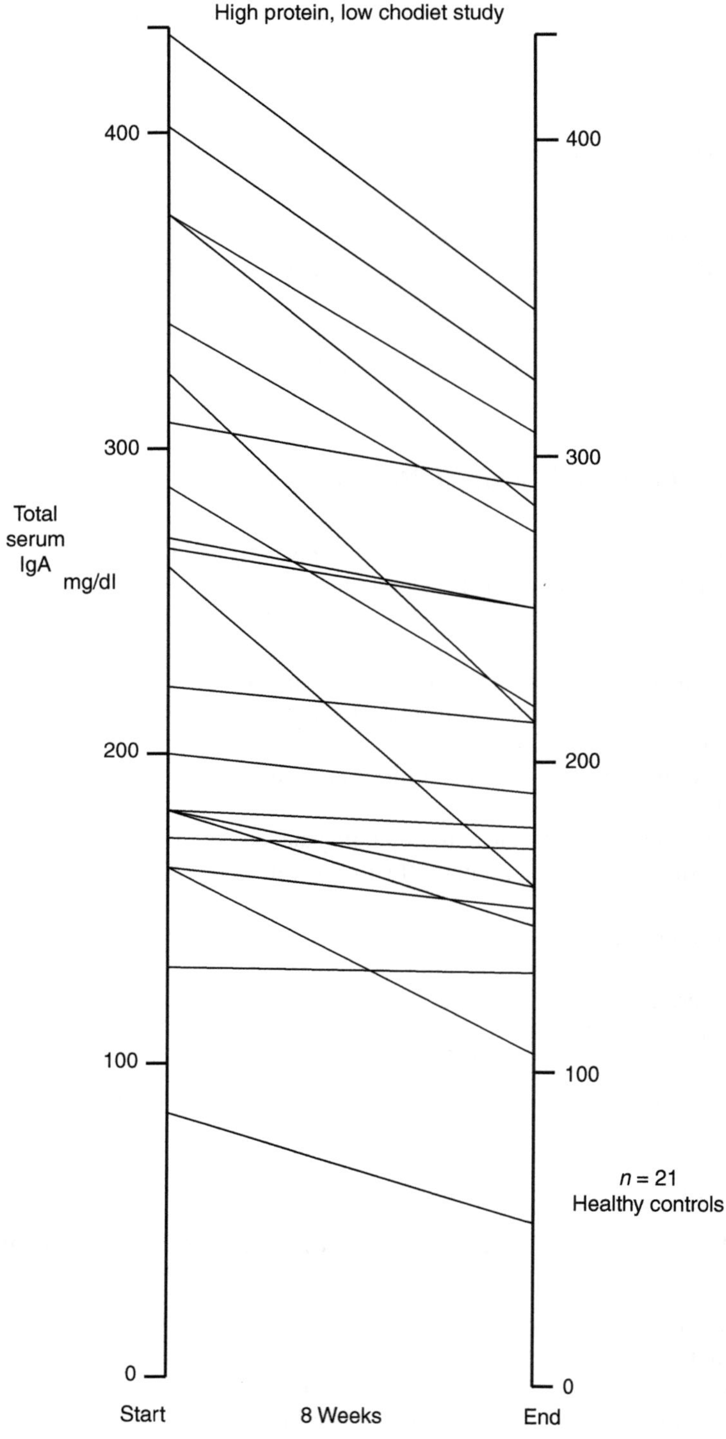

Fig. 20.1 Total serum IgA concentrations measured in 21 healthy control subjects, before and after an 8-week 'low-starch diet'

Total serum IgA was measured at the end of the first week, and 11 individuals were found to have a total serum IgA in excess of 250 mg/dl.

These 11 individuals then, undertook a 5-week 'low-starch diet' with a proposed mean starch reduction of 40 %.

Each individual received a personal 'iso-calorie, low-starch diet' protocol which was determined from their 1-week measured food intake study. Mono and disaccharides such as sucrose were not restricted and a list of appropriate 'starch exchangers' was provided.

The mean (± standard error) IgA fell from an initial 388 ± 23 mg/dl at the start of the diet to 259 ± 21 mg/dl ($t = 5.76$, $p < 0.001$) at the end of the 5-week diet period (Fig. 20.2).

C-reactive protein levels were not measured in this second group of controls.

It is clear from these two studies that total serum IgA is a simple and convenient method of measuring the immune response to bowel bacteria in subjects undergoing dietary starch restriction.

20.4 The 'Low-Starch Diet' in Ankylosing Spondylitis Patients

The 'low-starch diet' was attempted with patients attending the 'Ankylosing Spondylitis Research Clinic of the Middlesex Hospital'.

20.4.1 How Not to Do 'Coded Runs' Involving Diet Modification

Since many of the therapeutic studies involving drug therapy involved the use of double-blind and placebo-controlled investigations where the placebo usually was a tasteless white pill, it was thought some blind protocol should be introduced into this trial.

It is obvious that blind studies are impossible to carry out since the patients are aware of what they are eating. However, it was thought that some coding or blinding could be introduced into the study. Ankylosing spondylitis patients who had an 'even' hospital number would be told about the diet and supplied with the 'diet sheet', whilst patients who had an 'odd' hospitable number would not be told about the diet and would, it was hoped, act as 'controls'.

Within three or four outpatient sessions, the inevitable happened.

The ankylosing spondylitis patients with an 'odd' hospital number would come in and say, 'I was talking to the other patients whilst waiting outside, and they told me they are on this new diet. I would like also to try it'.

I had compromised the code. So it was decided to tell all ankylosing spondylitis patients about the diet, and the study would become an 'open trial'.

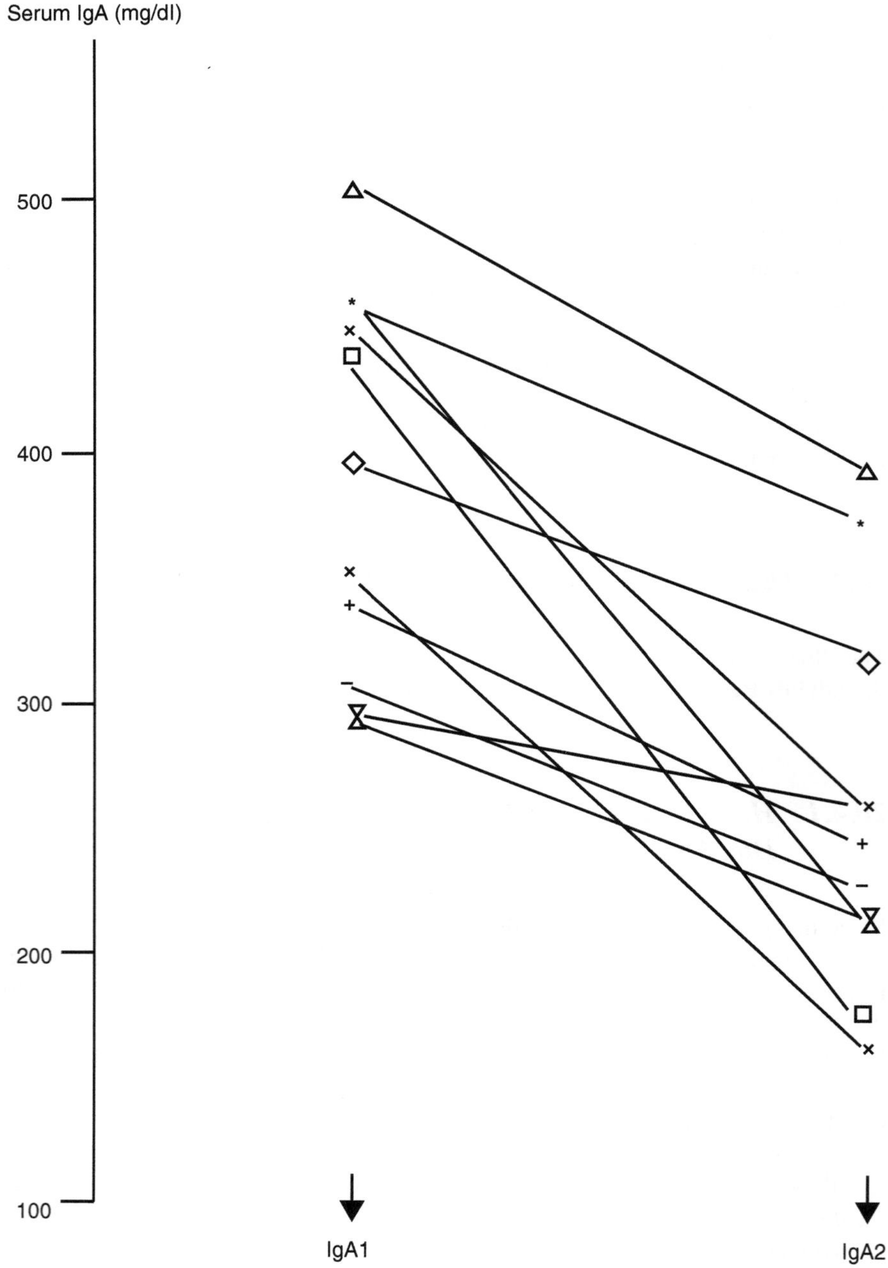

Fig. 20.2 Effect of 'low-starch diet' during a 5-week period on total serum IgA in 11 healthy control subjects whose initial serum IgA was greater than 250 mg/dl. IgA1 = Total serum IgA at beginning of diet; IgA2 = Total serum IgA after a 5-week period on a 'low-starch diet'

Each patient would be compared to his own clinical assessments and objective measurements of serum IgA, erythrocyte sedimentation rate, C-reactive protein levels and haemoglobin at the start of the diet and then followed over a period of time.

20.4.2 *Ankylosing Spondylitis Patients Partaking in the Diet Study*

A group of 74 randomly chosen ankylosing spondylitis patients in both active and inactive stages of the disease were asked to participate in the 'low-starch diet' for 10 months.

Ankylosing spondylitis was diagnosed using the New York criteria. The study included one patient with Crohn's disease, three non-HLA-B27 subjects and 4 individuals with psoriasis complicating their ankylosing spondylitis.

There were 51 male and 13 female patients and the mean (± standard error) age was 41.0 ± 1.4 years (range 22–67 years).

The ankylosing spondylitis patients attending the 'Ankylosing Spondylitis Research Clinic of the Middlesex Hospital' were mainly treated with the nonsteroidal anti-inflammatory drug (NSAID) phenylbutazone at varying doses.

Blood samples were taken routinely at each visit to check for erythrocyte sedimentration rate, C-reactive protein, haemoglobin and white cell count levels.

20.4.3 *Erythrocyte Sedimentation Rate and Haemoglobin Correlation*

A comparison of erythrocyte sedimentation rate and haemoglobin was carried out in the 74 ankylosing spondylitis patients before and after the diet (Fig. 20.3).

It can be seen that in all haemoglobin groups, the erythrocyte sedimentation rate came down significantly after 10 months on the diet.

The decrease was more marked in the two lowest groups, up to 11.9 G/dl haemoglobin and the 12.0–12.9 G/dl haemoglobin group.

The results indicate that the higher the haemoglobin group, the lower the average erythrocyte sedimentation rate in that group and also the smaller the decrease in erythrocyte sedimentation rate levels.

20.4.4 *C-Reactive Protein and Haemoglobin Correlation*

A similar type of result was observed when measuring C-reactive protein levels before and after the diet and correlating these values with haemoglobin measurements.

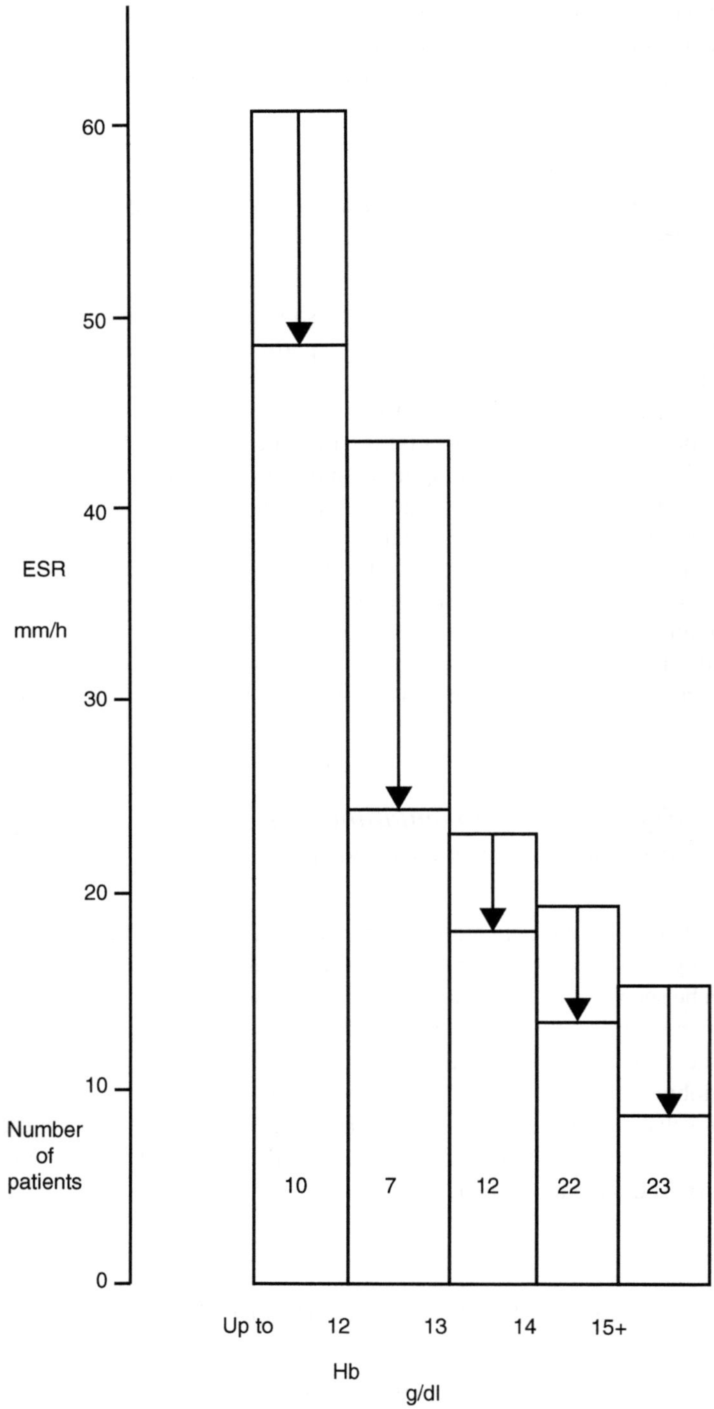

Fig. 20.3 Mean erythrocyte sedimentation rate values for five haemoglobin groups, before and after 10 months on a 'low-starch diet' in 74 ankylosing spondylitis patients

The highest C-reactive protein levels were seen in the group with low haemoglobin values. Again, there was a downward trend of C-reactive protein values after the diet except for a slight rise in the lowest haemoglobin group where the C-reactive protein did rise slightly.

This actually was due to one individual, whose C-reactive protein level rose after the diet (Fig. 20.4).

A very sharp drop in C-reactive protein levels was seen in the next group, the 12.0–13.0 haemoglobin group where the C-reactive protein level almost halved after the diet. Again as with the erythrocyte sedimentation rate study, when the haemoglobin levels increased, the C-reactive protein were seen to decrease and smaller reductions were observed after the diet in the higher haemoglobin groups.

20.5 'Low-Starch Diet' and Levels of Inflammation in Ankylosing Spondylitis Patients on the Diet

The 74 ankylosing spondylitis patients were divided into 2 groups according to their inflammatory status: those with an erythrocyte sedimentation rate below 15 mm/h and a second group with an erythrocyte sedimentation rate equal or above 15 mm/h at the start of the diet.

In the 43 ankylosing spondylitis patients, who had an erythrocyte sedimentation rate of 15 mm/h or above at the start of the diet, after 10 months, 40 individuals showed a decrease in their erythrocyte sedimentation rate, 2 patients worsened and one subject's erythrocyte sedimentation rate remained constant (Fig. 20.5).

The mean (± standard error) erythrocyte sedimentation rate for the whole group before the diet was 41.3 ± 9.8 mm/h; 10 months later, it was 27.7 ± 3.3 mm/h, and this difference is statistically significant ($t = 6.81, p < 0.001$).

In the group of ankylosing spondylitis patients whose erythrocyte sedimentation rate was below 15 mm/h at the start of the diet, the erythrocyte sedimentation rates remained unaltered (Fig. 20.6).

20.6 Discussion and Conclusions

Analysis of the data in these ankylosing spondylitis patients showed that there was a significant decrease in erythrocyte sedimentation rate, C-reactive protein and total serum IgA levels and an equivalent rise in haemoglobin values in those individuals who had a high initial total serum IgA equal or above 300 mg/dl at the start of the diet.

Almost all ankylosing spondylitis patients claimed that there was a significant reduction in pain, early morning muscle stiffness and rigidity.

A majority of subjects found in general that they could cope with the diet. However, a small number patients could not do without their 'starch' and relapsed on their diet.

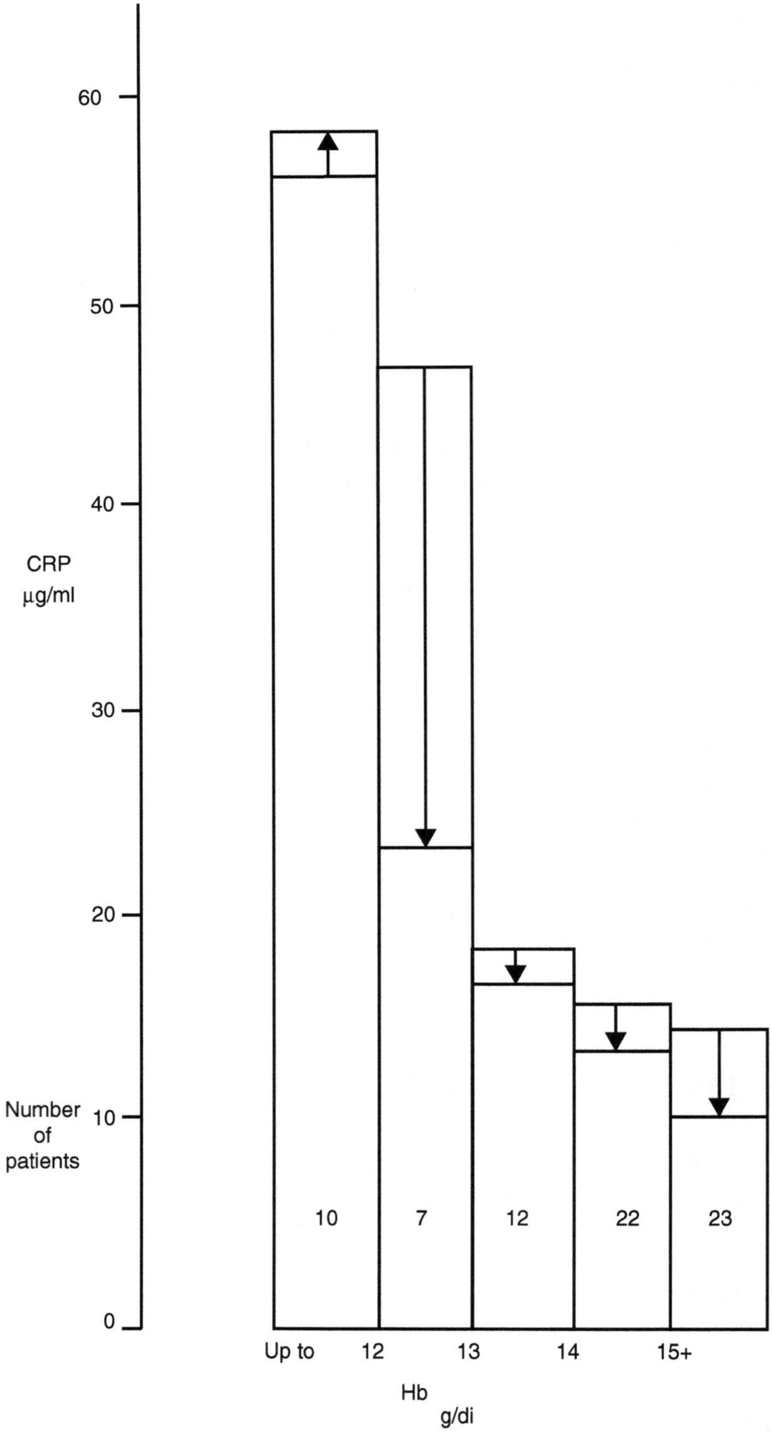

Fig. 20.4 Mean C-reactive protein values for five haemoglobin groups, before and after 10 months on a 'low-starch diet' in 74 ankylosing spondylitis patients

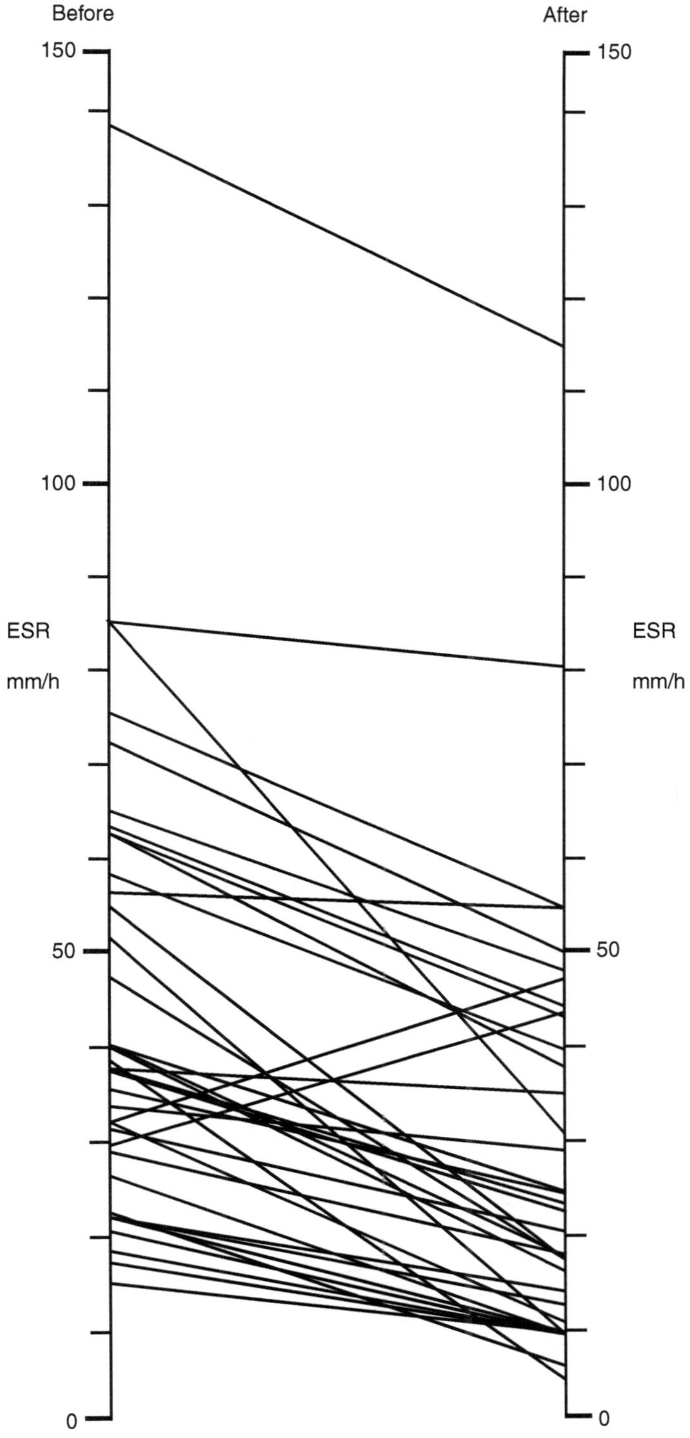

Fig. 20.5 Individual erythrocyte sedimentation rate values before and after 10 months on 'low-starch diet' in 43 ankylosing spondylitis patients, belonging to the group initially having initially an erythrocyte sedimentation rate level of 15 mm/h or above at the start of the diet

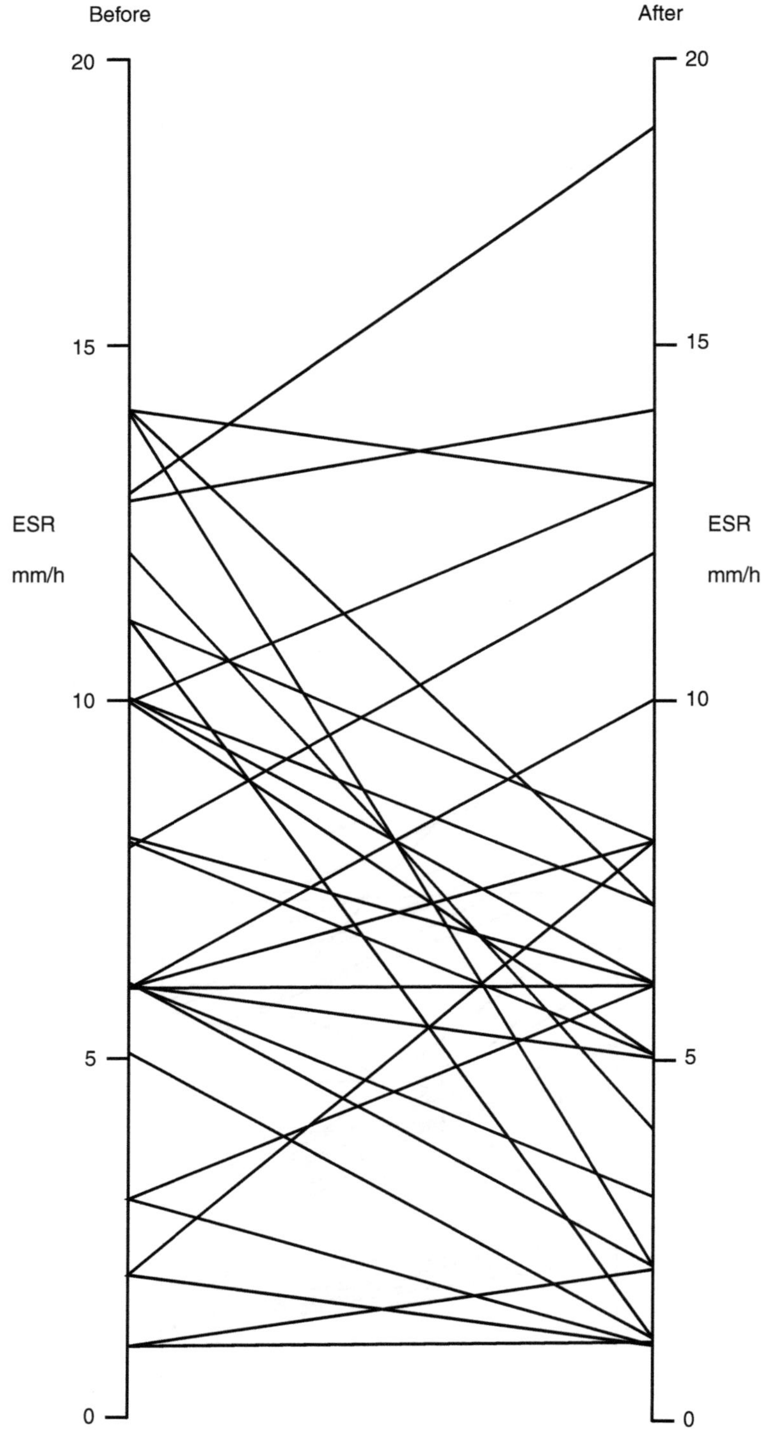

Fig. 20.6 Individual erythrocyte sedimentation rate values before and after 10 months on 'low-starch diet' in 31 ankylosing spondylitis patients, belonging to the group initially having an erythrocyte sedimentation rate level below 15 mm/h, at the start of the diet

These results have to be interpreted with caution, as the 'placebo' effect is well known in clinical trials when patients claim beneficial improvements.

It is for this reason that such dietary studies should be monitored with objective measurements such as erythrocyte sedimentation rate, C-reactive protein, total serum IgA and haemoglobin which are beyond the reach of the subjective enthusiasm of the patient or the clinician.

Further combination studies are required where the 'low-starch diet' is incorporated with established modalities of therapy, to see if benefits can be achieved in reducing side effects or even stopping the disease in its early stages before the irreversible bony changes have occurred in such patients.

20.7 A Patient Followed for 28 years. (Mrs. Beard's Story)

Mrs. Judith Beard, who is HLA-B27 positive, had her first symptoms of ankylosing spondylitis in 1969, when she was 20 years old. She was first seen in the 'Ankylosing Spondylitis Research Clinic of the Middlesex Hospital' in 1976 and over the subsequent 7 years had almost continuous, unremitting pains affecting large peripheral joints, thoracic cage and the whole of the spinal column, eventually leading to complete ankylosis.

During this period, her erythrocyte sedimentation rate was rarely below 20 mm/h (Fig. 20.7), and she acquired the radiological and clinical stigmata of advanced ankylosing spondylitis (Ebringer and Wilson 1996). She started on the 'low-starch diet' in 1983. She insists she would like to tell her own story.

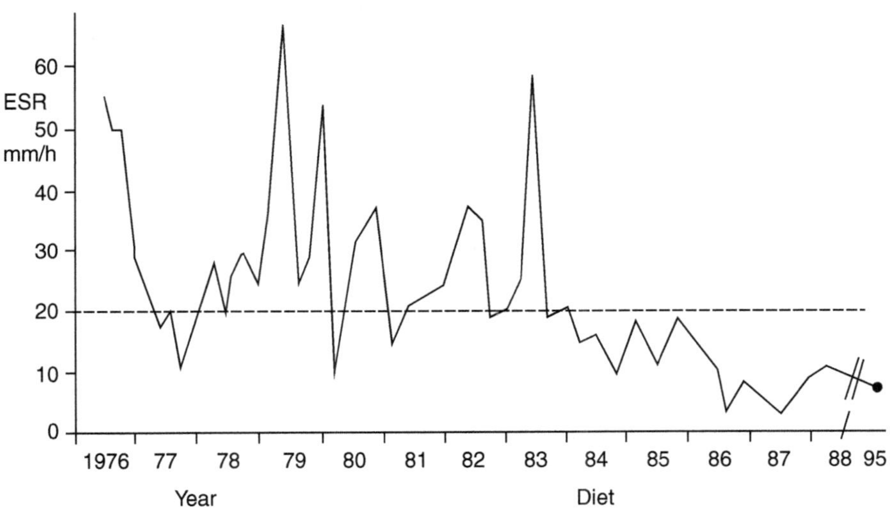

Fig. 20.7 Erythrocyte sedimentation rate (mm/h) in patient Mrs. Judy Beard from year 1976 till 1995. Period of diet from 1983 till the present day

Ms. Judy Beard writes:

It still surprises me that when I was told by the consultant rheumatologist at the Middlesex Hospital back in 1969, at the age of 20 that I had ankylosing spondylitis (AS), the news came as a huge relief. I had never heard of the disease but somehow I felt vindicated. The pain I had experienced over the previous five years was not down to "growing pains" nor was it a figment of my imagination for I had been told many times that there was nothing wrong with me that exercise could not cure. It had a name and it was treatable.

To be fair to the medics, diagnostic techniques of such conditions in the late 1960's were not as well advanced as they are now. It was thought in those days that AS was a disease of young men not women.

Nevertheless, at 15, I had low backache, more prominent at night and lasting for several hours. By 17, the pain started to travel from my back to my buttocks and thighs and sometimes I felt it on one side and sometimes on the other. At 19, I had developed muscle stiffness which was worse again during the night and I had acquired a slight stoop in my posture. The muscle stiffness eased in the mornings after exercising.

It was after graduating that my two university flatmates ganged up on me and made me promise to do something about myself when I relocated to London. That is how I came to be at the Middlesex Hospital.

On diagnosis I was prescribed phenylbutazone to reduce the backache and a course of physiotherapy to improve my mobility.

By the time I was 25 years old, the pains had spread to my shoulders, ribs and hips. It was then that the hospital confirmed that my ESR (erythrocyte sedimentation rate), a measure of inflammation was 55 units which indicated that the disease was very active. The upper normal level of ESR is 20 units.

It was in 1975, that I found out that I was HLA-B27 positive and that I had inherited the gene from one of my parents. This would explain why my mother's brother also had AS. I was treated with antibiotics, phenylbutazone and other non-steroidal anti-inflammatory drugs or NSAID's. Sometimes I felt better but at other times the pains came back. I do remember that in 1976 there was an exceptionally hot summer, and I had never experienced so much pain.

Two years later the pains and stiffness reached my neck which meant the whole of my spine was affected by the condition. I could not turn my head and had to rotate my whole body looking to the right and left when I crossed the street.

During my driving test, reversing round a corner proved to be the most difficult manoeuvre, but I passed. Nearly thirty years on, I was amused, when I took part in a fundraising day on a driving test site, to discover that I could reverse a medium-sized truck into a designated parking space without difficulty relying solely on its huge mirrors. The reason that I could do this was simply that I have had to depend heavily on mirrors ever since I passed my test all those years ago.

In 1983, Dr. Ebringer, who was then my consultant, suggested that I should try a "**low starch diet**". Initially I had 3 nutritious meals a day with fruit, vegetables, fish or meat but each had very little starch. The term "**low starch diet**" meant **no bread, no potatoes, no cakes, no pasta and no rice**. It was not always easy to stick to this regime but it is now a way of life – with the occasional lapse.

I began to feel better and my friends commented that they had noticed me "running upstairs" something which previously I had been unable to do. A year later my ESR was 15 and I had reduced the painkillers I was taking. The closest underground station to the Middlesex Hospital was Goodge Street on the Northern Line and on one visit to the hospital I walked up the 166 steps of the station, when the lifts were not working, rather than going to the next station and taking the escalator. Proud of this achievement, I mentioned it to Dr. Ebringer and it is written in my hospital notes of 1983.

In 1990 I spent three excellent weeks at the Royal National Hospital for Rheumatic Diseases in Bath. Five hours a day of concentrated physiotherapy and hydrotherapy made me much more mobile.

In 2000, I completed 25 years of attendance, every 4 to 6 months at the "Ankylosing Spondylitis Research Clinic" of the Middlesex Hospital. Since embarking on the "**low starch diet**" my ESR was never above 20 units in 41 outpatient visits. On two other occasions it was 22 and 23 units respectively.

This account is based on my hospital visits which focussed on the pains and discomfort of having this chronic condition. I am now 57.

I have had a good career and now have a demanding job as a director of a well known charity. My spine is fused and the changes are irreversible but I am reasonably straight and so far my general health is excellent perhaps because of my healthy diet. My stiffness improves the more exercises I do and as part of my regime I am glad to go walking every Easter with my local AS group.

I will never know whether anything could have been done to reduce the effects of the disease in its early stages and I don't dwell on that.

Having ankylosing spondylitis has given me a different life from the one I was expecting but I can honestly say that it has never stopped me doing anything that I have wanted to do.

20.8 A Sceptic Tries the 'Low-Starch Diet' (George's Story)

Carol Sinclair, the author of the book *IBS and the Low Starch Diet*, has given permission to quote Mr. George McCaffery's story.

Mr. George McCaffery writes: (With permission from C. Sinclair)

George first contacted me (Carol Sinclair) in 1999, to tell me that the "low starch diet" worked for AS. Without George I would probably never have heard the name ankylosing spondylitis, or discovered that I also had the disease. George has been on the diet as long as I have. He calls it the "secret diet", in his own words, "doctors keep it a secret". His story is remarkable and an inspiration to us all:

"Around the age of twenty-six I began to experience what I believed to be groin strains and thigh strains. My GP gave me pain killers/anti-inflammatory drugs and told me to rest. I eventually persuaded my GP to refer me to a specialist as these apparent injuries persisted and worsened.

At age twenty-eight I was seen by an orthopaedic specialist in Newcastle, who diagnosed a spinal instability needing a bone graft from my pelvis to my spine.

"I was admitted to the Freeman Hospital in Newcastle around 1978. I was prepared for theatre, that is shaved from toenails to ears and starved.

The morning of the operation the surgeon came to see me and asked how I was. He could not believe it when I told him I was feeling great. He lifted one leg at a time and dropped them – no problem. The stiffness had disappeared. He asked to get out of bed and touch my toes – no problem!

He then decided not to operate. Boy, am I pleased he called it off.!

Strange! I crawled into that bed and jumped out."

After this George went through a number of years sometimes feeling OK, sometimes feeling terrible. In 1982 he went to live in Singapore and began experiencing worsening pains and stiffness. His doctor in Singapore prescribed anti-inflammatory tablets which George describes as "great big pink things, as big as a door-stop." As well as the drugs, George was trying anything and everything.

"During this period I tried physiotherapy, a sports physician in Guildford who injected a solution radially through the muscles on either side of my spine (this is more painful than having AS but does not last as long), a blind mystic healer in Indonesia, acupuncture, massage..." You name it, George tried it.

"Around 1986 my GP in Singapore had some more X-rays taken and blood tests. He then told me I probably had something called ankylosing spondylitis, a progressive bone disease which had no cure but which could burn itself out. I should continue to take the anti-inflammatories. But I was having major problems with my stomach or back (sounds crazy doesn't it?)."

Still in search of a cure, George visited Guy's Hospital in London. "Someone had told me that a hospital in London was the place for AS, and Guy's was the only one I had heard of. I met a really good rheumatologist there, who told me the recommended treatment for AS was NSAID's (non-steroidal anti-inflammatory drugs) and, for longer term results, sulphasalazine.

He also mentioned that there was a school of thought that said diet may come into it. Of course I thought nothing of this. I had a bone disease, and what could diet have to do with it?

"Around 1988 someone told me they had read that a doctor at the Middlesex Hospital was doing research into AS. I phoned the Middlesex from Singapore. I was desperate at this time, in a lot of pain and contemplating having to give up work. I was told by a nurse in Rheumatology, "Oh, that will be Doctor Ebringer." Eventually I was able to speak to Dr Ebringer and told him of my situation, and asked if there were any research programmes I could be part of. I persuaded him to see me and came across in February 1988.

"Doctor Ebringer saw me (I crawled on to the table). He looked at my X-rays and sent me for blood tests. In March 1988 I went back and he told me, "You have AS. You are HLA-B27 positive and your ESR is 98." (ESR or erythrocyte sedimentation rate is a blood test which gives an index of inflammation and the upper limit of normal is 20 units). I said, "That's just great, Doc. I've already been told the first bit. I don't know what the other numbers mean. Just don't tell you can't do anything for me and to keep on taking the tablets!"

He said, "Not exactly, but I will tell you – you can help yourself." He then explained the "low starch diet/klebsiella theory" and gave me the "Middlesex Hospital AS Diet" sheet of what to eat and what not to eat.

"I have to say, at this point I was thinking, Oh no – a bloody quack! However, I said, 'OK, you tell me my problem is starch. Not another bit of starch will pass my lips!' (Probably a threat to expose his stupid theory.) I went on a bacon and egg diet as it was the only thing I could think of that didn't have any starch in it.

"Three days later, I woke up (I can remember exactly where I was, the Grand Hotel in Brighton) feeling great ! I phoned Ebringer, elated, and told him what was happening. He said, "Good. Stick with it."

"GOOD ! I couldn't believe it was that simple! Why had no one told me before?

"The rest is history. Once I found the problem, I could control it - look carefully at the contents of the things I ate. The psoriasis I had on my elbow and in my ears cleared up in a week or so. I kept visiting Dr. Ebringer's clinic in London whenever I passed through the country, and at the last count my ESR was eighteen.

"I now have a lot of friends who have AS through a website at www.kickas.org, which is a NSD (no starch diet) site, with a lot of people with similar experiences to mine from going on a low-starch diet."

George is being slightly modest here, because the rest of his history is that as a result of the low-starch diet he began to feel so well that he went on to become the managing director of a public company on the stock exchange in the UK. Then he started his own company in the USA, built it up, opened offices in other countries, and finally sold it recently for as he says, "a few million quid. Which I definitely could not have done without the secret diet."

20.9 Carol Sinclair and Her Book *The IBS Low-Starch Diet*

Carol Sinclair was born in New Zealand and worked in radio and television before becoming a writer of childrens' books.

She suffered from abdominal pains and bloating, as well as from backache for many years, before discovering that her symptoms disappeared on giving up eating starch. She is HLA-B27 positive.

Her abdominal pains were ascribed to 'irritable bowel syndrome' (IBS).

George McCaffery told her in 1998 that her book was similar to the 'low-starch diet' used in the Ankylosing Spondylitis Research Clinic of the Middlesex Hospital.

Her abdominal pains and bloating would come in waves sometimes lasting several days. Her mother believed in healthy eating and wholemeal bread, muesli and bran were present in almost every meal.

In 1986, almost at her wits' end with her symptoms, she listened to a TV documentary by Prof. John Hunter from Cambridge who claimed that eliminating wheat could successfully eliminate IBS symptoms.

She writes, 'I immediately gave up everything made from wheat, wholegrain and wheat bran and experienced a dramatic decrease in pains and bloating.'

Following her own discovery that she could control symptoms by reducing her starch intake, she wrote her book which contains many Low-starch recipes. The book has become a prized possession of many IBS and ankylosing spondylitis patients.

When she was seen at the Ankylosing Spondylitis research Clinic of the Middlesex Hospital, she was diagnosed as having pre-ankylosing spondylitis.

It has been claimed that some individuals having IBS symptoms go on to develop Crohn's disease, a condition affecting the small and large bowel, especially around the ileo-caecal region.

The question whether Crohn's disease and ankylosing spondylitis are associated is a common debating issue between gastroenterologists and rheumatologists.

References

Braun J, Brandt J, Listing J, Rudwaleit M, Sieper J. Biologic therapies in spondyloarthritis: new opportunities, new challenges. Curr Opin Rheumatol. 2003;15:394–407.

Dougados M, van der Linden S, Leirisalo-Repo M, Huitfeldt B, Juhlin R, Veys E. Sulfasalazine in the treatment of spondyloarthropathy: a randomized multi centre, double blind, placebo controlled study. Arthritis Rheum. 1995;38:618–27.

Ebringer A, Wilson C. The use of a low starch diet in the treatment of patients with ankylosing spondylitis. Clin Rheumatol. 1996;15 Suppl 1:61–5.

Feltelius N, Hvatum M, Brandtzaeg P, Knutson L, Hallgren R. Increased jejunal secretory IgA and IgM in ankylosing spondylitis: normalization after treatment with sulfasalazine. J Rheumatol. 1994;21:2076–81.

Kirwan J, Edwards A, Huitfeldt B, Thompson P, Currey H. The course of established ankylosing spondylitis and the effects of sulphasalazine over 3 years. Br J Rheumatol. 1993;32:729–33.

Kroessen S, Widmer AF, Tyndall A, Hasler B. Serious bacterial infections in patients with rheumatoid arthritis under anti-TNFα therapy. Rheumatology (Oxford). 2003;42:617–21.

Nissila M, Lahesmaa R, Leirisalo-Repo M, Lehtinen K, Toivanen P, Granfors K. Antibodies to *Klebsiella pneumoniae*, *Escherichia coli* and *Proteus mirabilis* in ankylosing spondylitis: effect of sulfasalazine treatment. J Rheumatol. 1994;21:2082–7.

Nissila M, Lehtinen K, Leirisalo-Repo M, Luukkainen R, Mutru O, Yli-Kerttula U. Sulfasalazine in the treatment of ankylosing spondylitis. A 26 week, placebo controlled clinical trial. Arthritis Rheum. 1988;31:111–6.

Ogrendik M. Treatment of ankylosing spondylitis with moxifloxacine. South Med J. 2007; 100:366–70.

Taggart A, Gardiner P, McEvoy E, Hopkins R, Bird H. Which is the active moiety of sulfasalazine in ankylosing spondylitis? A randomized controlled study. Arthritis Rheum. 1996;39:1400–5.

Van Tubergen A, Landewe R, van der Heijde D, Hidding A, Wolter W, Ascher M. Combined spa exercise therapy is effective in patients with ankylosing spondylitis: a randomized controlled trial. Arthritis Rheum. 2001;45:430–8.

Chapter 21
The Problem of Crohn's Disease and *Klebsiella*

21.1 Introduction: Crohn's Disease

Crohn's disease is characterised by a granulomatous inflammation affecting especially the terminal ileum, ileo-caecal region and ascending colon, sometimes extending to the rectum. It was first described in 1932, by Bernard Burill Crohn from the Mount Sinai Hospital in New York.

It starts most frequently between the ages of 20 and 40 years and affects both sexes equally.

Microscopically, inflammatory changes involve all coats of the bowel. Granulomas are seen in about 50 % of cases, and sometimes deep clefts or fissures open to the mucocal surface and may give rise to fistula formation.

Pain occurs especially on the right side. Recurrent episodes of colic due to attacks of subacute obstruction are a prominent feature in the life history of a patient with Crohn's disease. Diarrhoea affects some patients and associated features that can occur are skin rashes, arthritis and eye problems. In long-standing cases, there may be stricture formation which requires surgical intervention.

Interesting studies on the relationship between ankylosing spondylitis and the gut have come from a research team in Ghent

21.2 Ghent: Location and History

Ghent is located in the Flemish region of Belgium and has a population of approximately a quarter million.

In the Middle Ages, it became one of the largest and richest centres of Europe specialising in cloth making. Until the thirteenth century, it was the biggest city in Europe after Paris.

The Ghent altarpiece or Adoration of the Mystic Lamb is an early Flemish painting completed by the brothers Hubert and Jan Van Eyck in 1432 and is located in St. Bavo's Cathedral.

A. Ebringer, *Ankylosing Spondylitis and Klebsiella*,
DOI 10.1007/978-1-4471-4300-0_21, © Springer-Verlag London 2013

Charles V, Holy Roman Emperor and King of Spain, was born in this city, although after the 'Revolt of Ghent' in 1539, he punished the nobles by obliging them to walk barefoot with a rope noose round their necks. Since then, the people of Ghent are known as 'Stroppendragers' or noose bearers.

After the battle of Waterloo, it became part of the Netherlands and in 1817 established its own university.

Professors Mielants and Veys from Ghent have been studying ankylosing spondylitis and its link with the gut for many years.

21.3 The Link Between Ankylosing Spondylitis and Crohn's Disease

The Ghent group has been producing for two decades extensive clinical and laboratory evidence that in over 50 % of ankylosing spondylitis patients, microscopic gut lesions resembling Crohn's disease can be readily demonstrated. Ileocolonoscopy with biopsy of caecum, ileo-caecal valve and terminal ileum was performed on 232 patients with seronegative spondyloarthropathies and on 65 control patients. Inflammatory gut lesions were found in 57 % patients with ankylosing spondylitis. The controls had a normal gut (Mielants et al. 1988).

This finding would suggest that exogenous factors causing inflammation in the gut lead to an inflammatory mechanism inducing joint and tendon inflammation. Support for this hypothesis was provided by the results of a repeat ileocolonoscopy one or two years later, disclosing a strong association between the presence of inflammation in the gut on biopsy and persistence of joint inflammation.

The gut inflammation in ankylosing spondylitis is frequently subclinical and suggests that it is somehow involved in the pathogenesis of the disease.

Histologically, the lesions were predominantly of the chronic type and in most cases indistinguishable from early Crohn's disease. They conclude; in some cases, the inflammatory gut lesions could be bacterial in origin, although which microbe is involved was not discussed.

In ankylosing spondylitis, the majority of patients had chronic inflammatory lesions, Crohn's-like lesions being more common in HLA-B27 negative ankylosing spondylitis patients with axial involvement alone.

The question arises what environmental factor could link ankylosing spondylitis patients to the gut lesions resembling Crohn's disease.

Some studies from Birmingham in England could provide another approach to this problem.

21.4 Birmingham: Location and History

Birmingham is the second largest city in the UK after London.

During the Middle Ages, it was a market town; however, during the Industrial Revolution, it was at the forefront of many developments in science, technology and economic organisation. By 1791, it was hailed as the first manufacturing town in the world.

The first iron ore blast furnace and the first cotton mill were developed in the 1750s in Birmingham.

The city was finally represented in Parliament in the 1830s after the rotten boroughs had been eliminated.

The city suffered heavily during the Second World War, but it has been rebuilt and memories of the 'Birmingham Blitz' are fading with the passing away of the older generations.

Professor Bob Allen, Dr. Ibbotson and Dr. Felicity Pease from Birmingham University have been working on aetiological factors in Crohn's disease.

21.5 Antibodies to *Yersinia* and *Klebsiella* but Not *Pseudomonas* in Crohn's Disease Patients

In this study, 60 patients with Crohn's disease and 20 patients with ulcerative colitis were investigated for antibodies to *Yersinia* 0.3, *Yersinia* 0.9, *Klebsiella aerogenes* and *Pseudomonas maltophilia* by ELISA.

The diagnosis of Crohn's disease was made on clinical, histological and radiological criteria.

Elevated levels of antibodies were found against *Yersinia* and *Klebsiella* bacteria but not against *Pseudomonas*, especially during active phases of the disease.

The Crohn's disease patients were reviewed after 9–12 months, and in those who achieved a clinical remission, there was a decrease in the titre of antibodies (Ibbotson et al. 1987).

This would appear to be the first report showing an elevation in antibody titres against *Klebsiella* bacteria in Crohn's disease patients.

21.6 IBD Patients from the Royal Free Hospital in London Have Antibodies to *Klebsiella*

Total antibody (IgG, IgA, IgM) antibody levels were measured against *Klebsiella pneumoniae*, *Proteus mirabilis* and *Escherichia coli* in IBD (inflammatory bowel disease) patients attending the Gastroenterology Department at the Royal Free Hospital in London. They were compared either to ankylosing spondylitis patients attending the 'Ankylosing Spondylitis Research Clinic of the Middlesex Hospital' or rheumatoid arthritis patients attending the Department of Rheumatology at the Royal Hampshire Hospital in Winchester.

There were 60 patients with rheumatoid arthritis, 35 patients with ankylosing spondylitis, 30 patients with ulcerative colitis and 30 patients with Crohn's disease and compared to 60 healthy controls. Antibody assays were carried out as previously described.

When tested against *Klebsiella*, significant elevations were found in ankylosing spondylitis ($p<0.001$), ulcerative colitis ($p<0.001$) and Crohn's disease ($p<0.001$) but no elevations in rheumatoid arthritis patients when compared to healthy controls (Fig. 21.1).

When tested against *Proteus*, significant elevations were found only in rheumatoid arthritis patients ($p<0.001$) but not in ankylosing spondylitis, ulcerative colitis or Crohn's disease patients when compared to healthy controls (Fig. 21.2).

There was no significant elevation in total antibodies (IgG, IgA, IgM) to *Escherichia coli* in any of the four groups tested when compared to controls (Fig. 21.3).

In this study, we were not able to separate antibodies to *Klebsiella* in ankylosing spondylitis patients when compared to inflammatory bowel disease patients having either ulcerative colitis or Crohn's disease (Tiwana et al. 1997).

However, we could clearly distinguish rheumatoid arthritis disease from ankylosing spondylitis, ulcerative colitis or Crohn's disease in that the rheumatoid arthritis patients had antibodies to *Proteus mirabilis* and that is consistent with previous studies in rheumatoid arthritis patients when tested against *Proteus mirabilis* (Ebringer 2012).

21.7 Coeliac Disease Patients from St. Thomas' Hospital Do Not Have Antibodies Against *Klebsiella*

In this second study, sera were collected from five patient groups: ankylosing spondylitis, Crohn's disease, ulcerative colitis, coeliac disease and normal blood donors. The study was carried out to characterise seven *Klebsiella pneumoniae* serotypes: K2, K3, K17, K21, K26, K36 and K50 in these five different patient groups (Tiwana et al. 1998).

The ankylosing spondylitis sera were obtained from the 'Ankylosing Spondylitis Research Clinic of the Middlesex Hospital'. The IBD groups were obtained from the Department of Gastroenterology, Royal Free Hospital, London.

There were 46 unrelated Crohn's disease patients. Active disease was defined by physician's assessment with a raised C-reactive protein and/or a Harvey-Bradshaw score >4 (Harvey and Bradshaw 1980). In the Crohn's disease group, there were 23 with terminal and ileal and colonic disease, 10 had colonic disease alone, and 13 had disease limited to the small bowel.

There were also 50 unrelated patients with active coeliac disease, attending the Gastroenterology Unit of St. Thomas' Hospital in London: 19 had newly diagnosed disease, 7 were undergoing a gluten challenge, and 24 patients had active disease whilst on treatment. In the coeliac disease group, 49 patients had positive anti-endomysial antibodies, as demonstrated by immunohistochemistry.

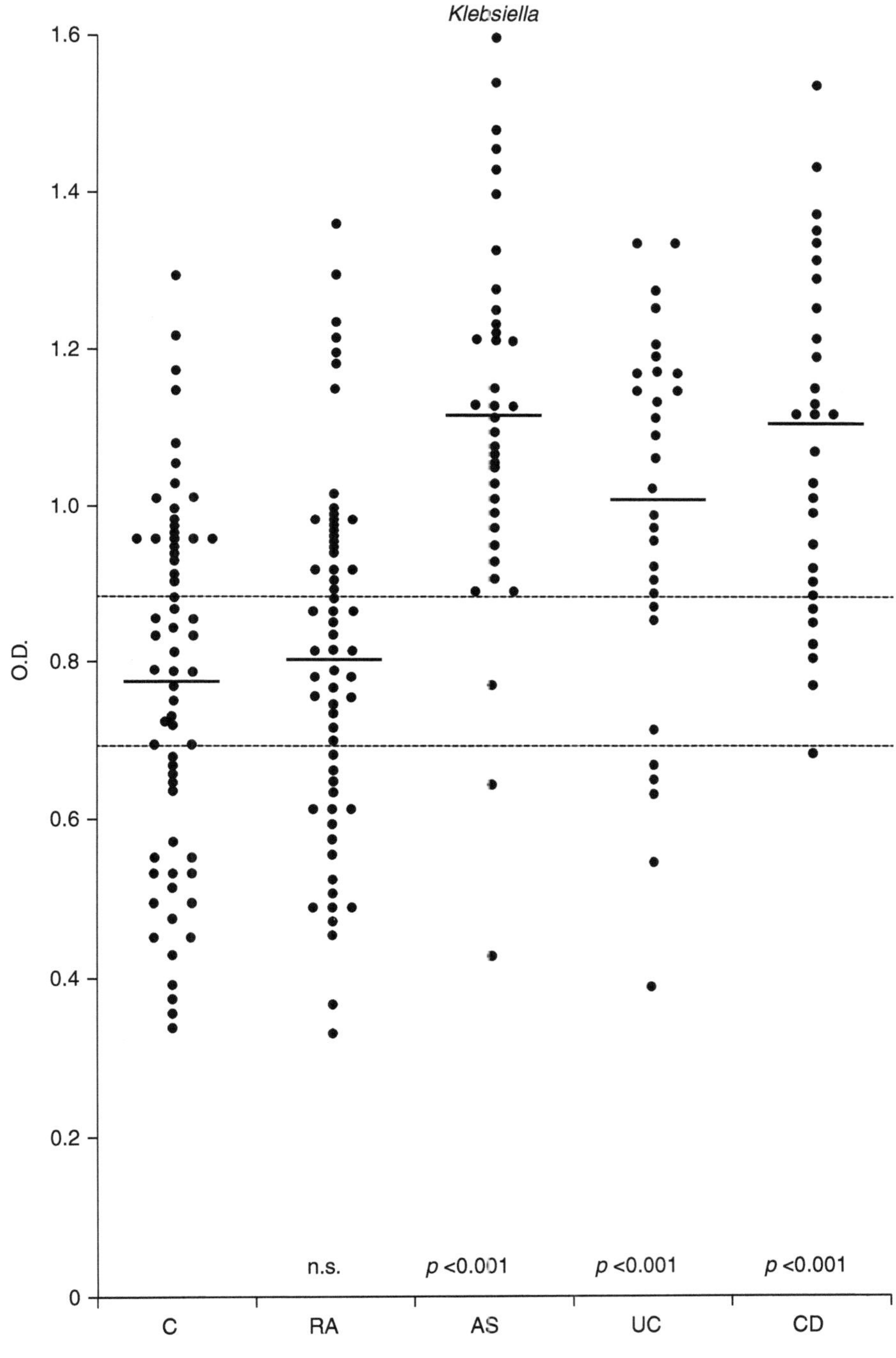

Fig. 21.1 Total immunoglobulin (IgG, IgA, IgM) levels against *Klebsiella* in controls (*C*), rheumatoid arthritis (*RA*), ankylosing spondylitis (*AS*), ulcerative colitis (*UC*) and Crohn's disease (*CD*) subjects (*dotted line* indicates 95 % confidence limits for mean of control – two tailed test; *OD* optical density, *n.s.* not significant

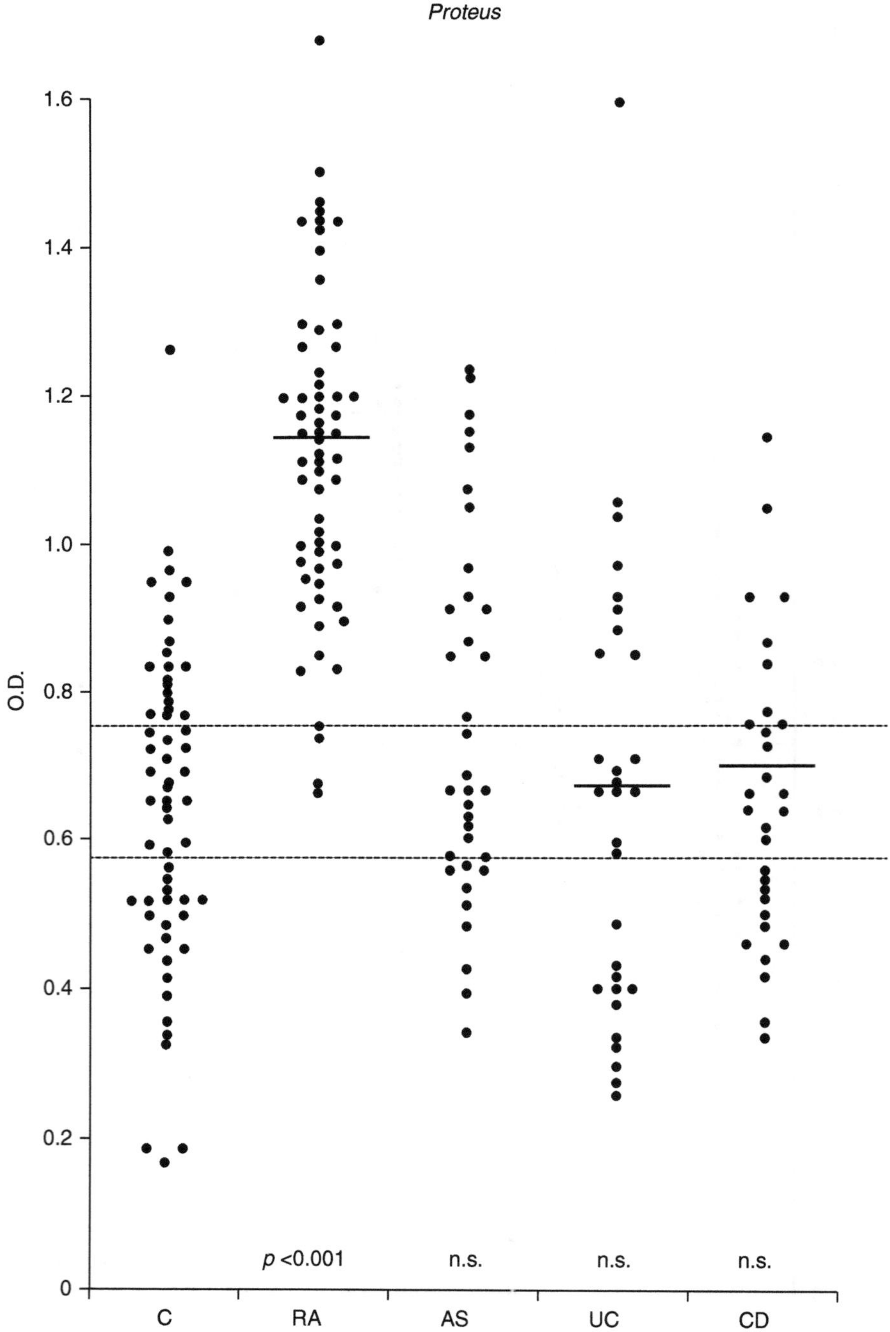

Fig. 21.2 Total immunoglobulin (IgG, IgA, IgM) levels against *Proteus* in controls (*C*), rheumatoid arthritis (*RA*), ankylosing spondylitis (*AS*), ulcerative colitis (*UC*) and Crohn's disease (*CD*) subjects (*dotted line* indicates 95 % confidence limits for mean of control – two tailed test; *OD* optical density, *n.s.* not significant

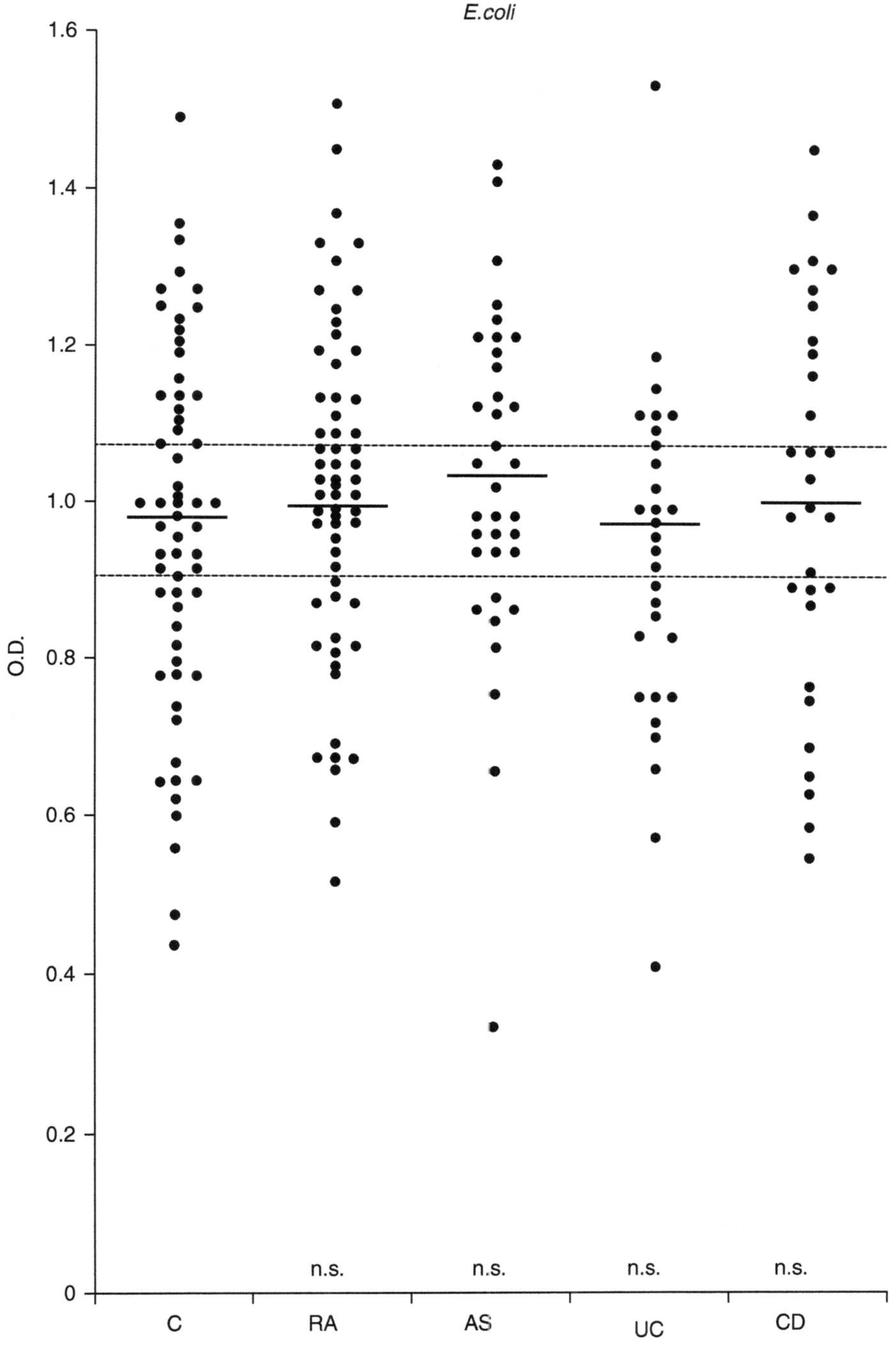

Fig. 21.3 Total immunoglobulin (IgG, IgA, IgM) levels against *Escherichia coli* in controls (*C*), rheumatoid arthritis (*RA*), ankylosing spondylitis (*AS*), ulcerative colitis (*UC*) and Crohn's disease (*CD*) subjects (*dotted line* indicates 95 % confidence limits for mean of control – two tailed test; *OD* optical density, *n.s.* not significant

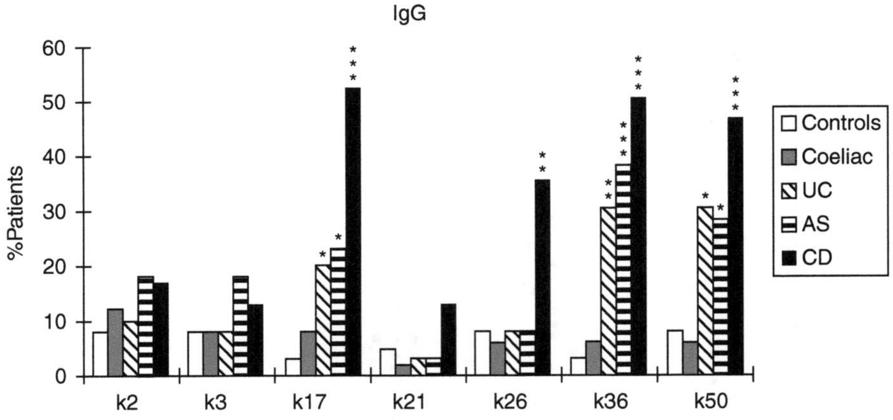

Fig. 21.4 Percentage of ankylosing spondylitis, Crohn's disease, ulcerative colitis and coeliac disease patients with antibodies (ELISA OD 630 nm) IgG elevated above the 95 % confidence limit of controls to whole bacterial preparations of *Klebsiella pneumoniae* serotypes K2, K3, K17, K21, K26, K36 and K50. An *asterisk* indicates statistical significance compared to the healthy control group $*p<0.05$, $**p<0.01$ and $***p<0.001$ using χ^2 test with Yates correction

Levels of IgG, IgA and IgM antibodies to each of the seven different *Klebsiella pneumoniae* were measured by ELISA, and the percentage of subjects with immunoglobulin levels above the 95 % confidence limit of the control population determined.

A significant percentage of ankylosing spondylitis patients showed raised IgG levels to whole *Klebsiella pneumoniae* species K17 ($\chi^2=5.60$, $p<0.05$), K36 ($\chi^2=13.20$, $p<0.001$) and K50 ($\chi^2=4.24$, $p<0.05$) compared with the healthy population (Fig. 21.4).

Furthermore, IgA antibody levels to K21 ($\chi^2=7.58$, $p<0.01$), K26 ($\chi^2=4.78$, $p<0.05$), K36 ($\chi^2=6.33$, $p<0.05$), K50 ($\chi^2=12.11$, $p<0.001$) (Fig. 21.5) and of IgM to K21 ($\chi^2=2.85$, $p<0.05$) were also found to be elevated in a greater number of ankylosing spondylitis patients when compared to controls (Fig. 21.6).

There was no significant elevation in anti-*Klebsiella* antibodies in coeliac disease patients compared to healthy, control subjects.

These results indicate that both ankylosing spondylitis patients and Crohn's disease patients have elevated levels of antibodies to *Klebsiella* bacteria. If anything, Crohn's disease patients have higher levels of antibodies to *Klebsiella* bacteria than ankylosing spondylitis patients.

When the same group of patients were tested with defined *Klebsiella* capsular extracts rather than whole bacteria, the same results were obtained; both ankylosing spondylitis patients and Crohn's disease had elevated levels of antibodies to *Klebsiella* components.

This raises the interesting question, whether the same microbe is involved in both diseases.

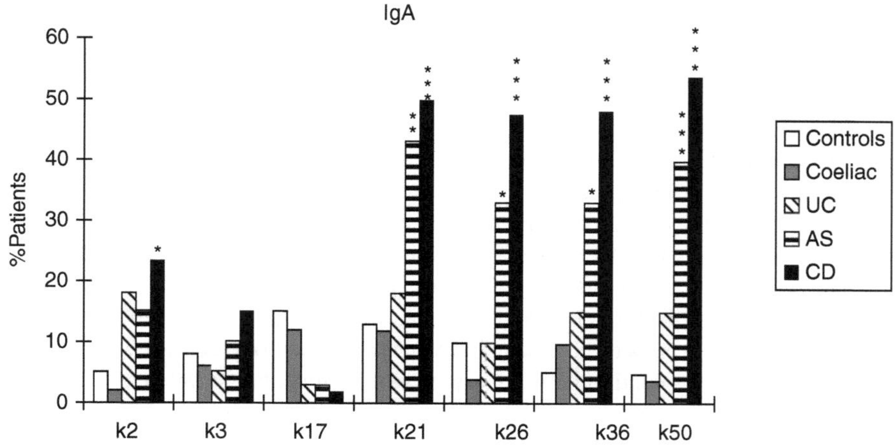

Fig. 21.5 Percentage of ankylosing spondylitis, Crohn's disease, ulcerative colitis and coeliac disease patients with antibodies (ELISA OD 630 nm) IgA elevated above the 95 % confidence limit of controls to whole bacterial preparations of *Klebsiella pneumoniae* serotypes K2, K3, K17, K21, K26, K36 and K50. An *asterisk* indicates statistical significance compared to the healthy control group **p*<0.05, ***p*<0.01 and ****p*<0.001 using χ^2 test with Yates correction

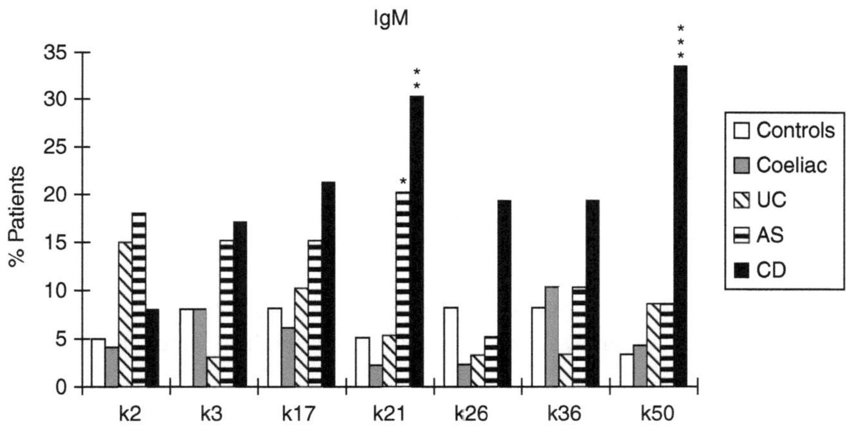

Fig. 21.6 Percentage of ankylosing spondylitis, Crohn's disease, ulcerative colitis and coeliac disease patients with antibodies (ELISA OD 630 nm) IgM elevated above the 95 % confidence limit of controls to whole bacterial preparations of *Klebsiella pneumoniae* serotypes K2, K3, K17, K21, K26, K36 and K50. An asterisk indicates statistical significance compared to the healthy control group **p*<0.05, ***p*<0.01 and ****p*<0.001 using χ^2 test with Yates correction

21.8 Antibodies to *Klebsiella* in Crohn's Disease and in Ankylosing Spondylitis Patients from Scotland

Antibodies to *Klebsiella* have been measured in ankylosing spondylitis and Crohn's disease in two centres in Scotland.

21.8.1 Glasgow

Antibodies to *Klebsiella pneumoniae* K43 was measured by ELISA in 64 patients with ankylosing spondylitis, 25 with rheumatoid arthritis, 30 with Crohn's disease and 20 with ulcerative colitis and compared to 35 healthy controls.

Significantly raised IgA antibody titres were seen in all groups when compared to the controls: ankylosing spondylitis ($p<0.0001$), rheumatoid arthritis ($p<0.01$), Crohn's disease ($p<0.05$) and ulcerative colitis ($p<0.05$) (Cooper et al. 1988).

The ankylosing spondylitis patients were divided into three groups of disease activity: active, probably active and inactive. Anti-*Klebsiella* IgA titres were elevated in all three groups of disease activity when compared to controls.

There was no correlation between erythrocyte sedimentation rate and C-reactive protein levels and the IgA anti-*Klebsiella* titre in the ankylosing spondylitis patients.

The titres of anti-*Klebsiella* IgG and IgM when compared to controls were not increased in the ankylosing spondylitis patients or any other group.

21.8.2 Edinburgh

The group from the Western General Hospital in Edinburgh have developed a technique of whole gut lavage which is a non-invasive, simple method of collecting intestinal secretions. Such a technique readily lends itself to the study of immune responses in diseases involving the gut (O'Mahony et al. 1991).

Elevated levels of serum IgA anti-*Klebsiella* antibodies were found in 14 active ankylosing spondylitis ($p<0.05$) when compared to healthy controls. There was a significant correlation in these 14 ankylosing spondylitis patients between serum IgA anti-*Klebsiella* antibodies and the erythrocyte sedimentation rate ($r=+0.72$, $p<0.005$) (O'Mahony et al. 1992).

In the patients with Crohn's disease, elevated levels of IgA anti-*Klebsiella* ($p<0.005$) and IgG anti-*Klebsiella* ($p<0.01$) antibodies were detected when compared to controls.

There was no elevation in IgM antibodies in all the groups.

Most control subjects had detectable IgA anti-*Klebsiella* antibodies in the gavage fluid.

High levels of intestinal IgM ($p<0.01$) and IgG antibodies ($p<0.0002$) to *Klebsiella* were detected in the Crohn's disease patients when compared to controls.

There was a trend in the whole gut lavage towards high levels of IgA antibody to *Klebsiella*, but it did not reach statistical significance.

It would appear that active ankylosing spondylitis patients have elevated levels of serum IgA antibodies to *Klebsiella*, but this is not specific since high antibody levels to *Klebsiella* are also found in Crohn's disease patients.

The high intestinal antibody levels in patients with Crohn's disease are not confined to *Klebsiella* as other groups have described elevated antibody levels to other bacteria such as bacteroides, *Escherichia coli* and *Yersinia*. Elevated levels of antibodies to *Saccharomyces cerevisiae* have been reported in Crohn's disease although their pathogenic significance is not clear (Giaffer et al. 1992).

21.9 Immune Response to Collagens in Patients with Crohn's Disease and Ankylosing Spondylitis

Crohn's disease is an inflammatory disorder associated with collagen deposition which leads to the formation of strictures (Graham et al. 1988). Immunochemical studies show that the collagens involved in Crohn's disease are of the types I, III and IV which are present in the lamina propria, mucularis mucosae and muscularis propia, respectively.

The aims of this study were to determine whether antibodies to collagens I, III, IV and V are increased in active Crohn's disease and ankylosing spondylitis patients when compared to controls.

Sera were obtained from 93 patients and healthy controls: 9 with early Crohn's disease (less than 2 years), 22 with Crohn's disease, 36 ankylosing spondylitis patients and 26 healthy controls.

The Crohn's disease patients were attending the Gastroenterology Outpatient Clinic at King's College Hospital.

The diagnosis of Crohn's disease was made using the standard St. Marks criteria with a Harvey-Bradshaw score > 3.

Levels of IgM, IgG and IgA antibodies to *Klebsiella pneumoniae* K50 were elevated in both ankylosing spondylitis and Crohn's disease patients when compared to controls.

Antibodies to collagen I (Fig. 21.7), collagen III (Fig. 21.8), collagen IV (Fig. 21.9) and collagen V (Fig. 21.10) were elevated in all three classes of immunoglobulins, IgM, IgG and IgA, in both Crohn's disease and ankylosing spondylitis

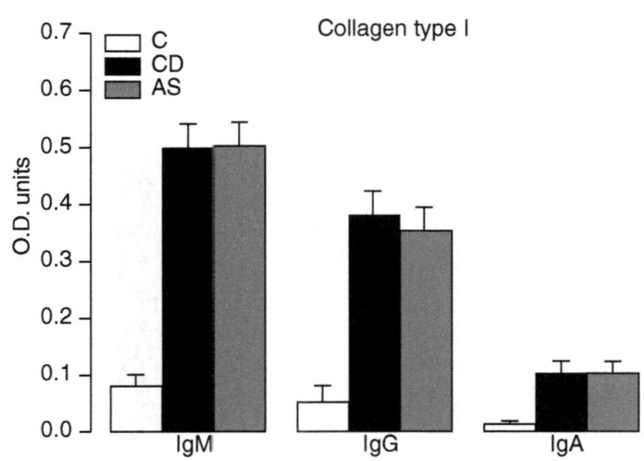

Fig. 21.7 Levels of IgM, IgG and IgA antibodies (mean ± standard to collagen type I in controls, Crohn's disease and ankylosing spondylitis patients)

Fig. 21.8 Levels of IgM, IgG and IgA antibodies (mean ± standard to collagen type III in controls, Crohn's disease and ankylosing spondylitis patients)

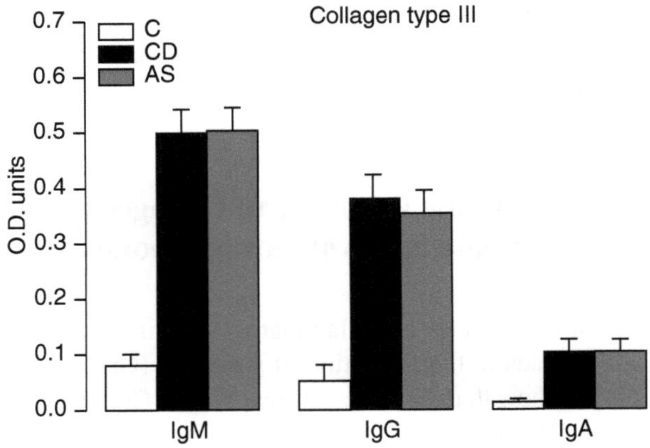

Fig. 21.9 Levels of IgM, IgG and IgA antibodies (mean ± standard to collagen type IV in controls, Crohn's disease and ankylosing spondylitis patients)

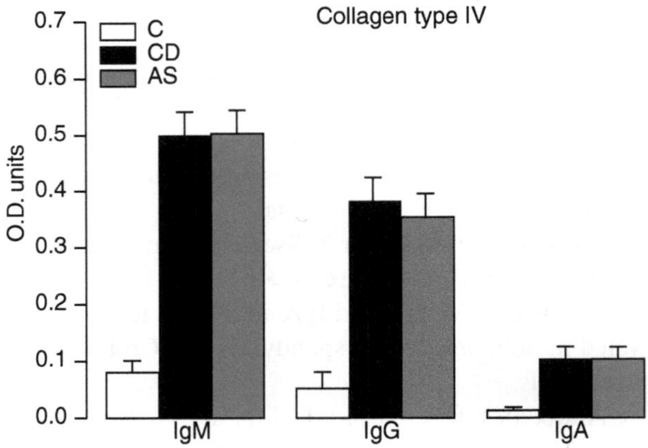

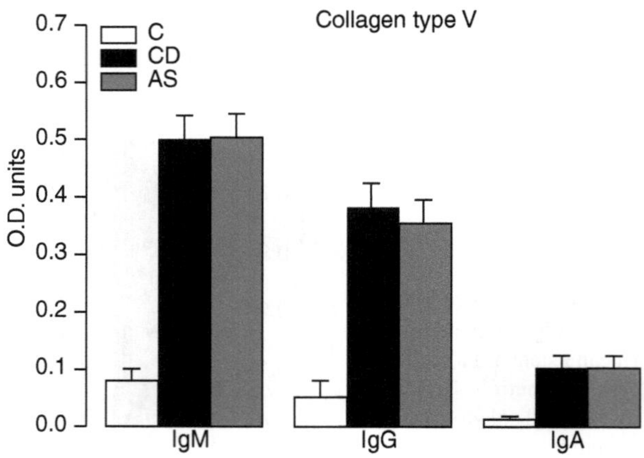

Fig. 21.10 Levels of IgM, IgG and IgA antibodies (mean ± standard to collagen type V in controls, Crohn's disease and ankylosing spondylitis patients)

patients, all at statistically significant values ($p < 0.001$) for 12 separate comparisons (Tiwana et al. 2001).

Molecular mimicry has been proposed as a mechanism involved in the pathogenesis of ankylosing spondylitis. There are not only similarities between HLA-B27 and pulD component of *Klebsiella* pullulanase but also with collagens.

There are similarities in amino acid sequences between the N-terminal end of the extracellular enzyme *Klebsiella* pullulanase (pulA) in the form of repeats of tripeptides (Gly-X-Pro) and collagen types I, III and IV.

Thus, the collagen antibodies detected in this study are acting as autoantibodies and producing pathological damage in both ankylosing spondylitis and Crohn's disease patients. Since these antibodies have been evoked by exposure to *Klebsiella* microbes, the inevitable conclusion arises that both diseases are caused by the same microbe.

In presence of HLA-B27, an antigen cross-reacting with pulD of *Klebsiella* pullulanase, autoantibodies against HLA-B27 are attacking HLA-B27 positive chondrocytes in the lumbar spine and causing spinal inflammation. Only small molecules, the size of an IgG, could penetrate the cartilage and attack the chondrocytes present in the lacunae.

In the absence of HLA-B27, autoantibodies are produced against collagens I, III, IV and V, whose antigens cross-react with pulA component of *Klebsiella* pullulanase and thereby produce strictures in the small bowel and cause Crohn's disease. Clearly, further studies are required to test this hypothesis. A case was reported from France of a Crohn's disease patient whose condition was exacerbated by *Klebsiella oxytoca* infections (Plessier et al. 2002).

21.10 Conclusion: Crohn's Disease Is Caused by *Klebsiella* in HLA-B27 Negative Individuals

Extensive studies, involving rheumatology and gastroenterology centres, indicate that there is a link between ankylosing spondylitis and the gut lesions found in Crohn's disease.

Immunological studies, involving six gastroenterology centres in the U.K.: Birmingham, Glasgow, Edinburgh, Royal Free Hospital, Middlesex Hospital and King's College Hospital, the last three in London, indicate that Crohn's disease patients have antibodies to *Klebsiella*, a microorganism associated with the development of the pathogenesis of ankylosing spondylitis. In these studies, it was impossible to separate ankylosing spondylitis from Crohn's disease patients.

One possible explanation is that the same microbe is involved in the causation of both diseases: in HLA-B27 positive individuals, it gives rise to ankylosing spondylitis, and in HLA-B27 negative individuals, it causes Crohn's disease.

Therapeutic implications also follow from this conclusion in that a 'low starch diet' should be beneficial not only to ankylosing spondylitis patients but also in patients suffering from Crohn's disease. These proposals should be critically examined by multi-centre studies.

References

Cooper R, Fraser SM, Sturrock RDF, Gemmell CG. Raised titres of anti-*Klebsiella* IgA in ankylosing spondylitis, rheumatoid arthritis and inflammatory bowel disease. Br Med J. 1988;296:1432–4.

Ebringer A. Rheumatoid arthritis and *Proteus*. Springer; 2012.

Giaffer MH, Clark A, Holdsworth CD. Antibodies to *Saccharomyces cerevisiae* in patients with Crohn's disease and their possible pathogenic significance. Gut. 1992;33:1071–5.

Graham MF, Diegelmann RF, Elson CO, Linblad WJ, Gotschalk N, Gay S, Gay R. Collagen content and types in the intestinal strictures of Crohn's disease. Gastroenterology. 1988; 94:257–65.

Harvey RF, Bradshaw JM. A simple index of Crohn's disease activity. Lancet. 1980;1:514.

Ibbotson JP, Pease PE, Allan RN. Serological studies in Crohn's disease. Eur J Clin Microbiol. 1987;6:286–90.

Mielants H, Veys EM, Cuvelier C, De Vos M. Ileocolonoscopic findings in seronegative spondyloarthropathy. Br J Rheumatol. 1988;27 Suppl 2:95–105.

O'Mahony S, Arranz E, Barton JR, Ferguson A. Appraisal of gut lavage in the study of intestinal humoral immunity. Gut. 1991;31:1341–4.

O'Mahony S, Anderson N, Nuki G, Ferguson A. Systemic and mucosal antibodies to *Klebsiella* in patients with ankylosing spondylitis and Crohn's disease. Ann Rheum Dis. 1992;51:1296–300.

Plessier A, Cosnes J, Gendre JP, Beaugerie L. Colites intercurrentes à *Klebsiella oxytoca* au cours de la maladie de Crohn. Gastroenterol Clin Biol. 2002;26:799–800.

Tiwana H, Wilson C, Walmsley RS, Wakefield AJ, Smith MSN, Cox NL, Hudson MJ, Ebringer A. Antibody responses to gut bacteria in ankylosing spondylitis, rheumatoid arthritis, Crohn's disease and ulcerative colitis. Rheumatol Int. 1997;17:11–6.

Tiwana H, Walmsley RS, Wilson C, Yiannakou JY, Ciclitira PJ, Wakefield AJ, Ebringer A. Characterization of the humoral immune response to *Klebsiella* species in inflammatory bowel disease and ankylosing spondylitis. Br J Rheumatol. 1998;37(5):525–31.

Tiwana H, Natt RS, Benitez-Brito R, Shah S, Wilson C, Bridger S, Harbord M, Sarner M, Ebringer A. Correlation between the Immune responses to type I, III, IV and V and *Klebsiella Pneumoniae* in patients with Crohn's disease and ankylosing spondylitis. Rheumatology. 2001;40:15–23.

Chapter 22
Ankylosing Spondylitis and 'Popper Sequences'

22.1 Introduction to 'Popper Sequences'

The cause of ankylosing spondylitis has been investigated by the methods of Sir Karl Popper (1902–1994) who claimed that a theory could not be proved by induction or any other methods but could be disproved.

A fact which was incompatible with a theory would thereby disprove it, and this approach has provided a powerful new method to investigate scientific problems (Popper 1972).

The 'Popper sequences' consist of four stages:

First is the 'scientific problem' (P1 = problem).
Second is the attempted solution or 'theory' (TT = tentative theory).
Third is the attempted falsification of the theory by 'experiments or observations' (EE = error elimination).
Finally, there is the generation of new knowledge which creates 'new problems' and 'new facts' (P2 = new problem).

Preliminary investigations have shown that 'Popper sequences' provide new ways of looking at scientific problems such as rheumatoid arthritis (Ebringer et al. 2010) or ankylosing spondylitis.

If the cause of ankylosing spondylitis can be found, then appropriate steps could be taken in the early stages of the condition so that both medical problems of the patients and financial costs to society can be minimised to the mutual benefits of both groups.

A. Ebringer, *Ankylosing Spondylitis and Klebsiella*,
DOI 10.1007/978-1-4471-4300-0_22, © Springer-Verlag London 2013

22.2 Components of a 'Popper Sequence'

The sequence of a 'Popper sequence' could be summarised as follows:

P(1) → **Problem**
↓
TT1 → **Tentative theory**
↓
EE1 → **Error elimination**
↓
P(2) → **New fact and new problem**

The second problem (P2) is different from the first; it is the result of the new situation that has arisen because of the tentative theories (TT1) and the error elimination (EE1) which consist of logical analysis or criticism and experimental investigations suggested by the 'tentative theories' (TT1).

22.3 First Popper Sequence

One of the greatest discoveries in the history of rheumatology was the simultaneous demonstration by research workers from London and Los Angeles that some 96 % of patients suffering from ankylosing spondylitis possessed or belonged to the HLA-B27 group, whilst the frequency of this marker in the general population of the UK or the USA was around 8 %.

This great disparity between the frequency of this 'major histocompatibility complex' marker, located on chromosome 6 and its low frequency in the general population, raised the possibility that it could provide some insight into the causation of this disease.

Any solution to the problem of ankylosing spondylitis should also explain the high frequency of this gene in this disease.

Patients with ankylosing spondylitis often experience symptoms of this disease for several years, before a final diagnosis is reached, and it has been suggested that this could be called an early phase of ankylosing spondylitis or pre-AS (Ebringer et al. 2005).

When ankylosing spondylitis and pre-AS are considered together, they could account for up to 1 % of the general population. It would appear that there are over 30 million individuals in the world who are HLA-B27 positive and suffer from either ankylosing spondylitis or pre-AS.

There are two ways of explaining this observation: either HLA-B27 molecules present some unknown antigens to immune cells, or the HLA-B27 molecule itself resembles or shows 'molecular mimicry' to some component of the bacteria or viruses present in the environment.

Since 'molecular mimicry' appeared to work in rheumatic fever and later in rheumatoid arthritis, we chose this approach to study the ankylosing spondylitis problem.

This leads to the first Popper sequence:

P(1) → **HLA-B27 is present in AS patients**

↓ ↓

TT(1) → **HLA-B27 resembles some microbe**

↓ ↓

EE(1) → **Inject HLA-B27 cells into a rabbit**

↓ ↓

P(2) → **Rabbit makes antibodies to *Klebsiella***

The result of the 'first Popper sequence' suggests that *Klebsiella* bacteria are somehow linked to HLA-B27. This raises the new problem (P2) that *Klebsiella* bacteria may be involved in the onset or origin of ankylosing spondylitis.

However, we are not sure whether this is a property of HLA-B27 lymphocytes, or the rabbit may have been inadvertently immunised or exposed to *Klebsiella* bacteria whilst in the animal house.

Therefore, this observation must be checked against HLA-B27 tissue typing sera, and this leads to the 'second Popper sequence'.

22.4 Second Popper Sequence

It is possible that the rabbit exhibiting anti-*Klebsiella* antibodies following immunisation with HLA-B27 lymphocytes may have been infected in the cage. Therefore, the fortuitous observation of anti-*Klebsiella* antibodies could be an artefact. The problem arises whether this observation is associated with human lymphocytes in general or can it be linked to the HLA-B27 specificity.

It was considered that to establish that *Klebsiella* microorganisms were somehow related to ankylosing spondylitis, they had to be linked to the HLA-B27 specificity by more reliable methods than xenogeneic rabbit immunisation.

The first clear demonstration of cross-reactivity between HLA-DR4 and *Proteus* occurred when allogeneic anti-HLA-DR4 tissue typing sera bound to *Proteus* antigens to a greater extent than HLA tissue typing sera specific for other HLA antigens.

Anti-DR4 tissue typing sera were found to bind to *Proteus mirabilis* to a significantly greater extent ($p<0.001$), whilst no such increased binding was observed with *Escherichia coli* microorganisms.

A similar approach was adopted to study this problem. HLA-B27 tissue typing sera were obtained from the Bristol Tissue Typing Centre.

P(2) → **HLA-B27 may crossreact with some *Klebsiella* antigens**

↓

TT(2) → **HLA-B27 tissue typing sera should bind to *Klebsiella* antigens**

↓

EE(2) → **Test anti-B27 tissue typing sera for the binding activity to *Klebsiella* antigens**

↓

P(3) → **HLA-B27 tissue typing sera bind preferentially to *Klebsiella* bacteria**

22.5 Third Popper Sequence

The possibility arises that ankylosing spondylitis patients have been infected by *Klebsiella* bacteria, which are normal constituents of the bowel flora and are mainly located in the large bowel, especially around the ascending colon.

The quantity of bacteria in the bowel is controlled by the 'gut-associated lymphoid tissues' which respond to antigens of the luminal bacteria and other components especially of undigested food.

When environmental antigens are acting across a mucosal surface, this leads to an elevation of total serum IgA.

The question arises whether total serum IgA is elevated in ankylosing spondylitis patients during active phases of the disease, and this forms the basis of the 'third Popper sequence'.

P(3) → **AS patients may be infected by *Klebsiella* across a mucosal surface**

↓

TT(3) → **Total serum IgA immunoglobulins should be elevated in AS patients**

↓

EE(3) → **Measure total serum IgA in AS patients**

↓

P(4) → **Active AS patients have elevated levels of total serum IgA**

Various independent studies have shown that concentrations of total serum IgA are increased significantly in active patients with ankylosing spondylitis.

These results suggest that bowel bacterial antigens have been acting across a mucosal surface.

If these antigens belong to *Klebsiella* bacteria, then ankylosing spondylitis patients should have elevated levels of antibodies against this microbe.

Antibodies to Gram-negative bacteria such as *Yersinia*, *Salmonella* or *Shigella* are elevated in patients with 'reactive arthritis', and these usually involve the IgA immunoglobulin.

In some patients who have had an enteric infection with these Gram-negative microorganisms, it is usually followed 6–8 weeks later by the development of an inflammatory arthritis, especially in the large joints such as hips, knees and ankles.

It is possible that *Klebsiella* infection or proliferation may not cause overt gastrointestinal symptoms, but if antibody levels become elevated, they may cause clinical symptoms and eventually lead to a disease like ankylosing spondylitis. This question leads to the 'fourth Popper sequence'.

22.6 Fourth Popper Sequence

There appears to be a link between HLA-B27 and the commensal bowel microbe *Klebsiella.* Total immunoglobulin studies suggest that the environmental agent is acting across a mucosal surface because total serum IgA levels are elevated in ankylosing spondylitis patients.

However, we do not know if ankylosing spondylitis patients have specific antibodies against this particular microbe.

Antibody levels against *Klebsiella* microorganisms have been measured by a number of techniques: Widal agglutination, ELISA, immunoblotting and immunofluorescence. In each case, the results were similar, in that active ankylosing spondylitis patients had significantly elevated levels of antibodies against *Klebsiella* microorganisms.

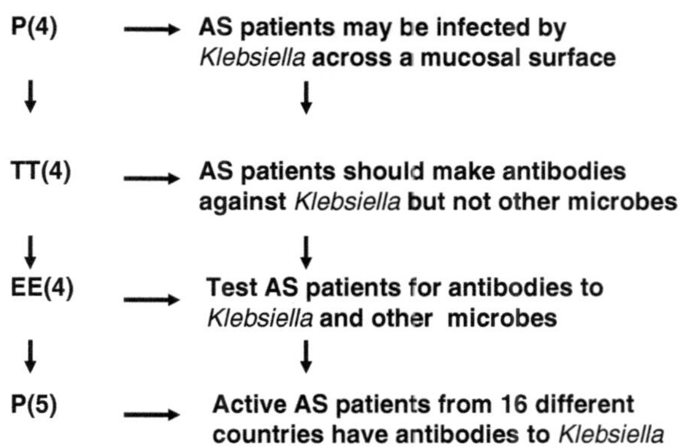

Table 22.1 The list of countries first reporting elevated levels of antibodies to *Klebsiella* in patients with ankylosing spondylitis, year of the report and publication reference

	Country	Year of study	Reference no.
1.	England	1983	Trull et al.
2.	USA	1987	Schwimmbeck et al.
3.	Scotland	1988	Cooper et al.
4.	Russia	1989	Nasonova et al.
5.	Slovakia	1989	Mateicka et al.
6.	China	1993	Yuan et al.
7.	Germany	1994	Sahly et al.
8.	Spain	1994	Collado et al.
9.	Turkey	1996	Ardicoglu et al.
10.	Japan	1997	Tani et al.
11.	Finland	1997a	Maki-Ikola et al.
12.	Sweden	1997b	Maki-Ikola et al.
13.	Taiwan	1998	Chou et al.
14.	Mexico	1998	Cancino-Diaz et al.
15	Netherlands	1998	Blankenberg-Sprenkels et al.
16.	India	2002	Madhavan et al.

The countries, years of the report and publication reference are summarised in the tabulated list (Table 22.1).

Although ankylosing spondylitis patients have antibodies to *Klebsiella* in many different countries, we still do not know how specific is this observation. Could other biological agents be also present in ankylosing spondylitis patients when they show elevated levels of antibodies to *Klebsiella*, and this brings us to the next and 'fifth Popper sequence'.

22.7 Fifth Popper Sequence

An examination was carried out to measure the levels of antibodies against *Klebsiella* in the serum of active ankylosing spondylitis patients compared to patients with other chronic diseases such as systemic lupus erythematosus, psoriatic arthropathy, rheumatoid arthritis, ulcerative colitis and Crohn's disease. However, apart from ankylosing spondylitis and Crohn's disease, none of the other groups with other rheumatic conditions had significant elevations in the anti-*Klebsiella* antibody levels.

P(5) → ***Klebsiella* antibodies may be present in AS patients but not in other diseases**

↓ ↓

TT(5) → ***Klebsiella* antibodies should not be present in other diseases**

↓ ↓

EE(5) → **Examine other diseases**

↓ ↓

P(6) → **Antibodies to *Klebsiella* confined to patients with AS and Crohn's disease but no other conditions**

The presence of antibodies to *Klebsiella* bacteria in patients with Crohn's disease raises interesting issues in the pathogenesis of both ankylosing spondylitis and Crohn's diseases.

It is possible that the same microbe is involved in both conditions, one in HLA-B27 positive individuals and the other one in HLA-B27 negative individuals. This hypothesis also provides an explanation as to what happens to HLA-B27 negative individuals who consume large quantities of starch. According to this theory, they would be more likely to develop Crohn's disease.

The next problem arises as to the mucosal site where these bacteria are located.

This brings us to the 'sixth Popper sequence'.

22.8 Sixth Popper Sequence

The location of the *Klebsiella* bacteria in active ankylosing spondylitis patients has so far not been resolved: Are these bacteria to be found in the respiratory tract or the gastrointestinal tract, two sites which have a mucosal surface and therefore would lead to an elevation in total serum IgA immunoglobulins, as shown in 'Popper sequence 3'. Antigens that act across a mucosal surface usually evoke predominantly IgA rather than IgG antibodies, and it is possible that the *Klebsiella* microbes might act across a mucosal surface.

P(6) → **AS patients are infected by *Klebsiella***

↓

TT(6) → ***Klebsiella* could be in the gastro-intestinal tract**

↓

EE(6) → **Test AS patients for *Klebsiella* bacteria in faecal cultures**

↓

P(7) → **AS patients have *Klebsiella* in faecal cultures as well as antibodies in serum**

There appear to be several studies which show positive faecal cultures for *Klebsiella* in active ankylosing spondylitis patients, although other groups have been unable to confirm these observations.

These six 'Popper sequences' have identified so far that HLA-B27 resembles some *Klebsiella* antigens. Furthermore, it would appear that antibodies to this microbe are present in ankylosing spondylitis patients, whilst no such antibodies are present in other chronic diseases, and the site of infection would appear to be the gastrointestinal tract especially around the ileo-caecal junction and ascending colon. This brings us to the next 'Popper sequence' whether *Klebsiella* is the only microbe present in ankylosing spondylitis patients or could antibodies be detected against other microbial agents.

22.9 Seventh Popper Sequence

Many studies have been carried out by different independent groups on antibodies against various microbial antigens, especially Gram-negative microorganisms (reviewed by Ebringer et al. 2006).

The results of these studies have shown that there were no significant elevations in the levels of antibodies against other *Klebsiella*-related or unrelated microbes including Gram-negative enterobacteria such as *Salmonella* or *Yersinia* and Gram-positive *Streptococcus* pathogenic bacteria.

In 10 out of 13 studies, anti-*Klebsiella* antibodies were shown to be present in ankylosing spondylitis patients at a statistically significant level ($p<0.001$) and the other 3 at lower levels of significance ($p<0.01$) or ($p<0.05$).

In one of the studies, anti-*Escherichia coli* were slightly elevated ($p<0.05$), but at the same time, the anti-*Klebsiella* titre was significantly elevated ($p<0.001$) in the ankylosing spondylitis patients.

P(7) → **AS patients are infected by *Klebsiella***
↓
TT(7) → **Other bacteria or viral agents should not be present in AS patients**
↓
EE(7) → **Test AS patients for other bacteria**
↓
P(8) → **Other bacteria not present in AS patients at the same statistical significance as *Klebsiella***

Furthermore, in another study involving ankylosing spondylitis patients from London, using an immunoblotting assay carried out in Finland, there was no elevation in anti-*Yersinia* antibodies when compared to Finnish patients suffering from *Yersinia* reactive arthritis.

It appears that *Klebsiella* bacteria are clearly involved in ankylosing spondylitis patients, but the pathological mechanism of joint damage and its link to HLA requires further examination.

We still do not know which component of HLA-B27 is associated with *Klebsiella* bacteria. This brings us to the 'eighth Popper sequence'.

22.10 Eighth Popper Sequence

The enzyme 'nitrogenase reductase' which is present in *Klebsiella* has a six amino acid homology with HLA-B27. This enzyme is not usually expressed in *Klebsiella* bacteria at a temperature of 37 °C but found mainly in soil bacteria at a temperature of 32 °C.

However, it is not clear whether the QTDRED sequence is somehow linked to other molecules in *Klebsiella* microbes.

P(8) → **QTDRED is present in HLA-B27 molecules**
↓
TT(8) → ***Klebsiella* homologue to HLA-B27**
↓
EE(8) → **Computer analysis of *Klebsiella***
↓
P(9) → **DRDE sequence in *Klebsiella* pullulanase-D**

The 'error elimination' (EE8) in this Popper sequence consists of carrying out a computer analysis of the components of the *Klebsiella* bacteria to see if they resemble or show 'molecular mimicry' to the QTDRED sequence.

A sequence DRDE was found in pullulanase-D which showed molecular mimicry with the DRED sequence present in HLA-B27 molecules.

The anatomical distribution of the lesions in ankylosing spondylitis involves the large joints and the lumbar spine. This brings us to the next Popper sequence.

22.11 Ninth Popper Sequence

If the collagens present in the large joints are targeted by antibodies, then this suggests that any aetiological agent proposed for the cause of ankylosing spondylitis must also explain the geography of the disease.

The chief site of pathology in ankylosing spondylitis is the lumbar spine and the large joints.

Gly-X-Pro tripeptide repeating sequences have been found in pullulanase-A components of *Klebsiella* microorganisms which show molecular mimicry with type I, III and IV collagens, and antibodies to such collagens have been described in ankylosing spondylitis patients.

These collagens are found predominantly in the tendons, spine, large joints and uvea.

Therefore, antibodies to *Klebsiella* pulA could have cytopathic properties against such collagens and would explain the distribution of the pathological sites in ankylosing spondylitis.

P(9) ⟶ **AS patients have antibodies to collagens**
↓ ↓
TT(9) ⟶ ***Klebsiella* may resemble some collagens**
↓ ↓
EE(9) ⟶ **Computer analysis of *Klebsiella***
↓ ↓
P(10) ⟶ **Gly-X-Pro sequences of pullulanase-A resemble I, III and IV collagens**

22.12 Tenth Popper Sequence

Ankylosing spondylitis is characterised by inflammatory episodes, and their occurrence can be monitored by the presence of an elevated erythrocyte sedimentation rate and/or elevated C-reactive protein levels.

It is important here to distinguish between clinical assessments of pain as measured by subjective 'analogue scales' whereby the patient indicates on a scale of 1–10, the degree of discomfort and pain felt, as opposed to an objective measurement of inflammation as given by an erythrocyte sedimentation rate or C-reactive protein level.

The usual levels which determine active disease and presence of biochemical inflammation is an erythrocyte sedimentation rate >30 mm/h (ESR) or a C-reactive protein level >15 mg/l.

The critical question arises whether such inflammatory episodes could be triggered by the high titres of anti-*Klebsiella* antibodies that have been identified in the ankylosing spondylitis patients.

The Popperian question arises whether such cytopathic effects can be demonstrated as an indication that anti-*Klebsiella* antibodies are the first triggers or agents in this disease.

This will provide an answer to the important question 'Do ankylosing spondylitis sera produce tissue damage?'

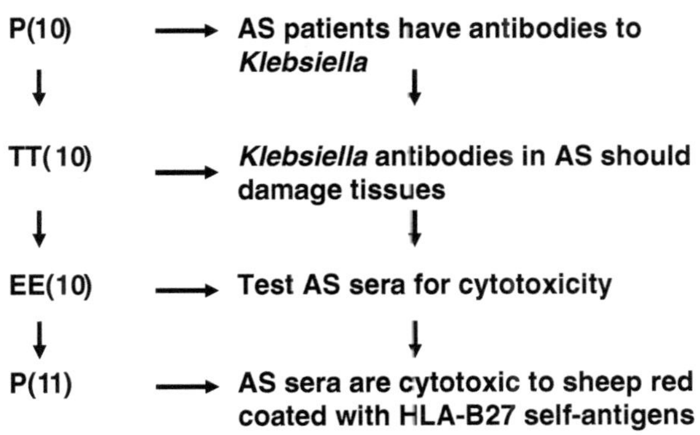

Sera from active ankylosing spondylitis patients were tested by a complement-mediated cytotoxicity assay. Sheep red cells were coated with HLA-B27 peptides or EQRRAA (HLA-DR1/4) or ESRRAL (*Proteus* haemolysin) peptides and compared to sera from patients with rheumatoid arthritis and healthy blood donors.

Ankylosing spondylitis sera were found to have cytotoxic activity against HLA-B27 peptides coated on sheep red cells but not against peptides involved in rheumatoid arthritis. However, the rheumatoid arthritis sera had cytotoxic activity against the rheumatoid antigens, the EQRRAA and ESRRAL, coated sheep red cells but not against the HLA-B27 coated sheep red cells. Thus, each disease acted as specificity control for the other condition. It is clear that active ankylosing spondylitis sera have specific cytopathic activity which could explain the inflammation in the entheses, lumbar spine, sacroiliac joints and uvea. The next question is what drives the production of such cytopathic autoantibodies, and this brings us to the next Popper sequence.

22.13 Eleventh Popper Sequence

In various independent studies throughout the world, ankylosing spondylitis patients were found to have elevated levels of antibodies to *Klebsiella* bacteria. Therefore, one possible way of reducing the numbers of *Klebsiella* microbes in the large bowel of ankylosing spondylitis patients is to reduce the quantity of substrates required for their growth.

Dietary starch provides an important substrate for the growth of gut microbes including *Klebsiella.*

Rats fed on starch increase the bulk of intestinal microflora, and *Klebsiella* bacteria grow preferentially on simple sugars. In American vegan subjects on a high starch diet, the number of *Klebsiella* bacteria in faecal specimens was elevated compared to subjects on an omnivorous diet.

Ileostomy fluids contain significant quantities of starch. A sizable proportion of starch escapes absorption from the small bowel and reaches the large bowel. This undigested starch forms an important substrate for the growth and proliferation of intestinal bacteria.

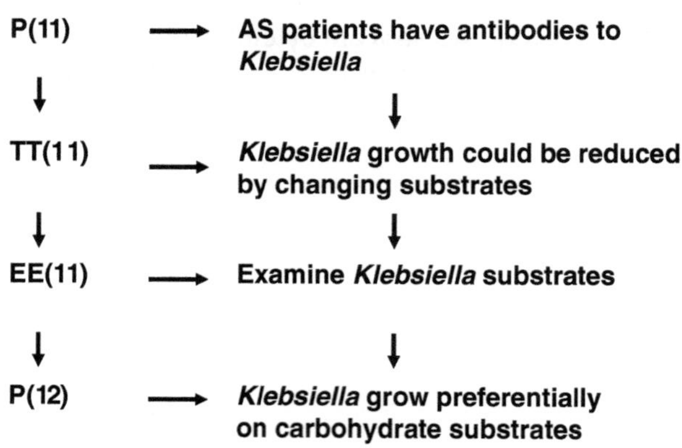

22.14 Twelfth Popper Sequence

It would appear that the quantities of carbohydrate substrates entering the large bowel across ileo-caecal junction are important in determining the number of *Klebsiella* microbes.

An important source of carbohydrate substrate comes from dietary starch. Dietary starch consists of approximately 20 % amylose and 80 % amylopectin.

Amylose is a linear polymer consisting of α(1–4) links between glucose residues, and these can be readily hydrolysed by amylases present in digestive enzymes. However, amylopectin is a branched polymer, consisting of linear sequences of amylase-like chains linked by α(1–4) bonds, but for every 10–15 residues, there is a α(1–6) side-chain, giving rise to a branched structure. The problem is that digestive enzymes cannot break down the α(1–6) links present in amylopectin. Following digestion, the amylopectin is debranched from the amylose side-chains ending up with a limit dextrin or 'hard starch' consisting of about 40 % of the original weight of the ingested starch. The terminal tips of such a molecule consist of α(1–6) glucose residues which cannot be cleaved by digestive enzymes.

However, the accumulated limit dextrin or 'hard starch' is available for the growth and propagation of gut bacteria, especially *Klebsiella*.

Klebsiella pullulanase is a powerful debranching enzyme which breaks or hydrolyzes the α(1–6) links and degrades the amylopectin remnants into monosaccharides and disaccharides, thereby making them available for bacterial growth.

This leads to the next Popper sequence.

In a 9-month study of ankylosing spondylitis patients on a 'low starch diet', the mean erythrocyte sedimentation rate (ESR) dropped, whilst there was no such reduction when the same patients were examined for 6 months before the onset of the diet.

The involvement of dietary starch leads to the next Popper sequence.

P(12) → **Pullulanase enzymes can degrade "hard starch" and provide substrates for the growth of *Klebsiella***

↓

TT(12) → **The disease activity in AS patients should be reduced by decreasing starch intake**

↓

EE(12) → **Test ESR in AS patients after a "low starch diet"**

↓

P(13) → **AS patients have a reduction in ESR following a "low starch diet"**

22.15 Thirteenth Popper Sequence

Ankylosing spondylitis has often been referred to as a disease of young men although it is recognised to occur in women.

The onset of the disease is usually in the late teens to twenties, and the male to female ratio has been estimated to be 3:1.

This early onset of the disease and sex ratio differs markedly from rheumatoid arthritis where it usually starts in the forties and fifties age groups and occurs more frequently in women.

Any theory trying to explain ankylosing spondylitis must also account for this early age of onset and male predominance.

So far we have proposed that the link with HLA-B27 leads to the identification of the bowel microbe *Klebsiella* which depends for its growth on the consumption of adequate amounts of dietary starch, and this leads to the next Popper sequence.

P(13)	→	**Onset of AS starts frequently in teens and twenties, especially in men**
↓		↓
TT(13)	→	**Onset may be linked to puberty, male hormones and muscle mass**
↓		↓
EE(13)	→	**Examine whether men consume more calories than women**
↓		↓
P(14)	→	**Men consume 40-50% more calories than women**

Ever since 1918, when Harris and Benedict from the Carnegie Institute in Washington published their equation for determining daily calorie requirements, there have been numerous studies showing that at puberty and thereafter, nutritional requirements in men increase sharply due to the development of hormonally induced muscle mass.

On average, men require 40–50 % more calories than women, the average daily recommended quantity in women being 2,000 calories compared to 3,000 calories in men, depending on degree of physical activity.

Clearly the extra 40–50 % calorie intake in some men may contain starch compounds which will contribute to an increased growth of *Klebsiella* bacteria near the ileo-caecal valve and ascending colon. This in turn will lead to the production of cytopathic antibodies which will attack targets in the spine and elsewhere, sites which contain cross-reacting antigens such as collagens I, III and IV as well as HLA-B27.

It would appear that the molecular mimicry theory involving HLA-B27 and *Klebsiella* can also account for the early onset of ankylosing spondylitis in young men.

22.16 Therapeutic Implications

The probable cause for the onset and development of ankylosing spondylitis has been identified through the demonstration of 13 'Popper sequences', each of which provided a new fact about the disease.

If any other theories were to be suggested, it would have to account for the 'new facts' uncovered by this Popperian analysis.

Current therapy of ankylosing spondylitis involves the use of agents such as methotrexate and anti-tumour necrosis factor (TNF) biologicals which significantly reduce the degree of inflammation. However, these methods do not treat the cause of the disease but the consequent inflammation produced by the cross-reacting bacterial autoantibodies following infection by *Klebsiella* microbes, when these antibodies bind to cross-reacting self-antigens, activate complement cascade and cause inflammatory tissue damage.

Another important problem with biologicals is the issue of safety, with an increased risk of infections as well as an increased incidence of malignancies.

The discovery that ankylosing spondylitis is triggered or caused by *Klebsiella* in the large bowel opens a new approach to the treatment of this disabling arthritic disease.

In future, the treatment of ankylosing spondylitis will not only involve the use of established modalities of therapy such as anti-inflammatory agents and various biologicals but also a protocol involving a reduced consumption of dietary components which increase the substrate for the growth of *Klebsiella* microorganisms. Controlled studies involving a 'low starch diet' appear to reduce erythrocyte sedimentation rate, a measure of biochemical inflammation in patients with ankylosing spondylitis.

Further studies are required to determine the effectiveness of 'low starch diet' in combination with existing methods of treatment. The effectiveness of existing methods of treatment could be improved together with the use of a 'low starch diet' in that deleterious side effects might be avoided with the delivery of lower doses of drugs.

In science, we are trying to get closer to the truth, but in medicine, the results of our investigations should help the patient as suggested by the Hippocratic oath.

Sufficient new evidence has been uncovered using Popperian methods of scientific research for anti-*Klebsiella* therapy to be assessed in the management of ankylosing spondylitis.

References

Ardicoglu O, Atay MB, Ataoglu H, Etiz N, Ozenci H. IgA antibodies to *Klebsiella* in ankylosing spondylitis. Clin Rheumatol. 1996;15:573–6.

Blankenberg-Sprenkels SHD, Fielder M, Feltkamp TEW, Tiwana H, Wilson C, Ebringer A. Antibodies to *Klebsiella pneumoniae* in Dutch patients with ankylosing spondylitis and acute anterior uveitis and to *Proteus mirabilis* in rheumatoid arthritis. J Rheumatol. 1998;25: 743–7.

Cancino-Diaz ME, Perez-Salazar JE, Dominguez-Lopez L, Escobar-Gutierrez A, Granados-Arreola J, Jimenez-Zamudio L, Burgos-Vargas R, Garcia-Latorre E. Antibody response to *Klebsiella pneumoniae* 60 kDa protein in familial and sporadic ankylosing spondylitis: role of HLA-B27 and characterization as a GroEL-like protein. J Rheumatol. 1998;25:1756–64.

Chou CT, Uksila J, Toivanen P. Enterobacterial antibodies in Chinese patients with rheumatoid arthritis and ankylosing spondylitis. Clin Exp Rheumatol. 1998;16:161–4.

Collado A, Gratacós J, Ebringer A, Rashid T, Martí A, Sanmartí R, Muñoz-Gomez J. Serum IgA antibodies in ankylosing spondylitis patients from Catalonia. Scand J Rheumatol. 1994;23:119–23.

Cooper R, Fraser SM, Sturrock RDF, Gemmell CG. Raised titres of anti-*Klebsiella* IgA in ankylosing spondylitis, rheumatoid arthritis and inflammatory bowel disease. Br Med J. 1988;296: 1432–4.

Ebringer A, Rashid T, Wilson C, Miškejova G. "Pre-ankylosing spondylitis" is a clinical entity: diagnostic criteria and therapeutic implications. Rheumatologia. 2005;18:91–6.

Ebringer A, Rashid T, Wilson C, Ptaszynska T, Fielder M. Ankylosing spondylitis, HLA-B27 and *Klebsiella*. An overview: proposal for early diagnosis and treatment. Curr Rheumatol Rev. 2006;2:55–68.

Ebringer A, Rashid T, Wilson C. Rheumatoid arthritis, *Proteus*, anti-CCP antibodies and Karl Popper. Autoimmun Rev. 2010;9:216–23.

Madhavan R, Porkodi R, Rajendran CP, Chandrasekaran AN, Umadevi KR, Alasmelu R. IgM, IgG and IgA response to enterobacteria in patients with ankylosing spondylitis in Southern India. Ann N Y Acad Sci. 2002;958:408–11.

Maki-Ikola O, Penttinen M, Von Essen R, Gripenberg-Lerche C, Isomaki H, Granfors K. IgM, IgG and IgA class enterobacterial antibodies in serum and synovial fluid in patients with ankylosing spondylitis. Br J Rheumatol. 1997(a);36:1051–3.

Mäki-Ikola O, Hällgren R, Kancrud L, Feltelius N, Knutsson L, Granfors K. Enhanced jejunal production of antibodies to *Klebsiella* and other *Enterobacteria* in patients with ankylosing spondylitis and rheumatoid arthritis. Ann Rheum Dis. 1997b;56:421–5.

Mateicka F, Kozakova D, Cebecauer M, Ondrasik M, Bosmansky K. Antibodies to *Klebsiella pneumoniae* in ankylosing spondylitis. Cas Lek Cesk. 1989;128:132–4.

Nasonova VA, Denisov LN, Belenkii AG, Balabanova RM, Iakovleva DB. Circulation of intestinal infection in the families of patients with rheumatic diseases and the state of humoral immunity to enterobacterial antigens. Vest Akad Med Nauk SSSR. 1989;6:56–60.

Popper KR. Objective knowledge. An evolutionary approach. Oxford: Clarendon Press; 1972.

Sahly H, Podschun R, Sass R, Bröker B, Kekow J, Gross WL, Ullmann U. Serum antibodies to *Klebsiella* capsular polysaccharides in ankylosing spondylitis. Arthritis Rheum. 1994;37: 754–9.

Schwimmbeck PL, Yu DTY, Oldstone MBA. Autoantibodies to HLA-B27 in the sera of HLA-B27 patients with ankylosing spondylitis and Reiter's syndrome: molecular mimicry with *Klebsiella pneumoniae* as potential mechanism of autoimmune disease. J Exp Med. 1987;166:173–81.

Tani Y, Tiwana H, Hukuda S, Nishioka J, Fielder M, Wilson C, Bansal S, Ebringer A. Antibodies to *Klebsiella, Proteus* and HLA-B27 peptides in Japanese patients with ankylosing spondylitis and rheumatoid arthritis. J Rheumatol. 1997;24:109–14.

Trull AK, Ebringer R, Panayi GS, Colthorpe D, James DC, Ebringer A. IgA antibodies to *Klebsiella pneumoniae* in ankylosing spondylitis. Scand J Rheumatol. 1983;12:249–53.

Yuan GH, Shi GY, Ding YZ. Antibodies to *Klebsiella pneumoniae* in ankylosing spondylitis. Zhonghua Nei Ke Za Zhi. 1993;32:467–9.

Index

DOI 10.1007/978-1-4471-4300-0, © Springer-Verlag London 2013

MIX
Papier aus verantwortungsvollen Quellen
Paper from responsible sources
FSC® C105338

If you have any concerns about our products,
you can contact us on
ProductSafety@springernature.com

In case Publisher is established outside the EU,
the EU authorized representative is:
Springer Nature Customer Service Center GmbH
Europaplatz 3, 69115 Heidelberg, Germany

Printed by Libri Plureos GmbH
in Hamburg, Germany